Oral Medicine

Guest Editors

VINCENT D. EUSTERMAN, MD, DDS
ARLEN MEYERS, MD, MBA

OTOLARYNGOLOGIC CLINICS OF NORTH AMERICA

www.oto.theclinics.com

February 2011 • Volume 44 • Number 1

SAUNDERS an imprint of ELSEVIER, Inc.

W.B. SAUNDERS COMPANY
A Division of Elsevier Inc.

1600 John F. Kennedy Boulevard • Suite 1800 • Philadelphia, Pennsylvania 19103-2899

http://www.theclinics.com

OTOLARYNGOLOGIC CLINICS OF NORTH AMERICA Volume 44, Number 1
February 2011 ISSN 0030-6665, ISBN-13: 978-1-4557-0480-4

Editor: Joanne Husovski
Developmental Editor: Natalie Whitted

Otolaryngologic Clinics of North America (ISSN 0030-6665) is published bimonthly by Elsevier, Inc., 360 Park Avenue South, New York, NY 10010-1710. Months of issue are February, April, June, August, October, and December. Business and Editorial Offices: 1600 John F. Kennedy Blvd., Suite 1800, Philadelphia, PA 19103-2899. Customer Service Office: 6277 Sea Harbor Drive, Orlando, FL 32887-4800. Periodicals postage paid at New York, NY and additional mailing offices. Subscription prices is $310.00 per year (US individuals), $590.00 per year (US institutions), $149.00 per year (US student/resident), $409.00 per year (Canadian individuals), $741.00 per year (Canadian institutions), $459.00 per year (international individuals), $741.00 per year (international institutions), $230.00 per year (international & Canadian student/resident). Foreign air speed delivery is included in all *Clinics'* subscription prices. All prices are subject to change without notice. **POSTMASTER:** Send address changes to *Otolaryngologic Clinics of North America*, Elsevier Health Sciences Division, Subscription Customer Service, 3251 Riverport Lane, Maryland Heights, MO 63043. **Telephone: 1-800-654-2452 (U.S. and Canada); 314-447-8871 (outside U.S. and Canada). Fax: 314-447-8029. E-mail: journalscustomerservice-usa@elsevier.com (for print support); journalsonlinesupport-usa@elsevier.com (for online support).**

Reprints. For copies of 100 or more of articles in this publication, please contact the Commercial Reprints Department, Elsevier Inc., 360 Park Avenue South, New York, NY 10010-1710. Tel.: 212-633-3812; Fax: 212-462-1935; E-mail: reprints@elsevier.com.

Otolaryngologic Clinics of North America is also published in Spanish by McGraw-Hill Interamericana Editores S.A., P.O. Box 5-237, 06500 Mexico D.F., Mexico.

Otolaryngologic Clinics of North America is covered in *MEDLINE/PubMed (Index Medicus), Current Contents/Clinical Medicine, Excerpta Medica, BIOSIS, Science Citation Index,* and *ISI/BIOMED.*

Printed and bound by CPI Group (UK) Ltd, Croydon, CR0 4YY

Transferred to Digital Print 2011

Contributors

GUEST EDITORS

VINCENT D. EUSTERMAN, MD, DDS
Assistant Professor, Department of Otolaryngology—Head and Neck Surgery, University of Colorado School of Medicine, Denver Health Medical Center, Denver, Colorado

ARLEN MEYERS, MD, MBA
Professor, Department of Otolaryngology, Dentistry and Engineering, University of Colorado Denver, Aurora, Colorado

AUTHORS

INDRANEEL BHATTACHARYYA, DDS, MSD
Associate Professor and Director Residency Program, Department of Oral and Maxillofacial Diagnostic Sciences, Oral and Maxillofacial Pathology, University of Florida College of Dentistry, Gainesville, Florida

AMIT CHATTOPADHYAY, BDS, MDS, FFPH, MPH, CPH, PGDHHM, PGDMLS, PhD
Epidemiologist, ARCAB, Gaithersburg, Maryland

HARDEEP K. CHEHAL, BDS
Assistant Professor, Department of General Dentistry, Oral and Maxillofacial Pathology, Creighton University School of Dentistry, Omaha, Nebraska

DONALD M. COHEN, DMD, MS, MBA
Professor, Department of Oral and Maxillofacial Diagnostic Sciences, College of Dentistry, University of Florida, Gainesville, Florida

JOEL B. EPSTEIN, DMD, MSD, FRCD(C), FDS RCS(Ed)
Professor, Department of Oral Medicine and Diagnostic Sciences, College of Dentistry; Department of Otolaryngology—Head and Neck Surgery, University of Illinois at Chicago, Chicago, Illinois

VINCENT D. EUSTERMAN, MD, DDS
Assistant Professor, Department of Otolaryngology—Head and Neck Surgery, University of Colorado School of Medicine, Denver Health Medical Center, Denver, Colorado

PETER J. GIANNINI, DDS, MS
Associate Professor of Oral and Maxillofacial Pathology, Department of Oral Biology; Director of Clinical and Translational Research, Cruzan Center for Dental Research, University of Nebraska Medical Center College of Dentistry, Lincoln, Nebraska

LOREN GOLITZ, MD
Professor, Department of Pathology, Director of Dermatopathology, University of Colorado Denver, Aurora, Colorado

ROBERT O. GREER Jr, DDS, ScD
Professor, Division of Oral and Maxillofacial Pathology, University of Colorado School of Dental Medicine; Professor, Departments of Pathology and Medicine, University of Colorado School of Medicine, Aurora, Colorado

NADIM M. ISLAM, DDS, MS
Assistant Professor, Department of Oral and Maxillofacial Pathology, Medicine and Radiology, Indiana University School of Dentistry, Indianapolis, Indiana

MARILYN E. LEVI, MD
Associate Professor, Department of Medicine, Division of Infectious Diseases, University of Colorado Denver, Aurora, Colorado

ARLEN MEYERS, MD, MBA
Professor, Department of Otolaryngology, Dentistry and Engineering, University of Colorado Denver, Aurora, Colorado

JACOB S. MINOR, MD
Resident, Department of Otolaryngology, University of Colorado at Denver, Denver, Colorado

GINAT W. MIROWSKI, DMD, MD
Adjunct Associate Professor, Department of Oral Pathology, Medicine, Radiology, Indiana University School of Dentistry, Indianapolis, Indiana

PALLAVI PARASHAR, BDS, DDS
Assistant Professor, Department of Diagnostic and Biological Sciences, University of Colorado Denver School of Dental Medicine, Aurora, Colorado

MEGAN PIRIGYI, BA
Medical Student, Department of Dermatology, Northwestern University Feinberg School of Medicine, Chicago, Illinois

SHERIF SAID, MD, PhD
Associate Professor, Department of Pathology, Director of Head and Neck Pathology, University of Colorado Denver, Aurora, Colorado

BETHANEE J. SCHLOSSER, MD, PhD
Assistant Professor, Department of Dermatology, Northwestern University Feinberg School of Medicine, Chicago, Illinois

KISHORE V. SHETTY, BDS, DDS, MS, MRCS
Private Dental Practice, Denver, Colorado

TOBY O. STEELE, MD
Department of Otolaryngology—Head and Neck Surgery, University of California Davis, Sacramento, California

Contents

The oral medicine specialist and oral pathologist are the disciplined sub-specialists in dentistry who deal with oral disease and related systemic conditions. Dental colleagues are an invaluable resource for the diagnosis and treatment of diseases unfamiliar to the otolaryngologist. This article reviews the process of history taking, the physical examination, head and neck examination, oral soft tissue anatomy, the oral examination, and screening and diagnostic testing.

Smokeless tobacco (SLT) has been smoked, chewed, and inhaled in various forms for hundreds of years. The primary oral, mucosal, and hard tissue changes associated with SLT use include SLT keratosis (STK); gingival inflammation, periodontal inflammation, and alveolar bone damage; and dental caries, tooth abrasion, and dysplasia and oral squamous cell carcinoma (SCC). Some high-risk STKs are human papillomavirus associated, and the highest level of transition of STK to dysplasia or oral SCC appears to be in those lesions that have a diffuse velvety or papillary texture clinically. There is minimal risk for oral cancer associated with SLT use.

Oral infections commonly originate from an odontogenic source in adults and from tonsil and lymphatic sources in children. Odontogenic infections arise from advanced dental caries or periodontal disease. Oral trauma, radiation injury, chemotherapy mucositis, salivary gland infection, lymph node abscess, and postoperative infection are potential nonodontogenic sources of infections that could potentially be life threatening. This article reviews the serious nature and potential danger that exists from oral infection and the antibiotics available to treat them are reviewed. Successful treatment requires an understanding of the microflora, the regional anatomy, the disease process, the treatment methods available, and interdisciplinary team collaboration.

Recurrent aphthous stomatitis is a common oral ulcerative disease, affecting 10% to 15% of the general US population. This article reviews the epidemiology and clinical presentations of recurrent aphthous stomatitis, including diagnosis and management.

Oral manifestations of hematologic and nutritional deficiencies can affect the mucous membranes, teeth, periodontal tissues, salivary glands, and perioral skin. This article reviews common oral manifestations of hematologic conditions starting with disorders of the white blood cells including cyclic hematopoiesis (cyclic neutropenia), leukemias, lymphomas, plasma cell dyscrasias, and mast cell disorders; this is followed by a discussion of the impact of red blood cell disorders including anemias and less common red blood cell dyscrasias (sickle cell disease, hemochromatosis, and congenital erythropoietic porphyria) as well as thrombocytopenia. Several nutritional deficiencies exhibit oral manifestations. The authors specifically discuss the impact of water-soluble vitamins (B2, B3, B6, B9, B12, and C), fat-soluble vitamins (A, D, and K) and the eating disorders anorexia nervosa and bulimia nervosa on the oral mucosa.

Burning mouth syndrome is a complex disorder of unclear etiology that is most prevalent in perimenopausal women. It is often accompanied by dysguesia and subjective xerostomia. Recent evidence implicates both central and peripheral neuropathies, possibly representing a phantom pain syndrome in some patients. Ensuring that the patient's oral burning is not secondary to some other local or systemic factor is central to appropriate management. Current standard therapies include clonazepam, paroxetine, and cognitive behavioral therapy, and several promising new alternatives are described.

Cancers of the oral cavity account for approximately 3% of malignancies diagnosed annually in the United States. As with other upper aerodigestive tract cancers, 5-year survival rates for oral cavity cancers decrease with delayed diagnosis. Cancers of the oral cavity are thought to progress from premalignant/precancerous lesions, beginning as hyperplastic tissue and developing into invasive squamous cell carcinoma. Despite the general accessibility of the oral cavity during physical examination, many malignancies are not diagnosed until late stages of disease. To prevent malignant transformation of these oral precursor lesions, multiple screening and detection techniques have been developed to address this problem.

Oral candidiasis is the most common fungal infection in both the immunocompetent and the immunocompromised populations. This article reviews the clinical presentations of the different forms of oral candidiasis, as well as the diagnosis and management.

THE CLINICS ARE NOW AVAILABLE ONLINE!

Access your subscription at:
www.theclinics.com

Preface

Oral Disease

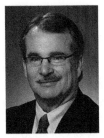 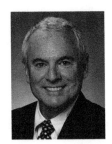

Vincent D. Eusterman, MD, DDS   Arlen Meyers, MD, MBA
Guest Editors

We are privileged to serve as guest co-editors for this issue of the *Otolaryngologic Clinics*, which is devoted to diseases of the oral cavity. It is intended to update the otolaryngologist–head and neck surgeon on important topics in the diagnosis and treatment of oral disease. Many nonmalignant diseases of the oral cavity including inflammatory, infectious, immunologic, congenital, and neoplastic diseases are often treated by our dental colleagues. Dentists, oral pathologists, oral medicine specialists, and oral and maxillofacial surgeons spend a good deal of their lives in the diagnosis and treatment of oral disease. The oral cavity is an often misunderstood and frequently overlooked by the medical profession. Otolaryngologist–head and neck surgeons, head and neck pathologists, and in some centers the dermatologist are taking bigger roles as the oral medicine specialist in the medical profession. This journal is a collaborative effort by both dental and medical professionals in these varied fields to help us better understand and manage oral disease with the most current information available to us. This publication is intended to refamiliarize us with many oral diseases we encounter in our practices. We also hope to stimulate further research as there are many oral diseases discussed here for which there are no accepted effective treatments.

Oral lesions are often transient, representing a local reaction that disappears before a diagnosis can be made; yet other times oral disease may represent a serious systemic illness like leukemia. It is important for the oral health professional to study these processes because we are often the last to see the patient and make the diagnosis. A thorough patient history and comprehensive head and neck examination is at the core of the evaluation and is essential for accurate diagnosis and effective treatment. We hope you enjoy this edition on oral medicine.

Otolaryngol Clin N Am 44 (2011) ix–x
doi:10.1016/j.otc.2010.10.004
0030-6665/11/$ – see front matter © 2011 Elsevier Inc. All rights reserved.

We are deeply indebted to all our colleagues for sharing their knowledge and experience to help make this issue possible. We also would like to thank our editor Joanne Husovski of Elsevier for her professionalism and support and our wives Jane and Kathleen for their patience and understanding during the preparation of this journal.

Vincent D. Eusterman, MD, DDS
Department of Otolaryngology-Head and Neck Surgery
University of Colorado School of Medicine
Denver Health Medical Center
777 Bannock
Denver, CO 80204, USA

Arlen Meyers, MD, MBA
Department of Otolaryngology, Dentistry, and Engineering
University of Colorado Denver
12631 East 17th Avenue, B205
Aurora, CO 80045, USA

E-mail addresses:
vincent.eusterman@dhha.org (V.D. Eusterman)
arlen.meyers@ucdenver.edu (A. Meyers)

History and Physical Examination, Screening and Diagnostic Testing

Vincent D. Eusterman, MD, DDS

KEYWORDS

- Oral mucosal disorders • Oral examination
- Oral cancer screening • Optical detection techniques
- Oral cancer biomarkers

INTRODUCTION

Oral diseases often reflect systemic health as well as local reactions to irritation. It is the role of the oral health professional to understand these disease processes for a timely diagnosis and treatment of potentially life threatening conditions. A precise history and physical examination and appropriate screening and diagnostic testing are at the center this process. This paper reviews this process and discusses the accuracy of screening and diagnostic testing for the patient with oral pathology. Newer oral cancer screening technology like salivary biomarkers and optical detection techniques are exciting developments in oral cancer detection and are discussed here. A more complete review should include the many excellent resources in oral medicine and oral pathology including Burket's *Oral Medicine* 11th edition, 2008,[1] and *Oral & Maxillofacial Pathology* by Brad Neville DDS, 3rd edition, 2008.[2]

HISTORY

A detailed patient history is the foundation for an accurate diagnosis. An incomplete history leads to a flawed diagnosis, unnecessary testing, a delay in disease management, and possibly a misdiagnosis. The surgeon has the responsibility to minimize patient risk by defining the patient's comorbidities and instituting appropriate measures and treatments. Previous medical records, including operative reports, radiographic and laboratory information pertaining to the patient's problem are important sources of information and should be used whenever possible to supplement an accurate history.

Financial disclosure: the author has nothing to disclose.
Department of Otolaryngology-Head and Neck Surgery, University of Colorado School of Medicine, Denver Health Medical Center, 777 Bannock, Denver, CO 80204, USA
E-mail address: vincent.eusterman@dhha.org

Otolaryngol Clin N Am 44 (2011) 1–29
doi:10.1016/j.otc.2010.10.001
0030-6665/11/$ – see front matter © 2011 Published by Elsevier Inc.

oto.theclinics.com

The chief complaint should be evaluated by determining onset, location, duration, intensity, frequency, progression, character, severity, triggers, factors that improve or worsen the condition, effect on function, and results of previous treatments. The symptoms of pain, burning, dry mouth, paresthesia, hypesthesia, swelling, texture, and visual abnormality evaluated with the patient's pertinent medical history gives the surgeon an initial level of concern regarding the urgency of the complaint.

The past medical and surgical history can often reveal pertinent information from childhood and adult illnesses, previous surgery, and anesthetic complications that can be critical in the patient's care. More often than not oral soft tissue disease represents infectious, traumatic, or a reactive systemic process rather than a neoplastic process. Therefore, additional comprehensive histories of autoimmune disease, allergic disease, cardiovascular disease, hypertension, diabetes, hyperthyroidism, infectious disease, as well as cancer are important considerations in developing an accurate diagnosis.

A drug allergy history should differentiate true allergies from side effects of medications. Latex protein allergens can rapidly incite anaphylactic shock in sensitive individuals; children with spina bifida are a high-risk group for latex allergy. Patients with soy or egg allergies may react to propofol, and patients allergic to shellfish may have contrast allergies. Patients with ester type local anesthesia allergies should avoid cocaine, procaine hydrochloride (Novocain), and tetracaine (Pontocaine). Ester class anesthetics have 1 letter i in the name; the amide class has 2 (lidocaine, mepivacaine). The medication history of current prescription and nonprescription medications, their dosages, schedules, and patient compliance should be reviewed and recorded.

The social and family history can indicate social, environmental, and genetic risk factors associated with certain diseases that can affect the diagnosis. Tobacco exposure, specifically cigarette, cigar, pipe and chewing tobacco history should be recorded. If possible, alcohol consumption should be quantified as type, frequency, and duration of use. Recreational drug use and lifestyle risk factors for communicable diseases like human immunodeficiency virus (HIV), hepatitis, and tuberculosis should be addressed. Exposures to hazardous materials, environmental toxins, and accidental radiation exposure may be important to discuss and document. Family history for genetic disorders, diabetes, heart disease, allergic and autoimmune diseases, and cancer can be important questions when looking for diseases that can have a genetic basis and have not been considered before.

Table 1 lists a recent history of the pertinent system disorders that may contribute to the chief oral complaint. It should include recent constitutional changes such as weight loss, fatigue, night sweats, rashes, heat and cold intolerance, and others that might give insight into the patient's problem.

PHYSICAL EXAMINATION

This physical examination section is limited to a comprehensive head and neck examination. References for examination of systems other than the head and neck can be found in *Bates' Guide to Physical Examination and History Taking*[3] or other guides to the physical examination. During the comprehensive head and neck examination it is important to look, listen, and feel the site being examined. Manual and bimanual palpation of high-risk areas, especially the tongue base, tonsils and floor of mouth (FOM), salivary glands, and thyroid may detect primary cancers early before they become metastatic. Listening to the patient's voice and speech are important in consideration of tumor location. A hot potato voice may represent an oropharyngeal tumor and a raspy hoarse voice might suggest a laryngeal neoplasm. The examination proceeds in 3 phases: (1) obtaining vital signs; (2) examination of the head, neck, and the oral cavity; (3) obtaining radiographic and laboratory studies. Additional special examinations of other organ systems may be necessary for patients whose signs and symptoms are suggestive of a systemic cause. A detailed physical examination of a patient of the opposite sex should be done in the presence of a medical assistant of the same gender as the patient. History taking helps the clinician to develop a rapport with the patient to allow the patient to feel comfortable and confident during the examination. Explaining what you are about to do helps put the patient at ease; it is also a time to educate the patient about the early signs and symptoms of head and neck cancer. The examination must be done using universal precautions, protective gloves, eyewear, and a mask if indicated. The clinician should have adequate equipment and supplies on hand for an efficient and professional examination, such as a good light source, mirrors, tongue blades, 2×2 gauze pads, topical decongestants, anesthesia, suction, flexible nasopharyngoscope, pneumatic otoscope, and a nasal speculum.

HEAD AND NECK EXAMINATION
General Appearance

Changes in appearance such as weight loss, anorexia, and fatigue could indicate malignancy.

Head and Neck

Inspect the head and neck for facial tone or palsy, skin changes, discoloration, pigmentation, ulceration, asymmetry, neck range of motion in flexion, extension, and lateral bending. Palpate the facial bones for asymmetry, masses, scalp abnormalities, swelling, and temporal wasting. Palpate the cervical chain lymph nodes. These are divided into large and smaller anatomic triangles or into lymph node regions (levels). The latter are endorsed by the American Head and Neck Society and the American Academy of Otolaryngology - Head and Neck Surgery. Level IA are the submental nodes, level IB are the submandibular nodes. Level II is part of the upper jugulodigastric chain above the hyoid bone (**Fig. 1**A). Level II is divided into IIB above and IIA below the spinal accessory nerve. Level III extends from the hyoid to the cricoid and level IV from the cricoid to the clavicle (see **Fig. 1**B). Level V is the posterior triangle and is separated into VA (spinal accessory nodes) above and VB (transverse cervical and supraclavicular nodes) below (see **Fig. 1**C). The parotid (or preauricular), retroauricular, and suboccipital node regions are denoted P, R, and S but are not part of this classification system. Infection produces mobile and tender nodes, whereas malignancy produces asymptomatic and fixed nodes. Auscultation of the neck with the bell of the stethoscope of a thyroid goiter can indicate Graves disease, carotid bruits, or the sounds of airway obstruction over the larynx and trachea.

Thyroid

Inspect the thyroid gland first then proceed to palpation. The normal thyroid gland is often difficult to feel. Palpation can be from the front or for the heavy neck by standing behind the patient. Palpate the entire gland. Have the patient turn toward the examining side to relax the sternocleidomastoid muscle. During palpation of the lobe ask the patient to swallow, this elevates the gland upward and may help identify a nodule. Note the characteristics of any nodules or abnormality as cystic or hard and record tender areas. If the inferior pole of the gland is difficult to palpate it may suggest substernal extension of the thyroid gland.

Table 1
Review of systems

System	Review
General	General health, blood pressure, weight change, appetite, weakness, fatigue, fever, night sweats, sleeping pattern, unexplained falls
HEENT	Head: headache or facial pain, head injury; change in vision, pain, inflammation, infections Eyes: double vision, scotomata, blurring, tearing, glaucoma Ears: hearing loss, tinnitus, deafness, ear pain, or discharge; light-headedness, dizziness Nose: nasal obstruction, bleeding, discharge, sinusitis, allergies Throat: dental problems, ulcers or sores in the mouth, bleeding, dryness, tumors; saliva gland diseases, bad breath or taste in mouth, denture fit, hoarseness, dysphagia, sore throat, swollen glands in the neck, neck masses, thyroid disease, neck pain, or decreased motion
Breasts	Masses, change in contour or skin color, nipple discharge, pain
Respiratory	Cough, sputum color, hemoptysis, dyspnea, wheezing, pleurisy, asthma, bronchitis, emphysema, pneumonia, tuberculosis, chronic obstructive pulmonary disease, night sweats, nocturnal dyspnea
Cardiovascular	Cardiac: heart disease, arrhythmias, hypertension, angina, rheumatic fever, murmur, palpitations, dyspnea, orthopnea, paroxysmal nocturnal dyspnea, edema, myocardial infarction, congestive heart failure, swelling feet or ankles, bacterial endocarditis, electrocardiogram or other test results. Heart surgery and prosthetic heart valve patient is at risk for sub-acute bacterial endocarditis (SBE) Vascular: claudication, varicosities, blood clots, extremity swelling or color change in cold weather, redness, or tenderness. Vascular diseases common to head and neck include hemangioma, arterial/venous/lymphatic malformations, Kaposi sarcoma, Sturge-Weber syndrome, hereditary hemorrhagic telangiectasia or Osler-Weber-Rendu (see **Fig. 3A**)
Gastrointestinal and hepatic diseases	Dysphagia, globus, heartburn, appetite, nausea, bowel habits, stool size and color, pain on defecation, bleeding, hemorrhoids, constipation, diarrhea, food intolerance, jaundice, liver or gall bladder problems, hepatitis, cirrhosis, peptic ulcer disease. Inflammatory bowel disease (IBD)/ulcerative colitis and Crohn disease are associated with increased risk of aphthous stomatitis in both, cobblestone mucosa, lymphadenopathy, and periodontitis in active Crohn disease. Immunosuppressants used to treat IBD including steroids, azathioprine (Imuran), cyclosporine (Neoral), and methotrexate can aggravate infection and may cause gingival hyperplasia
Urogenital	Urinary frequency, retention, polyuria, dysuria, nocturia, urgency, pain/burning, bleeding, infections, flank pain, stones colic, suprapubic pain, incontinence, chronic renal failure, dialysis

Endocrine	Thyroid disease, goiter, exophthalmus, heat or cold intolerance, excessive sweating, thrust or hunger, tremor, palpitations, polyuria, polydipsia, mood swings, depression, visual changes, thin hair, constipation, dry skin, change in hat, glove or shoe size, diabetes mellitus, adrenal disorders, steroid therapy, lactation, pregnancy. intravenous bisphosphonates (Aredia, Bonefos, Didronel, or Zometa) for hypercalcemia and bone pain associated with metastatic breast cancer, prostate cancer, and multiple myeloma are at high risk for bisphosphonate-associated osteonecrosis of the jaw especially after dental extraction (see **Fig. 14A**)
Neurologic	Headaches, strokes, seizures, attention, speech, memory, judgment, dizziness, weakness, imbalance, blackouts, paralysis, numbness, tingling, tremors, incontinence, seizure disorders, cerebrovascular disease, orofacial neurologic disorders (glossodynia, trigeminal neuralgia, Costen syndrome, burning mouth syndrome, and others)
Hematologic	Anemia, purpura, bruising or bleeding, anticoagulant therapy, past transfusions and reactions, hematologic malignancies, leukemia (see **Fig. 14B** and C), lymphoma (Hodgkin and non-Hodgkin lymphoma), transplantation, hemostasis during surgery, infection risk (HIV, hepatitis), hematologic disease may cause oral lesions (see article on this topic in this issue)
Infectious	Viral infections: HSV-1 and HSV-2, chicken pox, varicella zoster, herpangina, coxsackievirus (hand foot and mouth disease), Epstein-Barr (NPC), hepatitis (A,B,C), HIV, human papilloma virus. Fungal infections: *Candida albicans*, histoplasmosis, mucormycosis, aspergillosis, blastomycosis, coccidiomycosis. Bacterial infections: previous systemic infection, methicillin-resistant *Staphylococcus aureus*, vancomycin-resistant *Staphylococcus aureus*, tuberculosis, previous odontogenic infection, pseudomembranous colitis, oral infections by sexually transmitted disease
Cutaneous	Rashes, lumps, sores, ulcers, decubitus, pruritus, dryness, color change, hair/nails change, change in size/color of moles. Sun exposure history. May have oral manifestations of systemic disease. Oral mucosa pigmented lesions are: endogenous, bilirubin from cirrhosis, iron in hemochromatosis or melanin deposition in Addison disease, Peutz-Jeghers syndrome, McCune-Albright syndrome, Von Recklinghausen disease; exogenous, heavy metal in lead and bismuth toxicity, chromophilic bacteria or fungi in black hairy tongue, foreign material deposits in amalgam tattoo. Mucosal melanoma are dark brown to bluish black and must be differentiated from other oral pigmentation
Musculoskeletal	History and location of muscle or joint pain, redness, weakness, decreased motion, trauma, stiffness, arthritis, gout, backache, or prosthetic joint. High-risk infection in prosthetic joints occurs in new joints (<2 years), prior joint infection, hemophilia, diabetes mellitus, rheumatoid arthritis, and patients on immunosuppressive therapy. Temporomandibular joint is affected by arthritis and is a common source of ear pain. Bone diseases such as osteoporosis can cause thinning of the cortical plate, loss of trabeculation, loss of edentulous ridge, delayed healing of extraction sites, and thinning of maxillary sinuses that may refer pain to the teeth. Other systemic resorptive bone diseases that affect the oral cavity include vitamin D deficiency, osteomalacia (malabsorption syndromes, chronic renal failure), hyperparathyroidism, fibrous dysplasia, McCune-Albright syndrome, Paget disease, histiocytosis, multiple myeloma
Psychiatric	Nervousness, instability, tension, insomnia, mania, memory loss, mood swings, disorientation, depression, suicide ideation. Psychiatric disease and psychotropic medications can cause xerostomia

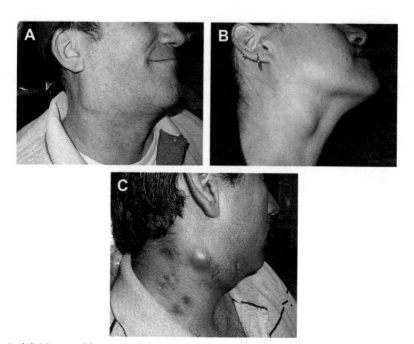

Fig. 1. (A) 38-year-old man with level II lymphadenopathy with histology consistent with Castleman disease. (B) 29-year-old woman with isolated level III adenopathy consistent with *Mycobacterium tuberculosis*. (C) 34-year-old man with HIV infection and a level V adenopathy from recurrent histoplasmosis abscess.

Salivary Glands

The second most common extra oral mass after lymphadenopathy is a salivary gland neoplasm. Parotid neoplasms are palpated in the preauricular and infra-auricular regions. Sublingual and submandibular gland masses are often tender and are more effectively evaluated by bimanual palpation.

Eyes

The cranial nerves II, III, IV, and VI can be tested here by examining extraocular movements and visual acuity by using a Snelen chart. Eye swelling, epiphora, or neural deficits could represent invasive cancer arising from the nose, sinuses or facial skin.

Ears

The external ears should be closely inspected noting color changes, ulcers, or deformities especially in the sun-exposed areas. Evaluate the external auditory canal for masses, drainage, or obstructing cerumen that may need to be removed to be able to see the tympanic membrane. Assess the integrity of the tympanic membranes by pneumatic otoscopy and hearing acuity with a finger rub or using tuning forks. Exclude ear pathology in the differential diagnosis for referred otalgia.

Nose

The nasal septum and anterior turbinates can be evaluated by anterior rhinoscopy using a headlight and nasal speculum. Nasal endoscopy allows examination of the posterior portions of the nasal cavity and the nasal pharynx. The scope is passed after applying local anesthetic spray to the nose. It is helpful to view the nose in its native state before and after decongestant use to determine soft tissue obstruction.

Throat

Note the position of the trachea in the anterior neck; deviation may suggest a neck mass or lung abnormality. The oral and pharyngeal examinations are discussed less later.

Temporomandibular Joint

Temporomandibular joint (TMJ) disease can be best identified by TMJ palpation during opening and closing. Examine both joints simultaneously by gently placing the middle finger anterior to the tragus. Tenderness on opening and closing can localize the problem to the TMJ. Maximum opening distance, opening symmetry, popping, clicking, or grinding should be noted. Ear pain after normal ear and TMJ examinations may be referred from cranial nerves IX and X and represent an upper airway carcinoma. Patients at risk for throat cancer should undergo nasopharyngoscopy before treatment of a suspected temporal mandibular disorder.

Cranial Nerves

The cranial nerve (CN) examination (**Table 2**) begins when the patient walks in the room. Eye movement and vision assessment clears CN II–VI and VI. Olfactory nerves can be checked by a simple alcohol sniff test[4] using a 70% isopropyl alcohol disposable pad. Motor assessment of CN V, VII, XI, and XII is by simple jaw, face, shoulder, and tongue movement. Afferent and efferent gag reflex tests CN IX and X. CN VIII can be tested by finger rub or more sophisticated tuning fork testing.

Table 2
Cranial nerve examination

Cranial Nerve	Examination
Olfactory (I)	Test with coffee, vanilla, peppermint, alcohol sniff test, or University of Pennsylvania Smell Identification Test
Optic (II)	Visual fields (Snelen chart), pupillary light reflex, swinging flashlight
Oculomotor (III)	Ptosis, nystagmus, pupillary size (PERRLA), eye movement, accommodation reflex
Trochlear (IV)	Eye movement, superior oblique
Trigeminal (V)	Light touch, pain, temperature, corneal reflex, jaw movement toward side of lesion
Abducens (VI)	Eye movement, lateral rectus
Facial (VII)	Motor: facial muscles, close eyes, wrinkle forehead, smile and show teeth Sensory: taste testing
Auditory (VIII)	Hearing acuity, Rinne test, Weber test, balance function testing
Glossopharyngeal (IX)	Mostly sensory to tonsils, pharynx, posterior tongue, loss of gag reflex (afferent limb)
Vagus (X)	Uvula away from side of lesion, hoarseness, dysphagia, loss of gag reflex (efferent limb)
Spinal accessory (XI)	Shrug shoulders, turn head right and left
Hypoglossal (XII)	Movement deviates toward side of lesion, tongue atrophy or fasciculations

ORAL SOFT TISSUE ANATOMY

The oral examination evaluates the lips, oral cavity, and oropharynx. The oral cavity is the anterior two-thirds of the tongue, the gingiva, buccal mucosa, FOM, hard palate, and retromolar trigone. The oropharynx is the posterior one-third of the tongue, soft palate, tonsils, and the lateral and posterior walls of the visible pharynx.

The oral soft tissues are covered by 3 types of mucosa: nonkeratinized, keratinized, and specialized. Nonkeratinized mucosa is nonmasticatory mucosa, the unattached lining mucosa on lips, cheeks, FOM, ventral tongue, soft palate, and the alveolar mucosa that is not firmly attached to underlying bone. This mucosa can be stretched or compressed and has a basal layer, an intermediate layer, and a superficial layer that does not produce keratin. This is the common site of the aphthous ulcer formation (**Fig. 2**A).

Keratinizing mucosa is masticatory mucosa that is the attached to gingiva around the teeth and hard palate, and is the common site for herpetic ulcer formation. It occurs in parakeratin and orthokeratin forms. Both forms of keratinized epithelium have basal layers, a prickle cell layer (bulk of the epithelium), a granular layer (kerato-hyaline granules), and a superficial keratin of varying thickness. Parakeratin contains nucleated keratinocytes, whereas the less common orthokeratin contains none. Hyperkeratosis is a microscopic diagnosis of the thickening of the stratum corneum, often associated with a qualitative abnormality of the keratin[5] and can be the result of an irritant or vitamin A deficiency.

Specialized mucosa is papillae on the dorsum and lateral tongue. The filiform papillae are most numerous and guide food in swallowing, and contain no taste buds. In addition to normal filiform papillae in **Fig. 3**A, the patient has small angiomas consistent with her diagnosis of Osler-Weber-Randu. The child in **Fig. 3**B exhibits

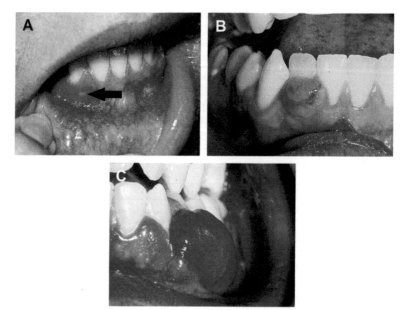

Fig. 2. (*A*) Aphthous ulcer formation (*arrow*) on nonkeratinized (unattached) mucosa. (*B*) Pyogenic granuloma (lobular capillary hemangioma) on keratinized (attached) mucosa. (*C*) Similar in appearance to (*B*), this lesion is a peripheral giant cell reparative granuloma, which occurred bilaterally in this patient.

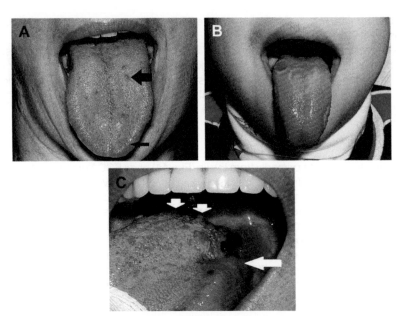

Fig. 3. (A) Normal-appearing tongue, small arrow identifies fungiform papillae, and large arrow points to angiomas associated with Osler-Weber-Randu disease. (B) Geographic tongue (benign migratory glossitis) and anterior glossitis with prominent fungiform papillae gives a strawberry tongue appearance. (C) Posterior tongue with large arrow on folate papillae, small arrows on circumvallate papillae, and a lingual varicosity between the two.

filiform papillae atrophy from benign migratory glossitis. Note the anterior tongue appears similar to strawberry tongue, with fungiform hypertrophy and filiform atrophy giving the tongue an enanthema or bright red background. Strawberry tongue is seen in scarlet fever and can occur in Kawasaki disease. The fungiform papillae (see **Fig. 3**A and B) are red mushroom like structures over the dorsum of the tongue and contain taste buds. The folate papillae (see **Fig. 3**C) appear on the lateral boarders of the tongue and have taste buds. The large circumvale papillae (see **Fig. 3**C) also have taste buds and are 10 to 14 large, raised, round papillae in a V-shaped pattern at the boarder of the anterior two-thirds and posterior one-third of the tongue. In addition, lingual varices can be seen in this region and on occasion the surgeon may be asked to take a biopsy from one of these normal posterior tongue structures because of abnormal presentation.

ORAL EXAMINATION

The areas of greatest risk for oral cancer occur in a U-shaped zone from the tonsillar pillars and oropharynx to the anterior FOM. The relative incidence rates of oral squamous cell carcinoma (SCC) are: tongue (25%), lower lip (30%–40%), FOM (20%), and oropharynx/soft palate (15%).[6] The patient should first remove lipstick and dental appliances so that all oral surfaces can be evaluated. An external light source will allows hands-free examination for bimanual palpation, retraction, and visualization of the posterior tongue and FOM. Mucosal surfaces and salivary duct openings are dried with an air syringe or gauze to allow visualization of color, texture changes, and salivary flow. Early oral cancers present as persistent erythroplastic lesions.[7]

Clinicians should be on the lookout for red lesions as well as white (leukoplakia) lesions, ulcers, bleeding, and indurations.

The oral cavity and adenexa should be examined in a sequential and consistent manner to minimize the possibility of overlooking disease. Start with the upper and lower lip, proceeding to the buccal mucosa and gingiva. Evaluate the oral tongue, FOM, and hard palate. Examine the oral pharynx, tonsils, soft palate, posterior pharynx, and tongue base. Then evaluate the hypopharynx and nasopharynx with the aid of a mirror or nasopharyngoscope.

Lip

Lip cancer can originate primarily from the lip (**Fig. 4**A) or as SCC from the oral cavity or as basal cell carcinoma from the facial skin. Examine the lips visually for intraoral and extraoral lip color, consistency, and shape. The vermilion boarder should be sharp and smooth. Palpate the lip for masses, the gingivolabial sulci, then the gingival mucosa, and teeth. The lower lip may have thickening or leukoplakia from sun damage and can show loss of the vermilion boarder. Edentulous patients who lose vertical dimension (lower facial height) have over closure of the oral commissure and can develop angular cheilitis caused by *Candida albicans.* Recurrent herpes labialis (see **Fig 4**B) can produce target lesions or erythema multiforme of the extremities (see **Fig. 4**C).

Buccal Mucosa and Gingiva

Stretch the buccal mucosa with a mirror or tongue blade and visualize the gingiva, gingivobuccal sulcus, and buccal mucosa. Racial differences are often apparent; dark-skinned patients often have gingival mucosal pigmentation and buccal leukoedema (**Fig. 5**A), which is a benign hydration of the buccal mucosa that may appear as leukoplakia in the posterior regions. Linea alba (white line) is a horizontal line of raised

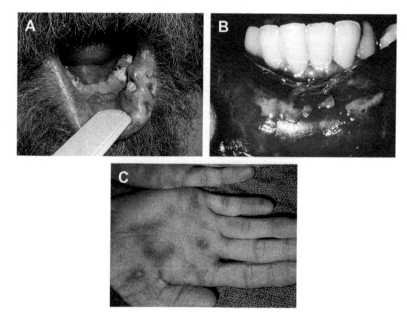

Fig. 4. (A) Left lip SCC arising from a previous small lip ulcer left untreated. (B) Lower lip herpetic lesion and erythemia multiforme (C) hand lesions as a result of the herpetic lip infection.

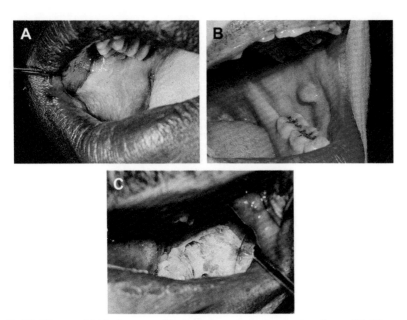

Fig. 5. (*A*) 38-year-old black man with right buccal mucosa leukoedema. (*B*) 31-year-old woman with chronic cheek bit trauma resulting in an irritation fibroma. (*C*) Oral mucosal aspirin burn injury from topical aspirin tablet use for adjacent tooth pain.

buccal mucosa adjacent to the occusal plane. This again is a benign hyperkeratosis from chronic dental irritation in the occusal plane and can also be seen in patients who are nervous cheek biters.[2] Irritation fibroma (see **Fig. 5**B) can occur from cheek bite trauma. Aspirin burn (see **Fig. 5**C) caused by topical analgesic can erode the cheek mucosa. The cheek exhibits white lesions such as lichen planus (see **Fig. 6**A) or less obvious hidden lesions representing invasive SCC (see **Fig. 6**B and C). The nonkeratinized (unattached) gingiva is a common site for aphthous ulcerative lesions (see **Fig. 2**A). Herpes virus type 1 in immune competent hosts commonly infects the keratinized (attached) gingiva. Pyogenic granuloma (lobular capillary hemangioma) (see **Fig. 2**B) and peripheral giant cell reparative granuloma (see **Fig. 2**C) can also be seen on the keratinized (attached) gingiva. The Stensen duct exits the buccal mucosa near the second maxillary molar and should be assessed for parotid flow by milking the parotid gland. Fordyce spots are small, painless, pale yellow ectopic sebaceous glands common to the posterior oral cavity and do not require biopsy. Examine the entire buccal mucosa from the labial commissure back to the anterior tonsillar pillar, then gently pinch the buccal mucosa between your fingers and thumb and feel for hidden masses.

Tongue

The dorsal tongue is examined when the tongue is protruded. Asymmetry in movement, irregularities, and color changes should be noted. The tongue usually deviates to the side of a hypoglossal nerve injury. The tongue is grasped with a 2 × 2 gauze sponge and drawn carefully forward. Black hairy tongue (lingua villosa nigra) (**Fig. 7**A) occurs as filiform papillae become elongated from abnormal desquamation. This can occur from a liquid diet, tobacco use, or after drinking bismuth subsalicylate (Pepto-Bismol). Absence of filiform papillae in the central tongue will produce medium rhomboid glossitis (see **Fig. 7**B). Neither of these conditions requires a biopsy. Dorsal

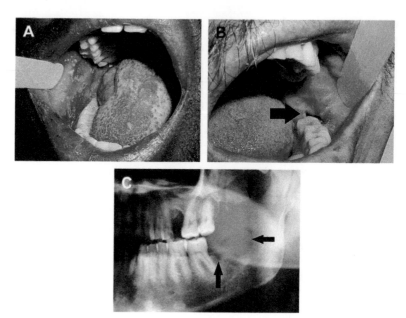

Fig. 6. (*A*) 26-year-old man with weight loss and oral lesions consistent with lichen planus. Note enlarged fungiform papillae on the anterior tongue. (*B*) 46-year-old male with no risk factors presents with an inconspicuous buccal sulcus hole (*large arrow*). (*C*) Pantographic film of patient in (*B*) with black arrows showing areas of bony invasion of the body and ramus by SCC.

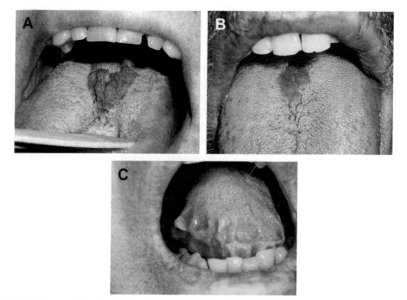

Fig. 7. (*A*) Elongated and pigmented filiform papillae consistent with black or brown hairy tongue. (*B*) Medium rhomboid glossitis, which responded to antifungal therapy. (*C*) Patient with multiple myeloma with macroglossia and dental indentations of the tongue and biopsies consistent with amyloid.

tongue atrophy can be the result of nutritional deficiencies (vitamin B_{12}, folate) or associated with oral manifestations of mucocutaneous disease. Tongue enlargement can suggest systemic disease as in the case of primary amyloidosis (see **Fig. 7C**). The lateral tongue surface is examined by extending the tongue and rotating it. Here there are few papillae and its mucosa is more erythematous. Posteriorly the folate papillae and lingual tonsil can be seen. The lingual tonsil is part of the Waldeyer ring of tonsil tissue and may appear enlarged and abnormal in the presence of infection. The lateral tongue and FOM are common sites for SCC, therefore any suspicious red or white lesion here should be considered for biopsy (**Fig. 8**). The ventral tongue has prominent vasculature and salivary duct openings. The Bartholin ducts arise from the sublingual gland and open in a soft tissue fold known as the plica sublingualis. The Wharton ducts from the submandibular gland open next to the lingual frenulum near the midline. Obstruction of the sublingual mucous ducts produces a bluish FOM with cystic-like swelling or ranula (**Fig. 9A**). Wharton duct obstruction from salivary stones (sialolithiasis) produces inflammation (sialodochitis) in the FOM (see **Fig. 9B**). Both may require surgical intervention.

Floor of Mouth

The FOM is the horseshoe-shaped area between the ventral tongue and the mandibular alveolar ridge, extending to the insertion of the anterior tonsillar pillar into the tongue. It is best seen anteriorly by elevating the tongue to the roof of the mouth. Posterior examination requires elevating the tongue medially and superiorly with a mirror or tongue blade. The FOM, submandibular gland, sublingual gland, and level I lymph nodes are evaluated by bimanual palpation. Torus mandibularis (see **Fig. 9C**) are common benign exostosis found in the FOM that complicate denture fabrication

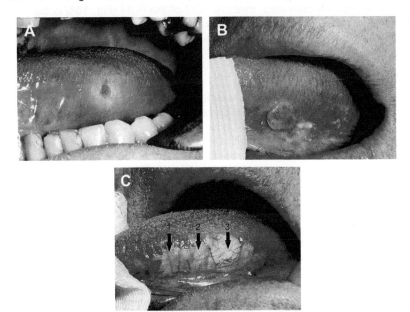

Fig. 8. SCC of the lateral tongue. (*A*) Benign-appearing nonhealing ulcer of the lateral tongue which was consistent with SCC. (*B*) Lateral tongue with a suspicious posterior erythroplakia that was mild dysplasia; the anterior sessile mass was positive for SCC. (*C*) Three lesions on the lateral tongue that represent leukoplakia (*1 arrow*), invasive SCC (*2 arrow*) and verrucous carcinoma (*3 arrow*).

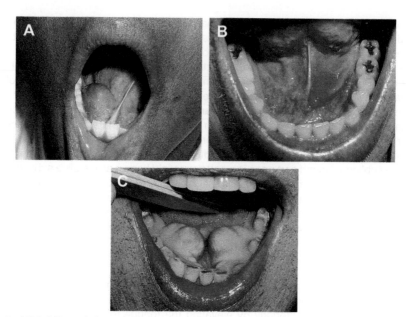

Fig. 9. (*A*) Sublingual duct obstruction in right FOM consistent with ranula formation. (*B*) Left Warthon duct obstruction and inflammation form sialolithiasis. (*C*) This patient presents with anterior FOM boney exostosis or torus mandibularis.

but are otherwise left untreated. Invasive SCC of the FOM (**Fig. 10**A) is common in patients with alcohol and tobacco risk factors. Extra time should be spent evaluating the lateral tongue and FOM because of their hidden nature and risk for cancer especially in the patient with risk factors.

Hard Palate

The hard palate is viewed by tipping the patient's head back. The minor salivary glands here are sites for neoplasia and should be carefully inspected (see **Fig. 10**B). Common benign palatal lesions include torus palatinus (see **Fig. 10**C), stomatitis nicotina or smoker's palate, and oral candidiasis. Dentures may cause a common red velvety erythema or papillary hyperplasia, a benign condition not considered erythroplakia. Upper denture edges can produce tissue redundancy known as epulis fissuratum. An ill-fitting denture is associated with oral cancer[8] and removing the denture during palate examination can help identify suspicious growth (**Fig. 11**A). Hard palate injury may undergo a benign reparative hyperplasia known as necrotizing sialometaplasia (see **Fig. 11**B). The histologic features of these ulcers, known as pseudoepitheliomatous hyperplasia, can imitate carcinoma but are benign. Pseudoepitheliomatous hyperplasia may also be seen in granular cell tumor of the tongue and North American blastomycosis of the larynx.

The Oropharynx

The oropharyngeal examination includes the soft palate, palatine tonsils, posterior and lateral pharyngeal walls, and base of the tongue. This examination is a continuation of the oral cavity examination and the 2 are often completed simultaneously. The oropharynx is the site of human papilloma virus (HPV) infection possibly because of a weakness at the embryonic junction between the oral ectoderm and pharyngeal

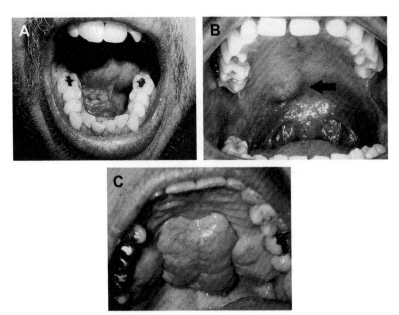

Fig. 10. (*A*) Anterior right FOM ulcerative SCC in a patient with oral cancer risk factors. (*B*) Right palatal mass (*arrow*) consistent with a minor salivary gland pleomorphic adenoma. (*C*) This patient has a large midpalatal exostosis or torus palatinus and adjacent maxillary alveolar exostosis.

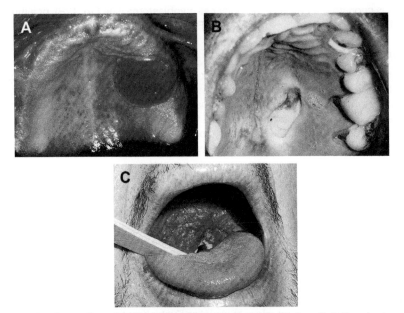

Fig. 11. (*A*) Left maxillary alveolar ridge SCC in a patient who had an ill-fitting denture. (*B*) Left palatal ulcer with pseudoepitheliomatous hyperplasia on biopsy and a diagnosis of necrotizing sialometaplasia. The lesion resolved without treatment. (*C*) Hard and soft palate SCC; biopsies were positive for high-risk HPV.

endoderm, an area known as the buccopharyngeal membrane. Recent increases in oropharyngeal cancer are related to HPV-16 and -18 infections in this area (see **Fig. 11C**).

Palatine Tonsil and Soft Palate

The tonsil, soft palate, and oropharyngeal examination requires depression of the posterior tongue, usually by asking the patient to say "Ahhh," or by mirror or tongue blade retraction. The tonsils and the tonsillar pillars and tonsillar fossa should be evaluated for symmetry and soft tissues abnormalities. Palpation of the palatine tonsil should be considered in cancer evaluation. The soft palate and uvula should be evaluated for masses or mucosal abnormalities. The uvula should be midline or this could represent vagal nerve palsy or peritonsillar space infection or parapharyngeal space mass.

Posterior and Lateral Oropharyngeal Wall

The posterior and lateral oropharyngeal walls can be seen with tongue depression with a tongue blade and soft palate elevation by saying "Ahhh." For adequate evaluation of this region, flexible nasopharyngoscopy should be considered.

Base of Tongue

Inspect the base of the tongue using a laryngeal mirror or flexible nasopharyngoscopy. Visualization is aided by pulling on the tongue with a 2×2 gauze sponge. Administration of 10% benzocaine spray to the tongue base will help reduce pain and gagging. Palpate the dorsum and lateral margins and lingual tonsils with a gloved finger. Masses at the tongue base vary. Some lesions include benign disease such as osseous choristoma (**Fig. 12A**), granular cell myoblastoma (see **Fig. 12B**), or a mucous retention cyst arising in the vallecula (see **Fig. 12C**).

Hypopharynx and Larynx

A thorough inspection of the hypopharynx and larynx is a critical component of the oral, head and neck cancer examination in patients with dysphagia, hoarseness, globus, or who have risk factors for hypopharyngeal or laryngeal cancer. A systematic evaluation for mucosal malignancy of the tongue base, vallecula, epiglottis, larynx, postcricoid and pyriform sinus areas is accomplished with a laryngeal mirror, flexible nasopharyngoscope, or a laryngeal stroboscope.

Nasopharynx

Examination of the nasopharynx can be done through an oral or nasal approach. The patient opens widely and breathes through the mouth, which causes the soft palate to rise. A tongue blade depresses the middle portion of the tongue. A small warmed nasopharyngeal mirror is extended over the tongue blade and into the oropharynx pointing upward. Ask the patient to now breathe through the nose to allow the soft palate to draw forward so that the examiner can see the nasopharyngeal region reflecting in the mirror. Inspect the posterior choanae and posterior part of the nasal septum. Inspect the turbinates and note the mucosa on the upper surface of the soft palate. Slowly rotate the mirror to visualize Eustachian tube openings, the pharyngeal tonsil, and walls of the nasopharynx. Look for masses, ulcerations, or discolorations. If your patient is unable to tolerate this procedure, consider a topical anesthetic or proceed to flexible nasopharyngoscopy.

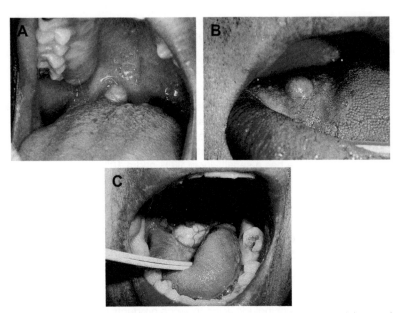

Fig. 12. Posterior tongue and tongue base lesions. (*A*) Osseous choristoma. (*B*) Granular cell myoblastoma. (*C*) Large mucous retention cyst arising from the vallecula producing dysphagia and sleep disturbance.

FLEXIBLE NASOPHARYNGOSCOPY

The flexible nasopharyngoscope has become an essential instrument for detecting head and neck cancers. The nasal cavity, nasopharynx, a portion of the oropharynx, hypopharynx, and larynx can all be thoroughly inspected using this scope. Following topical nasal vasoconstriction and anesthetic sprays, the nasopharyngoscope is carefully passed transnasally into the nasopharynx. The nasal cavity and nasopharynx are evaluated for mucosal lesions, masses, or structural abnormalities. The scope is gently advanced down into the oropharynx and hypopharynx. Examine all of the laryngeal structures as you would for the mirror examination. Then slowly remove the scope.

MIRROR EXAMINATION

Traditionally the laryngeal mirror has been the instrument of choice for examining the hypopharynx and larynx. Ask the patient to sit up straight and slightly protrude the chin upward and forward. Next have the patient open widely and protrude the tongue. Grasp the tip of the tongue with gauze and gently pull it forward. The patient should be concentrating on breathing in and out through the mouth. Carefully insert a warmed laryngeal mirror into the oropharynx, using the back of the mirror to elevate the soft palate. If the patient cannot tolerate this maneuver without gagging, consider 10% benzocaine topical anesthetic spray. Once the mirror is in place, the tongue base, vallecula, pharyngeal walls, and pyriform sinuses are evaluated for abnormalities. The epiglottis shape, position, and mucosal surfaces are closely inspected for abnormalities. The larynx and vocal cords are brought into view by having the patient say a high-pitched "e." Examine the arytenoids, aryepiglottic folds, false vocal cords, and true vocal cords for abnormalities. Assess the mobility of the true vocal cords by having the patient breath in (abduction) and phonate (adduction). If the mirror examination is insufficient and the patient is at high risk for laryngeal or hypopharyngeal cancer, a flexible nasopharyngoscope should be used to complete the examination.

SCREENING AND DIAGNOSTIC TESTING

There are limitations of any screening test or diagnostic test. Tests discriminate between the presence or absence of disease or a predictor of disease. The frequency with which a test indicates the presence of a disease is the sensitivity; specificity is the frequency with which a test indicates the absence of the disease.[9] A test that identifies a disease 90% of the time has a sensitivity of 90% and a 10% false-negative rate. A test that identifies the absence of disease 80% of the time has a specificity of 80% and has a 20% false-positive rate. The significance of choosing a test with a certain sensitivity or specificity corresponds to the accuracy of the test result.

Screening is looking for cancer before the patient has symptoms; finding a cancer at the early stage makes it easier to treat and improves outcome. Unfortunately by the time the oral symptoms appear cancer may be metastatic. Screening examinations in high-risk patients have shifted from the alcohol and tobacco abuser to those who have multiple partners or who participate in high-risk sexual activities or patients who have previously had oral cancer.

Risk factors for oral cancer include using tobacco products (cigarettes, cigar, pipes, smokeless, and chewing tobacco), heavy alcohol use, betel nut chewing, human papillomavirus infection (HPV-16 and HPV-18), sunlight exposure (lower lip) and being male. Most oral cancers occur in people older than 45 years, more often in blacks than in whites. Even though the total number of new cases and deaths from oral cancer has decreased slowly in the past 20 years, the number of new cases of oral cancer (especially of the tongue) has been increasing in adults less than 40 years of age.

Clinical Oral Examination

The clinical oral examination (COE) is considered a screening test with sensitivity ranging from 60% to 97%. A meta-analysis showed an overall sensitivity of 85% (95% CI 0.73, 0.92) and specificity of 97% (95% CI 0.93, 0.98) indicating a satisfactory test performance for an oral examination.[10] The visual detection of premalignant oral lesions has remained problematic, in contrast to skin lesions such as melanoma, where visual screening has been shown to have sensitivity and specificity of 93% and 98%.[11] One explanation for this discrepancy is that precancerous and early cancerous lesions are often subtle and rarely demonstrate the clinical characteristics observed in advanced cases: ulceration, indurations, pain, or associated cervical lymphadenopathy.[12] Besides their clinical subtlety, premalignant lesions are highly heterogeneous in their presentation and may mimic a variety of common benign or reactive conditions. Furthermore, there is a growing realization that some premalignant and early cancerous lesions are not readily detectable to the naked eye. Therefore, additional screening aids for oral cancer are needed.[10]

Toluidine Blue Test

The toluidine blue test (tolonium chloride) is a blue cationic (basic) dye used in histology. Alkaline solutions of the dye bind to nucleic acids and proteins in oral lesions but not normal mucosa. One percent acetic acid, a mucolytic agent is applied or rinsed first. Next a small amount of 1% toluidine blue solution is applied to the lesion and surrounding oral mucosa. The patient rinses with water and any tissue that stains is positive and a biopsy should be taken immediately.[13] Toluidine blue staining identifies high-risk primary oral premalignant lesions that may be treated before they progress to invasive carcinoma.[14]

Light Visualization Technology

Distinguishing premalignant and malignant lesions from benign mucosa may be difficult by simple observation and resulting delay could mean a poorer prognosis. Noninvasive technology that highlights oral premalignant and malignant lesions in a highly sensitive and specific manner could help clinicians in early diagnosis and treatment of these conditions. Several light visualization technologies (ViziLite, MicroLux, Orascoptic, and VELscope) have been approved by the US Food and Drug Administration for real-time cancer screening. Special light absorption and reflection properties makes healthy tissue and abnormal tissue appear differently. Dental reimbursement code CDT-5 D0431 is used here for oral cancer screening procedures that apply to the adjunctive light screening devices. Medical reimbursement code 2009 ICD-9-CM V76.42 is used for screening for malignant neoplasms of the oral cavity and CPT 82397 is used specifically for a chemiluminescent assay. Intraoral chemiluminescent visualization uses the emission of white light from a chemical source. ViziLite Plus (Zila Pharmaceuticals, Phoenix, AZ, USA) uses a low-energy, blue-white, light stick that reflects off abnormal cells after a 30-second acetic acid rinse. The light enhances visualization of hyperkeratosis as acetowhite lesions, which are seen as a white glow on the epithelial surface. TBlue a toluidine blue-based dye, can be used in conjunction with ViziLite to increase accuracy. A multicenter study by Epstein and colleagues[15] in 2006 reported that the effect of chemiluminescent light on visualization of mucosal lesions did not seem to improve visualization of red lesions, but red lesions with white had enhanced brightness and sharpness.

MicroLux/DL (AdDent Inc, Danbury, CT, USA) and Orascoptic systems (a Kerr Company, Middleton, WI, USA) use a diffused, blue-white, light-emitting diode (LED) light source. The patient rinses with acetic acid for 60 seconds and then the examiner looks for acetowhite lesions. In a study of 50 patients, McIntosh and colleagues[16] in 2009 showed MicroLux/DL had a sensitivity of 77.8% and a specificity of 70.7%, with a positive predictive value of 36.8%. He concluded that although MicroLux/DL seems useful at enhancing lesion visibility, it was a poor discriminator for inflammatory, traumatic, and malignant lesions.

Intraoral direct fluorescence visualization involves a hand-held device that emits a cone of blue light that excites various molecules within the mucosa. The light energy is absorbed and re-emitted as a visible fluorescence. Abnormal tissues attenuate the light and appear dark brown to black.[12,17,18] VELscope (LED Dental, White Rock, BC, Canada) emits a blue light into the oral cavity that penetrates the stratified squamous epithelium, inducing fluorescence in normal cells. Dysplastic and malignant cells will interrupt the light and cause a loss of fluorescence, delineating a dark area of abnormality. Poh and colleagues[12] describe dark areas of cancer (**Fig. 13**) and premalignancy compared with normal tissue using direct fluorescence visualization. More studies must be performed to evaluate the role of the VELscope in screening. Lingen concluded, "There is currently no hard data to support the contention that these technologies can help the clinician to identify premalignant lesions before they are detectable by COE alone. Nevertheless, studies to determine their utility in this setting are anticipated in the near future."[10]

Brush Cytology

OralCDx Laboratories, Inc (Suffern, NY) produces OralCDx Brush Test, a noninvasive oral brush biopsy kit made up of a sterile biopsy brush, 2 fixative packages, a glass

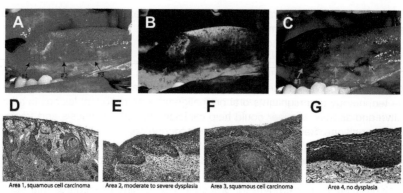

Area 1, squamous cell carcinoma   Area 2, moderate to severe dysplasia   Area 3, squamous cell carcinoma   Area 4, no dysplasia

Fig. 13. Clinical characterization and corresponding histology within an oral cancer field at right lateral tongue of a 52-year-old male former smoker. (*A*) White light image of a clinically visible nodular lesion (#1) and an ill-defined change (#2 and #3) anterior to the nodular tumor area. (*B*) The same field under a fluorescence visualization (FV) device showed an area of dark brown change of FV loss at the nodular lesion (#1) and an additional area (#2 and #3), 25 mm anterior to the nodular area (#1). (*C*) Uptake of toluidine blue in areas #1 and #3 but absent in area #2. (*D–G*) Photomicrographs showed varying degrees of histology change of the field: (*D*) (#1) invasive SCC, (*E*) (#2) moderate to severe dysplasia, (*F*) (#3) invasive SCC, and (*G*) (#4) no dysplasia at the surgical boundary, 10 mm away from FV boundary (hematoxylin-eosin staining, original magnification, 40×). (*Reproduced from* Tsui IFL, Garnis C, Poh CF. A dynamic oral cancer field: unraveling the underlying biology and its clinical implication. Am J Surg Pathol 2009;33(11):1732–8; with permission.)

slide and slide holder, a prepaid mailer box, a test requisition form, billing and reimbursement information. It requires no topical or local anesthetic. The circular brush is applied to the suspicious area and rotated 5 to 10 times. The material is transferred to a glass slide, preserved, and dried. The slide is then mailed to a laboratory where a pathologist examines the cells to determine the final diagnosis. In a prospective, randomized, controlled study, Hohlweg-Majert evaluated the advantage of computer-assisted analysis of the oral brush biopsy compared with synchronous scalpel biopsy in the early detection of oral lesions. The sensitivity for the detection of abnormal cells by means of OralCDx was 52%, specificity 29%, and the positive predictive value 63%. According to these findings, the use of oral brush biopsy as a standardized, minimally invasive method of screening oral lesions should be reconsidered.[19]

Given the lack of evidence on the effectiveness of adjunctive cancer detection techniques, clinical examination and histopathologic confirmation with biopsy remain the gold standard for the detection of oral cancer. More randomized controlled studies are needed to confirm the positive cost-benefit relationship and the true usefulness of these new diagnostic methods in oral mucosal pathology.[20]

Biomarkers

Biomarkers are biologic molecules that are indicators of a physiologic state and also of change during a disease process. Their usefulness in oral squamous cell carcinoma (OSCC) is the ability to provide early detection and monitor progression in this patient population. Genomics and proteomics have been the source of recent study. Genomics is the discipline of mapping and sequencing genes and studying their function and relationships. Proteomics is a blend of protein and genome and is the study of the full set of proteins in a cell type or tissue, and the changes under various conditions. Both proteomic[21] and genomic[22] approaches are currently being used to characterize diagnostic biomarkers in saliva. Saliva baseline protein and mRNA expression levels are needed to interpret changes that may indicate disease states. In the past, several molecular markers have been used to detect OSCC with varying degrees of specificity and sensitivity. DNA markers include TP53, microsatellite instability, the presence of papillomavirus, and Epstein-Barr virus genomic sequences.[23] It is known that mRNA is not always translated into protein[24] and the amount of protein produced for a given amount of mRNA depends on the gene it is transcribed from and on the current physiologic state of the cell. Proteomics confirms the presence of the protein and provides a direct measure of the quantity present. Saliva was once considered a hostile environment to find cancer markers because of the decomposing bacteria and cellular debris. Recently the human salivary proteome has been completely identified as 1166 proteins. It is thought that by screening for a combination of biomarkers, the sensitivity and specificity of cancer detection will be enhanced compared with screening for single tumor markers.[21] Using salivary proteomics, Hu and colleagues[25] in 2008 identified 5 candidate biomarkers in patients with OSCC and the combined use of these biomarkers yielded a receiver operating characteristic value of 93%, sensitivity of 90%, and specificity of 83% in detecting OSCC. Current saliva-based technology is making new headway in salivary transcriptome,[26] salivary soluble CD44,[27] salivary proteomics,[25] and microRNA (miRNA).[28] Blood biomarker research in oral cancer screening includes identification of specific mRNA[29] and interleukin-6.[30] Microfluidics and micro- and nanoelectromechanical systems (MEMS and NEMS) such as the hand-held Oral Fluid NanoSensor Test (OFNASET by GeneFluidics, Inc, Monterey Park, CA, USA) is being developed for saliva-based diagnostics. The routine measurement of proteins, DNA, mRNA, electrolytes, and small molecules in saliva using MEMS/NEMS is envisioned.[31] As the technologies required for biomarker identification and detection advance, the functional value of saliva as a diagnostic fluid will become more important for the improvement of oral health.

DIAGNOSTIC TESTING
Laboratory

Anemia
The World Health Organization defines the normal hemoglobin threshold ranges from 11 g/dL in children to 13 g/dL in adult men. Modern counters measure red blood cell (RBC) count, hemoglobin concentration, mean corpuscular volume (MCV), and RBC distribution width, and are used to calculate hematocrit, mean corpuscular hemoglobin (MCH) and mean corpuscular hemoglobin concentration (MCHC), which are then compared with values adjusted for age and sex. Microcytic anemia (MCV <80) such as iron-deficiency anemia can cause glossitis, angular cheilitis or stomatitis, or dysphagia from esophageal webs (Plummer-Vinson syndrome). Macrocytic anemia (MCV >100) can result from vitamin B_{12} and folate deficiency.

Neutrophilia
Neutrophilia is an absolute neutrophil count greater than 7500 cells/mm^3. Physiologic causes include exercise and stress; infectious causes include bacterial, fungal, or viral infections. Inflammatory causes include surgery, burn injury, myocardial infarction, or pulmonary embolus. Metabolic disorders (diabetic ketoacidosis, uremia, and eclampsia) include acute hemorrhage or hemolysis. Myloproliferative diseases such as myelocytic leukemia cause abnormal neutrophils. Drugs (steroids, epinephrine, or lithium), malignant tumors, or hereditary neutrophilia may produce increases in the total neutrophil count.

Neutropenia

Neutropenia is a decrease in the absolute number of neutrophils to less than 1500 cells/mm³. Major causes include drugs in chemotherapy, such as cyclophosphamide, 5-fluorouracil, azidothymidine, other drugs, such as phenothiazines, sulfonamides, and phenytoin, some infections, hematologic diseases, and autoimmune disorders.

Leukemia

Diagnosis is based on a CBC and bone marrow evaluation. The disease is a bone marrow cancer, acute or chronic, of the lymphocytic cell line (acute and chronic lymphocytic leukemia) or myelogenous cell lines (acute and chronic myelogenous leukemia). Platelet counts from 25,000 mm³ to 60,000 mm³ are at sufficiently low levels to result in spontaneous bleeding. Most patients have white blood cell (WBC) counts of greater than 10,000 mm³. Common head and neck manifestations are cervical lymphadenopathy, laryngeal pain, gingival bleeding, oral ulceration, and gingival enlargement (**Fig. 14**B). Fever was the most common symptom in patients with all types of leukemia.[32]

Diabetes mellitus

Diabetes mellitus is associated with several oral disorders including gingivitis, peridontitis, salivary dysfunction, dental caries, oral mucosal diseases (lichen planus, recurrent aphthous stomatitis), candidiasis, xerostomia, burning mouth, and taste and neurosensory disorders.[33] The current preferred screening tests are limited to fasting plasma glucose (FPG), random plasma glucose (RPG), oral glucose tolerance test (OGTT), and glycosylated hemoglobin (HbA$_{1C}$).[34] The sensitivity and specificity

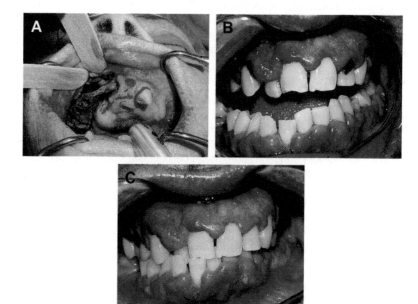

Fig. 14. (A) Patient taking intravenous bisphosphonate for metastatic breast cancer developed bisphosphonate-associated osteonecrosis after right upper molar extraction and required maxillectomy to keep necrosis from advancing into the orbit. (B) Patient with acute myelomonocytic leukemia with gingival hypertrophy before oral hygiene. (C) Improvement in gingival inflammation in same patient 48 hours after dental prophylaxis and initial chemotherapy.

relates to the glucose concentration. An FPG of greater than 110 mg/dL has sensitivity of 85.2% and specificity of 88.5%. An RPG of 130 mg/dL or greater has a balanced sensitivity (63%) and specificity (87%), based on diagnosis by OGTT. The OGTT, although inconvenient and rarely used, remains the gold standard for diagnosis of diabetes with 100% specificity. HbA_{1C} testing can be done in both fasting and nonfasting states and represents glucose control for a period of months rather than a single point value. When participants had both an HbA_{1C} greater than 6.1% and an FPG of 110 mg/dL or greater, the HbA_{1C} sensitivity was 71.6% and specificity 95.7%.[34]

Vitamin B_{12} and folate deficiency

Vitamin B_{12} and folate are B complex vitamins that are necessary for normal RBC formation, tissue and cellular repair, and DNA synthesis. Children do not have as extensive hepatic reserves of vitamin B_{12} and folate as adults and have rapidly progressing symptoms. A deficiency in either vitamin B_{12} or folate can lead to macrocytic anemia, with weakness, light-headedness, and shortness of breath. A vitamin B_{12} deficiency can result in varying degrees of neuropathy with tingling and numbness in the hands and feet and mental changes that range from confusion and irritability to severe dementia. Patients may also have impaired sense of smell, syncope, and may have an increased risk of myocardial infarction and stroke.

HIV

The HIV virus is detected by a screening enzyme-linked immunosorbent assay (ELISA) test, which is confirmed by a Western blot test. Tests can be done on blood, urine, and saliva. A large study on HIV testing in 752 US laboratories reported a sensitivity of 99.7% and specificity of 98.5% for enzyme immunoassay.[35] Viral load is a quantitative RNA viral test using polymerase chain reaction (PCR); the value is between 50 and 1,000,000 copies/mL, and less than 50 copies/mL is considered undetectable.

CD4 counts between 500 and 1500 per milliliter of blood are considered normal; counts less than 200 are considered AIDS.

Hepatitis

Hepatitis is inflammation of the liver from several causes. The viral hepatitis panel includes A, B and C viruses. Viral hepatitis B and C pose serious risks to health care workers; hepatitis B is discussed here. Testing for hepatitis B virus (HBV) is directed toward antibodies produced in response to HBV infection (anti-HBc, anti-HBs, IgM anti-HBc, IgG anti-HBc, anti-HBe); antigens produced by the virus (HbsAg, HBeAg), and viral DNA detection (HBV-DNA). Susceptible patients have no antigens or antibodies. Patients with acute infection have surface antigen, core and IgM antibodies but no surface antibody. Patients with chronic infection have surface antigen, core antibodies but no IgM and no surface antibody. Anyone with surface antigen (HbsAg) present is infective. Anyone with surface antibody (anti-HBs) present is immune (**Table 3**).

Coagulopathy

The best screening test for coagulopathy is a good history.[36] Initial laboratory evaluation includes CBC, platelets, peripheral blood smear, prothrombin time (PT) and partial thromboplastin time (PTT). Normal platelets range from 150,000 to 450,000 cells/µL. Thrombocytopenia can be detected from a CBC; a peripheral smear can help rule out pseudothrombocytopenia and identify abnormal platelets.[37] Traditionally, platelet function was measured by bleeding time, however the Platelet Function Analyzer-100 (Dade Behring Inc, Newark, DE, USA) has been shown to be superior in detecting von Willebrand disease, with a sensitivity of 89% and a specificity of

Table 3
Interpretation of hepatitis B serology

Tests	Results	Interpretation
HBsAg	Negative	Susceptible
Anti-HBc	Negative	
Anti-HBs	Negative	
HBsAg	Negative	Immune because of natural infection
Anti-HBc	Positive	
Anti-HBs	Positive	
HBsAg	Negative	Immune because of hepatitis B vaccination
Anti-HBc	Negative	
Anti-HBs	Positive	
HBsAg	Positive	Acutely infected
Anti-HBc	Positive	
IgM anti-HBc	Positive	
Anti-HBs	Negative	
HBsAg	Positive	Chronically infected
Anti-HBc	Positive	
IgM anti-HBc	Negative	
Anti-HBs	Negative	

90%.[38,39] PT is 10 to 12 seconds and measures extrinsic pathway factor VII and common pathway factors V, X, prothrombin and fibrinogen. Vitamin K is required for the synthesis of the critical factors of these pathways; liver disease and warfarin prolong the PT. The PT is now expressed in the international normalized ratio, a ratio of the patient's prothrombin time divided by a reference control. The activated PTT measures the intrinsic and common pathways (all factors except VII and XIII). PTT is altered in hemophilia A (factor VIII deficiency) and B (factor IX deficiency), and with use of the anticoagulant heparin.[1] An excellent discussion on coagulation factor inhibitor (blocking antibodies) vessel wall disorders (scurvy) and other disorders may be found in *Burket's Oral Medicine*.[1] Several new platelet function analyzers have been developed recently for screening for platelet function abnormalities and monitoring antiplatelet therapy; most have been designed as point-of-care instruments that are rapid, simple to use, and easy to interpret. These include modified thromboelastography, VerifyNow, Plateletworks, impact cone and plate(let) analyzer, and vasodilator-stimulated phosphoprotein phosphorylation assay. These newer technologies have yet to be extensively studied; therefore, their precision, reliability, and clinical usefulness remain unproved.[40]

CBC

CBC measures the cells that circulate in the bloodstream: WBCs (leukocytes), RBCs (erythrocytes), and platelets (thrombocytes). The WBC count is generally between 4300 and 10,800 cells/mL. The differential can be helpful to determine bacterial (neutrophil), viral (lymphocyte), or parasitic (eosinophil) infection; basophils and monocytes can also be helpful in identifying many disease states. The RBCs are evaluated for the amount of hemoglobin in grams/deciliter (low in anemia) and the packed cell volume or the hematocrit. The RBC indices, MCV, MCH, and MCHC, are useful in determining causes for anemia and other diseases such as thalassemia. Platelet disorders are congenital or acquired and are classified into quantitative and qualitative platelet disorders.[1]

CULTURE STUDIES

Gram staining is performed on the specimen at the time of culture. Although infections can be caused by aerobic or anaerobic bacteria or a mixture of both, brain, dental, and lung infections have a high probability of being caused by anaerobic bacteria. Anaerobic organisms have a characteristic appearance. *Bacteroides* are irregular-shaped gram-negative rods, *Fusobacterium* are pale gram-negative spindle-shaped rods, and *Clostridium* are large gram-positive rods that form spores. Anaerobes can live only in the absence of oxygen and are destroyed when exposed to the atmosphere in a matter of seconds. These cultures should be placed in an oxygen-free environment at 35°C (95°F) for at least 48 hours before the culture plates are examined for growth. Aerobic, fungal and *Mycobacterium* cultures are commonly performed in infections of the head and neck and require oxygen to grow; therefore a special environment during culture is not necessary. The oral cavity has indigenous aerobic and anaerobic flora, aerobic gram-negative rods, and fungi. The anaerobic organisms of oropharyngeal flora are pathogenic. The presence of aerobic gram-negative rods and fungi generally represent colonization and antibiotic coverage need not routinely be directed at these organisms. On the other hand, the antibacterial spectrum of an agent used for head and neck prophylaxis should include coverage for pathogenic oral flora, namely the gram-positive aerobic cocci (especially streptococci) and anaerobic bacteria.[41] *Mycobacterium* does not retain stain because of high lipid content in its wall, and is neither gram-positive nor gram-negative; a Ziehl-Neelsen stain (acid-fast) is required. Fungal specimens can be evaluated clinically by mixing with 10% potassium hydroxide and examining under magnification for the presence of fungal elements. Fungal cultures are then inoculated on to Sabouraud dextrose agar (SDA) with antibiotics for fungal culture and observed for 3 weeks. Fungi are identified from rate of growth, color, texture, pigmentation of fungal colony, and their morphologic features on microscopy. Viral swab specimens from the head and neck are placed in viral transport medium at 2 to 8°C. Diagnostic laboratory testing for virus infections are confirmed by cell culture, which causes cell changes specific for the type of virus involved. Acute viral infections are detection with virus-specific IgM antibodies in blood, which is produced for weeks. Chronic or previous viral infections are detected by virus-specific IgG antibodies, which are produced indefinitely. Viral antibody and antigens can be detected by ELISA. Viral nucleic acids (DNA, RNA) can be detected with PCR or by nucleic acid hybridization with virus-specific probes. Other techniques of viral detection include electron microscopy and hemagglutination assay.

PATHOLOGY
Fine-needle Aspiration

Fine-needle aspiration (FNA) cytology for an abnormal neck mass is reliable and inexpensive. A 23-gauge needle on a 10-mL disposable syringe is inserted into the questionable mass and cells are aspirated with negative pressure using multiple passes. A smear is made on a glass slide, which is then placed in 95% ethyl alcohol and followed by the Papanicolaou staining technique. The success depends on the accuracy of sampling and on the skill and experience of the tissue pathologist who will be examining the cells. Repeat aspiration is suggested and excision biopsy is occasionally considered. Frable and Frable[42] in 1982 reviewed 567 patients with neck masses and found the sensitivity and specificity of FNA to be 85% to 90%. Stevens and colleagues[43] showed pooled estimates of FNA for thyroid nodules to have sensitivity of 94% and specificity of 81%. This means that about 10% will have false-negative results and approximately 20% will be falsely positive. Ultrasound and computed tomography (CT) guidance can increase the accuracy of the FNA.[44] Aspirate results are based on 1 of the 4 types: 1, inadequate/insufficient; 2, benign; 3, atypical/indeterminate (suspicious of malignancy); 4, malignant.

Punch Biopsy

A punch biopsy ranges from 1 to 8 mm in diameter. The appropriate diameter for most inflammatory skin conditions is 4 mm. Ideally the biopsy should include the full thickness of skin and subcutaneous fat to fully identify the disease process. Smaller punched incisions often require only silver nitrate cautery and are left to heal without suturing.

Biopsy

Suspicious mucosal lesions that persist more than 3 weeks after removal of local irritants such as traumatic oral conditions, infection, or inflammation should undergo biopsy. The oral biopsy remains the gold standard for diagnosing a premalignant lesion or invasive carcinoma. If the biopsy results in dysplasia (low to high grade) the patient is at risk for progression to cancer and requires long-term monitoring and medical or surgical treatment. A clinical photograph of the lesion before biopsy is important as it documents the size, characteristics, and location of the original lesion. Future considerations for re-excision for malignancy, additional margins, or for directing accurate radiotherapy are improved with photographic documentation. The incisional or excisional biopsy procedure is done in the office under local anesthesia. A core biopsy is another method of tissue diagnosis that is used instead of FNA biopsy, or vice versa. The core biopsy preserves the cellular relationship of the tumor, which can help in diagnosis. Core biopsy is a more invasive procedure than FNA, as it involves making a small incision (cut) in the skin. A 14-gauge Vim-Silverman needle or the 16-gauge automated Biopty needle is passed through the incision and several narrow samples of the tissue are taken. Ultrasound guidance may be needed to locate the lump or area to be sampled. Core biopsy is also done under local anesthetic.

RADIOLOGY

Medical radiology of the head and neck includes the plain film, CT generally for bone assessment, magnetic resonance imaging for soft tissue evaluation, positron emission tomography initially used for head and neck cancer surveillance, now being used to improve accuracy of head and neck staging in newly diagnosed cancer,[45] barium swallow for functional swallow and aspiration evaluations, radionuclide imaging generally for thyroid and lymphatic assessment, and ultrasound for soft tissue evaluation and localization for FNA biopsies. Robitschek and colleagues[44] showed significant improvement in FNA sensitivity in the head and neck when using ultrasound.

Dental radiology includes the periapical film (PAX) to visualize periapical pathology, bitewing films to identify occlusal and interpromimal dental caries, occlusal films most commonly to identify submandibular sialolithiasis, the panorex (panoramic radiograph or orthopantomogram) is a two-dimensional view of the bones and dentition of the upper and lower dental arches. Cone-beam computed tomography is a recent addition to the dental practice, a helical three-dimensional CT scan for hard tissue imaging with high diagnostic quality and lower radiation doses than conventional CT scans.[46]

REFERENCES

1. Greenberg MS, Glick M, Ship JA. Burket's oral medicine. 11th edition. Hamilton (Ontario): BC Decker; 2008.
2. Neville BW, Damm DD, Allen CM, et al. Oral and maxillofacial pathology. 3rd edition. St. Louis (MO): WB Saunders; 2009.
3. Bickley LS, Szilagyi PG. Bates' guide to physical examination and history taking. 10th edition. Philadelphia: Lippincott Williams & Wilkins; 2008.
4. Davidson TM, Murphy C. Rapid clinical evaluation of anosmia: the alcohol sniff test. Arch Otolaryngol Head Neck Surg 1997;123(6):591–4.
5. Kumar V, Fausto N, Abbas A. Robbins & Cotran pathologic basis of disease. 7th edition. Philadelphia: W.B. Saunders Company; 2004. p. 1230.
6. Sapp JP, Eversole LR, George PW. Contemporary oral and maxillofacial pathology. 2nd edition. St Louis (MO): Mosby; 2004.
7. Mashberg A, Samit A. Early diagnosis of asymptomatic oral and oropharyngeal squamous cancers. CA Cancer J Clin 1995;45(6):328–51.
8. Vaccarezza GF, Antunes JL, Michaluart-Júnior P. Recurrent sores by ill-fitting dentures and intra-oral squamous cell carcinoma in smokers. J Public Health Dent 2010;70(1):52–7.
9. Saah AJ, Hoover DR. "Sensitivity" and "specificity" reconsidered: the meaning of these terms in analytical and diagnostic settings. Ann Intern Med 1997;126:91–4.
10. Lingen MW, Kalmar JR, Karrison T, et al. Critical evaluation of diagnostic aids for the detection of oral cancer. Oral Oncol 2008;44(9):10–22.
11. Whited JD, Grichnik JM. The rational clinical examination. Does this patient have a mole or a melanoma? JAMA 1998;279(9):696–701.
12. Poh CF, Zhang L, Anderson DW, et al. Fluorescence visualization detection of field alterations in tumor margins of oral cancer patients. Clin Cancer Res 2006;12(22):6716–22.
13. Helsper JT. Staining techniques: screening tests for oral cancer. Available at: http://caonline.amcancersoc.org. Accessed October 5, 2010.
14. Zhang L, Williams M, Poh CF, et al. Toluidine blue staining identifies high-risk primary oral premalignant lesions with poor outcome. Cancer Res 2005;65(17):8017–21.
15. Epstein JB, Gorsky M, Lonky S, et al. The efficacy of oral lumenoscopy (ViziLite) in visualizing oral mucosal lesions. Spec Care Dentist 2006;26(4):171–4.
16. McIntosh L, McCullough MJ, Farah CS. The assessment of diffused light illumination and acetic acid rinse (Microlux/DL) in the visualisation of oral mucosal lesions. 2009. Available at: http://www.oraloncology.com. Accessed October 5, 2010.
17. Lane PM, Gilhuly T, Whitehead PD, et al. Simple device for the direct visualization of oral-cavity tissue fluorescence. J Biomed Opt 2006;11(2):024006.
18. Poh CF, Ng SP, Williams PM, et al. Direct fluorescence visualization of clinically occult high-risk oral premalignant disease using a simple hand-held device. Head Neck 2007;29(1):71–6.
19. Hohlweg-Majert B, Deppe H, Metzger MC, et al. Sensitivity and specificity of oral brush biopsy. Cancer Invest 2009;27(3):293–7.
20. Trullenque-Eriksson A, Muñoz-Corcuera M, Campo-Trapero J, et al. Analysis of new diagnostic methods in suspicious lesions of the oral mucosa. Med Oral Patol Oral Cir Bucal 2009;14(5):E210–216.
21. Hu S, Loo JA, Wong DT. Human body fluid proteome analysis. Proteomics 2006; 6(23):6326–53.

22. Park NJ, Li Y, Yu T, et al. Characterization of RNA in saliva. Clin Chem 2006;52(6): 988–94.
23. Sidransky D. Emerging molecular markers of cancer. Nat Rev Cancer 2002;3: 210–9.
24. Dhingraa V, Gupta M, Andacht T, et al. New frontiers in proteomics research: a perspective. Int J Pharm 2005;299(1–2):1–18.
25. Hu S, Arellano M, Boontheung P, et al. Salivary proteomics for oral cancer biomarker discovery. Clin Cancer Res 2008;14(19):6246–52.
26. Li Y, St John MA, Zhou X, et al. Salivary transcriptome diagnostics for oral cancer detection. Clin Cancer Res 2004;10(24):8442–50.
27. Franzmann EJ, Reategui EP, Carraway KL, et al. Salivary soluble CD44: a potential molecular marker for head and neck cancer. Cancer Epidemiol Biomarkers Prev 2005;14(3):735–9.
28. Park NJ, Zhou H, Elashoff D, et al. Salivary microRNA: discovery, characterization, and clinical utility for oral cancer detection. Clin Cancer Res 2009;17: 5473–7.
29. Li Y, Elashoff D, Oh M, et al. Serum circulating human mRNA profiling and its utility for oral cancer detection. J Clin Oncol 2006;24(11):1754–60.
30. Malhotra R, Patel V, Vaque JP, et al. Ultrasensitive electrochemical immunosensor for oral cancer biomarker IL-6 using carbon nanotube forest electrodes and multi-label amplification. Anal Chem 2010;82(8):3118–23.
31. Wong DT. Salivary diagnostics powered by nanotechnologies, proteomics and genomics. J Am Dent Assoc 2006;137(3):313–21.
32. Hou GL, Huang JS, Tsai CC. Analysis of oral manifestations of leukemia: a retrospective study. Oral Dis 2008;3(1):31–8.
33. Ship JA. Diabetes and oral health: an overview. J Am Dent Assoc 2003;134: 4S–10S.
34. Cox ME, Edelman D. Tests for screening and diagnosis of type 2 diabetes. Clin Diabetes 2009;7:132–8.
35. Chou R, Huffman LH, Fu R, et al. Screening for HIV: a review of the evidence for the U.S. preventive services task force. Ann Intern Med 2005;143(1):55–73.
36. Manning SC, Beste D, McBride T, et al. An assessment of preoperative coagulation screening for tonsillectomy and adenoidectomy. Int J Pediatr Otorhinolaryngol 1987;13(3):237–44.
37. Ballas M, Kraut EH. Bleeding and bruising: a diagnostic work-up. Am Fam Physician 2008;77(8):1117–24.
38. Posan E, McBane RD, Grill DE, et al. Comparison of PFA-100 testing and bleeding time for detecting platelet hypofunction and von Willebrand disease in clinical practice. J Thromb Haemost 2003;90:483–90.
39. Hayward CPM, Harrison P, Cattaneo M, et al. Platelet function analyzer (PFA)-100 closure time in the evaluation of platelet disorders and platelet function. J Thromb Haemost 2006;4(6):312–9.
40. Seegmiller A, Sarode R. Laboratory evaluation of platelet function. Hematol Oncol Clin North Am 2007;21(4):731–42.
41. Johnson JT, Yu VL. Role of aerobic gram-negative rods, anaerobes, and fungi in wound infection after head and neck surgery: implications for antibiotic prophylaxis. Head Neck 1989;11(4):371.
42. Frable MA, Frable WJ. Fine-needle aspiration biopsy revisited. Laryngoscope 1982;92(12):1414–8.
43. Stevens C, Lee JK, Sadatsafavi M, et al. Pediatric thyroid fine-needle aspiration cytology: a meta-analysis. J Pediatr Surg 2009;44(11):2184–91.

44. Robitschek J, Straub M, Wirtz E, et al. Diagnostic efficacy of surgeon-performed ultrasound-guided fine needle aspiration: a randomized controlled trial. Otolaryngol Head Neck Surg 2010;142(3):306–9.

45. Lonneux M, Hamoir M, Reychler H, et al. Positron emission tomography with [18F] fluorodeoxyglucose improves staging and patient management in patients with head and neck squamous cell carcinoma: a multicenter prospective study. J Clin Oncol 2010;28(7):1190–5.

46. Scarfe WC, Farman AG, Sukovic P. Clinical applications of cone-beam computed tomography in dental practice. J Can Dent Assoc 2006;72(1):75–80.

Oral Manifestations of Smokeless Tobacco Use

Robert O. Greer Jr, DDS, ScD[a,b,c,*]

KEYWORDS

- Smokeless tobacco keratosis • Squamous cell carcinoma
- Dysplasia • Dental caries • Periodontal disease

For hundreds of years, tobacco has been smoked, chewed, and inhaled in various forms.[1,2] The use of smokeless tobacco (SLT) in North America seems to have originated with American Indians, and before 1900, the dominant form of tobacco used in North America was in fact SLT rather than cigarettes. With the advent of cigarettes, SLT use declined, until the 1970s when there was resurgence in its use.[3] Some investigators have suggested that there was a 10% increase in the use of SLT from the early 1970s until 1986, when the US Surgeon General's first report on SLT usage was published.[4] There was a brief decline in sales in the United States after the issuance of this report, but there has been a steady growth in usage since then.[3] Until this resurgence, there was a paucity of information concerning longitudinal cross-sectional evaluation of SLT-induced oral lesions of any kind in juveniles, adults, or geriatric patients. Since then research into the use and health consequences of all forms of SLT occurred, related with certainty to not only an upsurge in usage but also the lack of standardized clinical and histopathologic criteria detailing the oral manifestations of SLT use.

SLT is a broad encompassing term that includes both chewing tobacco and snuff. Three types of SLT are commonly manufactured: loose-leaf chewing tobacco, moist snuff, and dry snuff.[5] Loose-leaf chewing tobacco is processed and manufactured in the United States largely from tobacco plants grown in the Midwest. The product consists of shredded flakelike aggregates of air-cured leaf tobacco that is flavored with sweetening agents. Loose-leaf tobacco usage, long been favored by men, has declined during the past 2 decades.[6]

In contrast, moist snuff usage has dramatically gained popularity in the United States over the past 2 decades, with sales increasing as much as 77% over the

[a] Division of Oral and Maxillofacial Pathology, University of Colorado School of Dental Medicine, 13065 East 17th Avenue, Mail Stop F844, Aurora, CO 80045, USA
[b] Department of Pathology, 12605 East 16th Avenue, Mail Stop F768, Aurora, CO 80045, USA
[c] Department of Medicine, University of Colorado School of Medicine, 12801 East 17th Avenue, Mail Stop 8117, Aurora, CO 90045, USA
* Corresponding author. Division of Oral and Pathology, University of Colorado School of Dental Medicine, 13065 East 17th Avenue, Mail Stop F844, Aurora, CO 80045.
E-mail address: Robert.greer@ucdenver.edu

Otolaryngol Clin N Am 44 (2011) 31–56
doi:10.1016/j.otc.2010.09.002
0030-6665/11/$ – see front matter © 2011 Elsevier Inc. All rights reserved.

15-year period, from 1985 to 2000.[7] Known as *snus* in Sweden, moist snuff is composed of finely ground tobacco that can be placed discreetly in the oral cavity, most often between the buccal vestibular mucosa and gingiva. The product can be extracted from a small round tin or carton and delivered to the mouth via what is known colloquially as a tobacco "pinch."

Moist snuff produces minimal juices when used and requires very little expectoration. Moist snuff products in the United States undergo fermentation, whereas moist snuff products from Sweden, which undergo high-heat treatment, do not. Fermentation tends to give moist snuff its unique flavor, but the fermentation process also enhances cancer-inducing bacterial associated by-products, such as tobacco-specific N' nitrosamines and certain nitrites.[6]

Dry snuff, also fermented and fire cured, was first inhaled nasally by users and later used in oral form, primarily by women in the Southern states of the United States. The product was in common usage in the late nineteenth and early twentieth centuries. However, since the mid-20th century dry snuff usage has declined dramatically.

Oral use of snuff is colloquially referred to as "snuff dipping."[8] In 1984, it was estimated that the number of moist snuff sales in the United States was approximately 37.5 million pounds.[8] Albert and colleagues,[9] in 2008, reported that moist snuff sales had increased to the point that the sales accounted for 71% of the SLT market. Dry snuff sales are generally considered to be less than 10 million pounds annually and on the decline.[6]

EPIDEMIOLOGY

The number of Americans who currently use SLT in any of its forms can only be estimated. Estimates have ranged from 6 million[10] to 22 million.[11] The American Cancer Society[12] has placed the usage figure at closer to 7 million, whereas the American Council for Drug Education places the figure at a largely unsubstantiated 47 million.

In addition to the United States and Sweden, SLT is also widely used in India. In the largest single study of SLT usage in India, which included the assessment of 255,194 individuals from 9 geographic areas, the usage was reported to range from 11% to 49%.[13]

Some Swedish studies have reported that 35% of men in the age group of 16- to 24-years were regular or occasional users of snuff.[14,15] However, the frequency of snuff use seems to decline with the increasing age of subjects in each of the countries referenced.

Investigators in the United States have long attempted to determine the prevalence and specific usage patterns of SLT. In 1985, a national representative geographic study revealed that 60% of men in the United States between the ages of 12 and 17 years had used some form of SLT within the previous year.[11] Of those who had used SLT, approximately one-third used the product one or more times per week.[11] Grady and colleagues[16] reviewed 8 surveys of adolescent and adult SLT users in the United States and Canada published between 1981 and 1983 and found that between 8% and 10% of the young men were regular users of SLT.

ORAL MANIFESTATIONS OF SLT USE

The principle changes seen in the oral cavity related to SLT use include oral mucosal lesions (MLs) typically defined as (1) SLT-induced keratoses (STKs); (2) gingival inflammation, periodontal inflammation, and alveolar bone damage; (3) dental caries, tooth abrasion, and staining of tooth structure; and (4) dysplasia and oral cancer.

STK

Most studies related to SLT usage and the production of STKs have limitations. Most fail to control for confounding determinants such as cigarette smoking and alcohol usage. Negative confounding in some studies is also a possibility, especially in those in which smoking rates are lower in SLT users than in nonusers. It would necessarily appear that the relative risk (RR) for oral cancer would turn out to be remarkably low for SLT users in such studies. Nonetheless, most of the studies that have been reported over a period of approximately 47 years, primarily in the United States and Scandinavia, show a consistent clinical pattern as it relates to changes in the oral mucosa when SLT is used. The earliest study, by Pindborg and Renstrup[15] in 1963, described the effect of snuff on oral epithelium. Since that time, approximately 50 studies, including a study in 1986 concerning the noncancerous effects of SLT by the US Surgeon General, have been reported.[4]

Table 1 summarizes 16 of the most significant studies in the United States and Europe, which have detailed the oral manifestations of SLT usage with an end point of STK. The studies have been broken down into the following categories: prospective, experimental, and cross-sectional.

The placement of SLT, regardless of the type, in direct contact with the oral mucosa produces a thickened layer of keratin on the oral epithelial surface that occurs directly in the anatomic site where the SLT is placed.[16–18] STKs occur at the site of SLT placement in 60% of SLT users within 6 months to 3 years of initiation of use.[8] The studies by Greer and Poulson[8] suggest that moist snuff, which is alkaline, tends to produce lesions that are more prominent and more readily identifiable than those that occur in relation to the use of dry snuff or loose-leaf tobacco. However, regardless of the form of the SLT used, lesions nearly always appear directly in the anatomic site where the product is placed.

A central problem in the experimental design of many studies that have accessed the oral mucosa changes associated with SLT use is that the end point, that is STK, often does not exclude the possibility that the same type of keratotic lesion being evaluated may also be present in non-SLT users. Greer and colleagues[19] have only recently helped to clear up this confounding issue by defining the specific histology of SLT lesions compared with benign alveolar ridge hyperkeratoses (ARK) control tissue samples, thereby defining a specific type of hyperkeratotic histologic appearance that is benign and unique to STKs.

Axéll and colleagues[20] were the first to develop standardized clinical guidelines for grading STKs in adult snuff dippers. Their studies were followed by that of Hirsch and colleagues[21] who reviewed the clinical, histomorphologic, and histochemical features of snuff-induced lesions in 50 habitual adult snuff dippers. Hirsch and colleagues graded STKs according to an original 4-point clinical scale devised by Axéll and colleagues. Hirsch and colleagues further reported that all the lesions they accessed were hyperkeratotic to some degree, all lesions had color variations ranging from white to brown to yellow, and the surface texture of all lesions evaluated showed a variation in the mucosal surface pattern that ranged from wrinkled to leathery to deeply furrowed. Twelve significant additional Scandinavia clinical studies of STK have complemented the investigations of Axéll and colleagues and Hirsch and colleagues.[22–33] Kallischnigg and colleagues[34] summarized the findings of 50 studies documenting the oral changes associated with SLT use in both Europe and the United States in a review article in 2008.

In studies conducted in the United States during 1980 to 1982, Greer and Poulson[8] developed a standardized method for grading STKs that represented a modification of

Table 1
SLT studies with STK as an endpoint

Primary Author	Study Duration	Sex	Age	Population	Unique Details of Study Design	Ending Determinant
Experimental studies						
Grasser & Childers,[38] 1977	10 d	M, F	18–47 y	214 soldiers	4 SLT users with oral leukoplakia told to stop SLT use	STK
Payne et al,[39] 1998	7 d	M	Mean 25 y	16 snuff users with oral lesions at habitual sites	Site of snuff placement altered	STK
Martin et al,[35] 1999	6 wk	M	17–34 y	3051 air force trainees	119 SLT users with oral leukoplakia ordered to stop SLT use	STK
Cross-sectional studies of populations unselected by SLT use						
Greer & Poulson,[8] 1983	2 y	M, F	14–19 y	1119 high school students	—	STK
Poulson et al,[37] 1984	18 mo	M, F	14 to 19 y, mean 16.7 y	445 high school students	—	STK
Offenbacher & Weathers,[40] 1985	Not stated	M	10–17 y, mean 13.8 y	565 grammar and high school students	—	STK
Wolfe & Carlos,[41] 1987	Not stated	M, F	14–19 y, mean 16 y	226 Native American children at boarding school	—	STK
Cummings et al,[42] 1989	1985	M	22–44 y, mean 29 y	25 baseball players and coaches	—	STK
Creath et al,[36] 1988	Not stated	M	11–18 y	995 adolescent football players	—	STK

Study	Year	Sex	Age	Population	Comments	
Stewart et al,[43] 1989	Not stated	M	10–18	114 middle and high school students	5588 men and women interviewed, 182 examined orally, no results for 68 women	STK
Ernster et al,[44] 1990	1988	M, F	20–29 y	1109 professional baseball players	—	STK
Tomar et al,[45] 1997	1986–1987	M, F	12–17	17,027 school students	NIDCR National Survey on Oral Health	STK
Sinusas et al,[17] 2006	1991–2000	M	Mean 26 y	190–259 baseball players and coaches examined each year	Men attending spring training. Multiple occasion attendance	STK
Cross-sectional studies of populations selected by SLT use and/or presence of oral lesions						
Smith, et al[46] 1970	Not stated	M, F	Mean 55 y	15,000 long-term snuff users	—	STK
Little et al,[47] 1992	Not stated	M	15–77 y	245 SLT users in a Kaiser Permanente Dental Care Program	223 age-matched non-SLT users included in study	STK
Greer et al,[11] 1986	Not stated	M, F	15–75 y	45 SLT users	Patients segregated into 3 age groups	STK

Abbreviations: F, female; M, male; NIDCR, National Institute of Dental Research.

the Axéll classification, ultimately dividing STKs into 3 categories: degree I, degree II, and degree III lesions. Degree I lesions were defined by these investigators as those STKs that were superficially keratotic with slight opaqueness and color similar to that of the surrounding mucosa and with only slight wrinkling and no obvious mucosal thickening. Degree II lesions were classified as those lesions that were also superficial keratoses, typically white with occasional reddish areas and with moderate wrinkling and no obvious or dramatic thickening. Grade III lesions were white lesions that showed intervening furrows of normal mucosal color, obvious mucosal thickening, and dramatic wrinkling. Examples of the 3 grades of STK are shown in **Figs. 1–3**. In addition to evaluating the clinical appearance of STKs associated with SLT use, Greer and Pulson[8] classified all lesions according to their texture, contour, and color. The vast majority of the 117 lesions that were ultimately evaluated and classified from a total of 1119 teenagers screened were white, corrugated, and raised.

The prevalence of STK has been found to increase with the increased frequency of SLT use or with the amount of SLT used.[8,11,18,35,36] One study of note reported a resolution of STKs. This study involved US Air Force trainees with STKs who were evaluated after 6 weeks of mandated discontinuance of SLT.

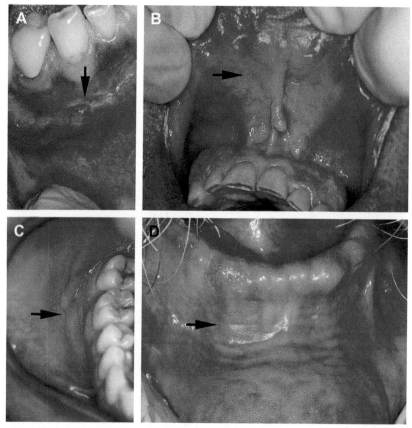

Fig. 1. (*A–D*) Grade I STK (*arrows*) demonstrating an area of superficial keratoses with opaqueness, slight wrinkling, and no dramatic mucosal thickening. (*Courtesy of* John McDowell, DDS, Denver, CO, USA.)

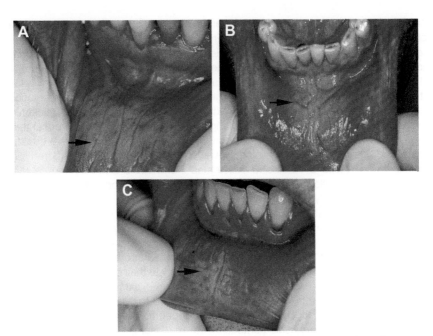

Fig. 2. (*A–C*) Grade II STK (*arrows*) demonstrating white keratotic areas with moderate wrinkling and the absence of significant thickening. (*Courtesy of* John McDowell, DDS, Denver, CO, USA.)

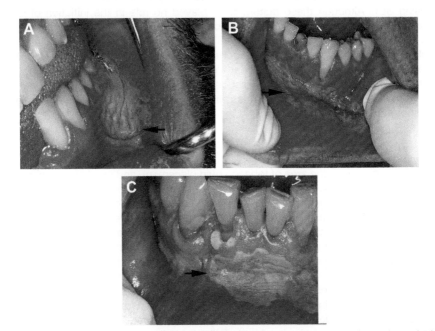

Fig. 3. (*A–C*) Grade III STK (*arrows*) demonstrating white keratotic areas with obvious thickening of the mucosal surface and dramatic wrinkling. (*Courtesy of* John McDowell, DDS, Denver, CO, USA.)

Although the initial investigations of Greer and Poulson[8] assessed oral tissue alterations associated with SLT use in teenagers, Greene and colleagues[18] completed a 3-year study of STKs in major and minor league baseball players and found that in a somewhat older population, in which the subjects were between the ages of 20 and 29 years, 4 different types of leukoplakic lesions could be identified: (1) STKs that had no or only very slight color change, with some obvious change in mucosal texture; (2) STKs that had a color and texture change with no mucosal thickening; (3) STKs that had a color and texture change, with mild or moderate mucosal thickening; and (4) STKs that had no semblance of normal mucosal color, severe texture change, and heavy mucosal thickening. However, this classification that offered slight modifications to those of Axéll and colleagues[20] and Greer and Poulson[8] is rarely used. Greene and colleagues[18] also found no focally erythroplakic component to the lesions in their study, as did Greer and Poulson.[8]

In a study of SLT use in India, Murti and colleagues[13] identified STKs in patients who chewed tobacco. However, the tobacco that was used was typically used in association with betel quid, a mixture of betel leaves, areca nut, slaked lime, and catechu. These investigators did not classify the lesions identified into any clinical grade.

Greer and colleagues[11] completed a follow-up study to their original study in 1983 of STK in teenagers with an assessment that involved an evaluation of STK in juvenile, adult, and geriatric patients. These investigators found that the 3 clinical classifications of SLT lesions that they had originally developed for teenagers, including alterations in the color, texture, and contour of the mucosal lining of the mouth, were equally applicable to adults and geriatric patients. The lesions the investigators identified in the adult population were site specific, just as in teenagers. However, there were associated confounding variables in both studies. Some subjects in each of the studies also used alcohol, and as high as 18% had smoked cigarettes in addition to using SLT. Although these factors likely played no role in the initiation of site-specific STK, their possible causative role cannot be ignored.

In addition to the 16 studies of STK in the United States outlined in **Table 1**,[8,11,17,35–47] Kallischnigg has reported on 21 similar European studies.[34] The European studies report findings similar to those from the United States, although the Kallischnigg review defined SLT-associated lesions documented by investigators in both the United States and Europe as simply MLs and suggested that the lesions were not necessarily SLT specific.

Histopathology of STK

STK occurs directly in the area of tobacco quid placement, and most lesions occur in the mandibular mucobuccal folds where the tobacco quid is held between the alveolus and the buccal or labial mucosal surface.[8] Other anatomic sites, most often the maxillary alveolar mucosa and buccal mucosa, can be affected. Although as many as 33 scientific articles published between 1963 and 2007 have described the clinical appearance of STK,[34] only a few studies describe the histopathology of such lesions. The largest studies describing such histopathologic changes have included evaluations of 45, 27, 77, 81, 92, and 142 tissue samples. These studies include a study by Greer and colleagues[11] in which 45 tissue samples were examined, the study by Greer and Eversole[48] in which 27 tissue samples were examined, the investigation by Greer and colleagues[49] in which 77 tissue samples were examined, the 81 STK samples studied by Greer and colleagues,[19] the studies of Grady and colleagues[16] in which 92 biopsy samples were examined, and the investigations of Daniels and colleagues[50] in which 142 samples were examined.

A remarkably consistent pattern has been documented by these investigators in cataloging the microscopic features associated with STK. The lesions evaluated in the aforementioned 6 studies were principally classified as degree I, degree II, or degree III lesions, using the clinical grading criteria established by Greer and Poulson.[8] Each category of lesion showed a distinct pattern of mild, moderate, or severe hyperkeratosis or parakeratosis along the epithelial surface. These histologic patterns can be seen in **Figs. 4–6**. The pattern of keratinization often demonstrates streaks of parakeratosis that extends above the epithelial surface, giving the lesion a focal wavy, "chevron," or church spire appearance (see **Fig. 5**). The chevron streaks often show parakeratinized streams of cells arranged in a latticelike pattern, resembling a pine tree. Between chevrons, the epithelial cells typically demonstrate vacuolated cytoplasm, and keratohyalin granules tend to be prominent. Chevron keratinization can be judged as either mild, moderate, or severe, and although the chevron pattern is not unique to STK because it has also occasionally been documented in lesions from pipe smokers and cigarette smokers, Greer and colleagues[19,37,48,49] found this specific form of church spire–like keratinization to be present in 93% of the samples they examined in 4 different studies. Matched control samples from cigar and cigarette smokers demonstrated chevron keratinization in only 30% of cases, and chevron keratinization was absent in 30 cases of matched control alveolar keratoses in the study by Greer and colleagues.[19]

The epithelium in most STKs does not demonstrate cytologic atypia, although basal layer hyperplasia, a form of altered cellular maturation, can be quite prominent.

Another histologic feature commonly associated with STK is the presence of dark cell keratinocytes.[11,49] This special form of keratinocyte is characterized by its strong affinity for basic dyes and by the electron density of the cell's cytoplasm and nucleus. Dark cell keratinocytes are not unique to SLT lesions and have been reported in other keratoses as well as normal epithelium.[11,49] The presence or absence of dark cell keratinocytes cannot be correlated with a specific grade of STK, and these keratinocytes do not appear to represent any form of premalignant alteration. On electron microscopic evaluation, dark cell keratinocytes appear almost exclusively in a basal or parabasal position in the epithelium. When compared with cheek biting controls or hyperkeratoses caused by denture trauma, the dark cell keratinocytes in STK can be identified 15 times more frequently.

Subepithelial Collagen Eosinophilia

Pindborg and Renstrup[51] in Sweden and Archard and Tarpley[52] in the United States reported finding a band of homogeneous eosinophilic material in the connective tissue of mucosal sites chronically exposed to SLT. Initially, these changes were thought to

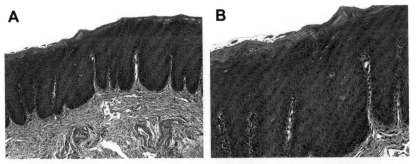

Fig. 4. (*A, B*) Low- and medium-power photomicrographs showing the histopathology of grade I STK. Note the corrugated parakeratotic surface and epithelial acanthosis (hematoxylin and eosin stain, original magnification *A,* × 100; *B,* × 200).

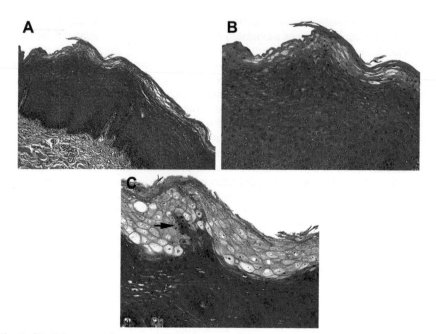

Fig. 5. (*A, B*) Low-, medium-, and high-power photomicrographs of grade II STK (hematoxylin and eosin stain, original magnification *A,* × 100; *B,* × 200). (*C*) A classic chevron parakeratotic streak, resembling the latticelike pattern of a pine tree (*arrow*) (hematoxylin and eosin stain, original magnification × 200).

be related to the use of a particular brand snuff, and neither investigative team was able to characterize this material as amyloid. Greer and colleagues[11] were able to find the eosinophilic band in only 2 of the 45 cases they studied, and the impression of these investigators was that the band represented a form of collagen sclerosis and that it was of extracellular origin. Further investigations of this special form of collagen eosinophilia have not been undertaken.

In addition to the band of homogenous eosinophilic material described by Pindborg and Renstrup,[51] the connective tissue in STKs can demonstrate salivary gland fibrosis and chronic sialadenitis (see **Fig. 6**). Dilated excretory ducts have been identified in STK and seem to be most common in grade III lesions. **Tables 2–4** delineate the

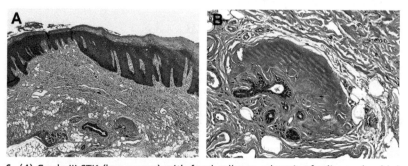

Fig. 6. (*A*) Grade III STK (low power) with focal collagen sclerosis of salivary gland lobular architecture (hematoxylin and eosin stain, original magnification × 40). (*B*) Medium-power photomicrograph showing glandular sclerosis (hematoxylin and eosin stain, original magnification × 200).

Table 2
Juvenile and young adult SLT users (15- to 25-years old)

Case	Age (y)	Salivary Gland Fibrosis	Dark Cell Keratinocytes	Eosinophilic Band	Chevron Keratinization	Basal Layer Hyperplasia	Koilocytosis
1	16	NE	+	—	+	—	—
2	16	NE	—	—	—	—	—
3	20	—	+	—	+	+	+
4	15	NE	+	+	+++	++	+
5	17	NE	NE	—	++	++	+
6	17	NE	—	—	+	—	+
7	13	NE	—	—	+	—	+
8	20	NE	—	—	+++	+	+
9	21	+++	+	—	+++	—	+
10	22	—	NE	—	++	+	—
11	21	—	—	—	++	+	—
12	17	NE	—	—	++	+	+
13	22	—	—	—	++	+	—
14	18	NE	+	—	+	++	+
15	25	++	+	—	++	+	+

Abbreviations: +, mild: sparsely distributed chevron spikes with multiple wide zones of flat parakeratin along epithelial surface; ++, moderate: intermittent chevron spikes with frequent narrow flat zones of parakeratin along epithelial surface; +++, severe: diffuse linear chevron spiking with rare flat zones of parakeratin along epithelial surface; NE, not evaluable.

histopathologic features of STK originally identified by Greer and colleagues[11] in their studies of juvenile, young adult, and adult SLT users.

Koilocytosis

An additional histologic feature common to the epithelium of biopsy samples from SLT users is koilocytotic change within epithelial cells (**Fig. 7**). Koilocytes represent the inclusion of intranuclear viruslike particles from human papillomavirus (HPV) in the epithelium. Koilocytes have been identified in uterine cervical carcinoma as well as in oral squamous cell carcinoma (SCC).[19,48,49] Greer and colleagues[11] found koilocytes to be present in 26 of 45 STK biopsy specimens they examined in a study of STK in 1986. When these tissue samples were immunohistochemically stained for the presence of HPV capsid antigen, 6 of the 26 cases were positive for the antigen. These studies, along with others by the same research group, were the first to suggest a possible link between HPV infection, STK, and oral SCC.[49,53,54]

Gingival and Periodontal Inflammation and Alveolar Bone Damage

A second significant clinical effect that has been reported in association with SLT use is gingival and periodontal inflammation and alveolar bone damage. However, there is a considerable divergence in findings reported in the United States and the Scandinavian literature concerning the subject. From 21 Swedish studies that Kallischnigg and colleagues[34] evaluated, only 1 study showed a relationship between gingivitis and snuff use[26] and no studies demonstrated a statistically significant relationship

Table 3
Adult users (26- to 54-years old)

Case	Age (y)	Salivary Gland Fibrosis	Dark Cell Keratinocytes	Eosinophilic Banc	Chevron Keratinization	Basal Layer Hyperplasia	Koilocytosis
16	46	NE	+	—	+++	+++	+
17	42	NE	—	—	+++	—	+
18	29	NE	+	—	++	—	+
19	50	+	—	—	+++	++	+
20	47	NE	—	—	+++	++	+
21	27	NE	+	—	++	—	—
22	28	—	—	—	+	—	—
23	51	NE	—	—	++	+	—
24	29	NE	+	—	++	+	—
25	30	NE	—	—	+++	+	—
26	54	NE	+	—	+++	++	—
27	41	—	—	—	++	+	+
28	38	NE	+	—	++	—	+
29	25	—	—	—	++	++	+
30	54	—	—	—	++	—	+

Abbreviations: +, mild: sparsely distributed chevron spikes with multiple wide zones of flat para-keratin along epithelial surface; ++, moderate: intermittent chevron spikes with frequent narrow flat zones of parakeratin along epithelial surface; +++, severe: diffuse linear chevron spiking with rare flat zones of parakeratin along epithelial surface; NE, not evaluable.

between the presence of calculus, plaque, pocket depth attachment loss, or alveolar bone loss and snuff use.

Studies in the United States, however, report high rates of gingival recession[40] and loss of periodontal ligament attachment[33,44] in SLT users. In all, a total of 8 studies from the United States strongly support that SLT use results in attachment loss, particularly gingival recession, (**Fig. 8**) and ultimately periodontal disease and bone loss.[36,40–42,44,55] It seems that the association between SLT and periodontal or gingival recession is related to the quantity of SLT used In the United States, initial gingivitis in the area of SLT placement seems to promote the ensuing and damaging SLT effect. Bastiaan[56] found routine gingivitis in the area of SLT contact in 31% to 92% of young adult SLT users. Greer and Poulson,[8] in their study of oral tissue alterations associated with SLT use by teenagers, also documented tobacco-associated periodontal deterioration or advanced periodontal disease.

Periodontal pathology is most likely related to long-term use of SLT and is more typical in adult population than in teenagers, as several investigations have reported.[11,33,37,40,41]

Although gingival and periodontal inflammation and bone damage can clearly be seen in association with SLT use, there have been no relevant studies completed that totally eliminate confounding variables, such as the use of other forms of tobacco; periodontal damaging systemic diseases, such as diabetes; or simply preexisting periodontal disease that may already exist in concert with SLT use. Therefore, although SLT can clearly cause damage to the periodontium, most commonly seen in the form of gingival migration and attachment loss, graded forms of that damage similar to the clinical grading schemes that have been devised for STK have not been established.

Table 4
Geriatric users (55 years and older)

Case	Age (y)	Salivary Gland Fibrosis	Dark Cell Keratinocytes	Eosinophilic Band	Chevron Keratinization	Basal Layer Hyperplasia	Koilocytosis
31	62G	NE	—	—	+++	+++	+
32	66G	NE	—	—	+	+	+
33	66G	NE	—	+	—	+	—
34	63G	—	—	—	+++	—	+
35	67G	NE	—	—	+++	—	+
36	69G	NE	+	—	+++	—	—
37	66G	++	—	—	—	+	—
38	63G	NE	+	—	+++	++	—
39	73G	—	+	—	++	++	+
40	74G	—	+	—	++	+	—
41	64G	—	+	—	++	+	+
42	72G	—	+	—	++	+	—
43	66G	—	—	—	+	—	—
44	55G	—	—	—	+	—	—
45	56G	—	—	—	++	—	+

Abbreviations: +, mild: sparsely distributed chevron spikes with multiple wide zones of flat para-keratin along epithelial surface; ++, moderate: intermittent chevron spikes with frequent narrow flat zones of parakeratin along epithelial surface; +++, severe: diffuse linear chevron spiking with rare flat zones of parakeratin along epithelial surface; NE, not evaluable.

Dental Caries, Tooth Abrasion, and Staining of Teeth

Dental caries in association with SLT use has been investigated extensively in 7 studies in the United States[8,37,40,44,55,57,58] and 3 important studies from Sweden.[32,59,60] These 7 studies in the United States showed minimal relationship between dental caries and SLT use. However, the use of loose-leaf chewing tobacco was specifically found to be associated with decayed teeth, decay in filled permanent

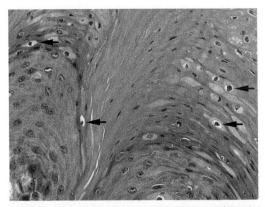

Fig. 7. High-power photomicrograph of markedly hyperparakeratinized grade III STK, demonstrating HPV-associated koilocytosis (*arrows*). This lesion ultimately transitioned to precancerous verrucous hyperplasia (hematoxylin and eosin stain, original magnification × 400).

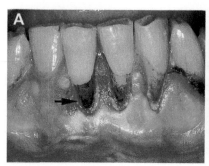
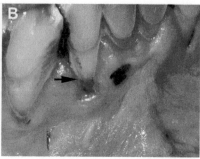

Fig. 8. (*A, B*) Periodontal damage in the form of significant gingival recession and loss of ligament attachment associated with grade I STK (*arrows*). (*Courtesy of* John McDowell, DDS, Denver, CO, USA.)

teeth, and caries of root surfaces in several studies.[8,37,40,44,55,57] The amount of dental caries increased with the number of packs of chewing tobacco used on a weekly basis and also with the number of years of use in a comprehensive study done by Tomar and Winn.[58] Two Swedish investigations[32,60] showed no relationship between SLT use and dental caries, whereas a third study[59] reported a slight increase in caries among snuff users. The overall evidence from both the studies in Sweden and the United States suggests that there is a relationship between the use of SLT and dental caries and that the risk increases significantly with the use of loose-leaf chewing tobacco.

It has been speculated that the relative lack of dental caries in heavy users of SLT may be because of the accelerated salivary flow that the tobacco stimulates, thus washing the bacteria necessary to induce caries away from tooth structure and in effect causing a physical cleanings action and a mild buffering action that inhibits the accumulation of plaque and carcinogenic material on the teeth. It has also been reported by Christen[2] that certain SLT products contain fluoride, which may be instrumental in the suppression of dental caries in SLT users as well.

Both tooth abrasion and severe staining of teeth (see **Fig. 8**) can be seen in association with SLT use. However, Greer and Poulson[8] reported only a single case of abrasion in their study of 117 teenage SLT users, which at the time of the study was thought to be chemical erosion of tooth structure. Whether or not abrasion is related to the presence of some agent other than tobacco in SLT or, in fact, is related merely to a constant placement of the SLT in the same anatomic site has not been established.

Rare instances of SLT-associated melanosis and prosthetic appliance stains associated with SLT use as well as delayed alveolar wound healing in association with SLT use after tooth extractions have been reported.[61] These changes appear to be as dependent on the amount of available plaque and calculus in the patient's mouth as they are to the amount of SLT used.

Oral Cancer and Dysplasia

The most significant issue to be debated in relation to the oral manifestations of SLT use is whether or not SLT plays a role in causing oral epithelial dysplasia, as seen in the clinical and biopsy histopathologic photographs of an SLT user in **Figs. 9** and **10**, or oral SCC, as seen in the clinical and biopsy histopathologic photographs of an SLT user in **Figs. 11** and **12**. In a study in 1986 of 45 STK biopsy specimens from juveniles, adults, and geriatric patients, with 15 patients assigned to each category, Greer and

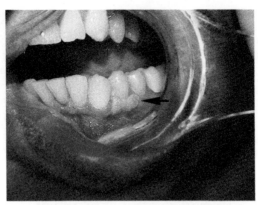

Fig. 9. STK showing moderate epithelial dysplasia microscopically. (*Courtesy of* John McDowell, DDS, Denver, CO, USA.)

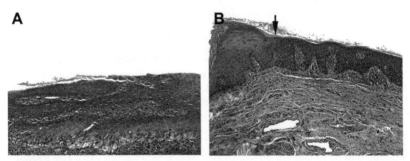

Fig. 10. Photomicrograph of mild epithelial dysplasia, in two grade II STKs. Note the marked basal layer hyperplasia (*A*) and the zone of dysplastic transition (*B*, *arrow*) (hematoxylin and eosin stain, original magnification *A*, × 200; *B*, × 100).

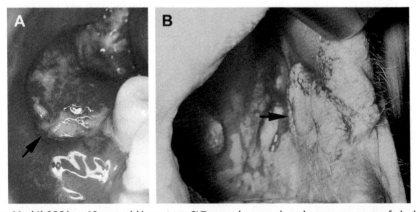

Fig. 11. (*A*) SCC in a 46-year-old long-term SLT user who was also a heavy consumer of alcohol (*arrow*). (*B*) SCC in a 77-year-old woman who had used dry snuff for 48 years (*arrow*). The patient admitted to being a moderate consumer of alcohol. Her lesions were initially multi-focal, presenting in 4 areas on the oral cavity, and the lesion shown was HPV-16 positive with PCR amplification of HPV-16 DNA. (*Courtesy of* John McDowell, DDS, Denver, CO, USA [A].)

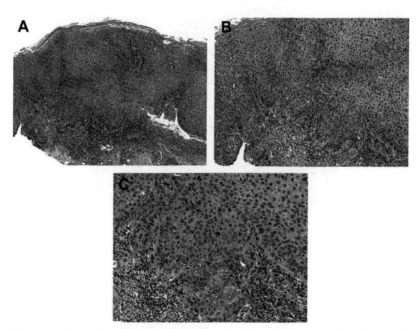

Fig. 12. Low- (*A*), medium-(hematoxylin and eosin stain, original magnification × 40) (*B*), and high-power (hematoxylin and eosin stain, original magnification × 100) (*C*) photomicrographs of SCC in a long-term SLT user and smoker (hematoxylin and eosin stain, original magnification × 200).

colleagues[11] found 1 instance of mild dysplasia in a 44-year-old man. The subject was also a smoker but did not use alcohol. Thus, it was not possible to determine if SLT alone accounted for the dysplastic epithelial change, even though the lesion biopsied was site specific for SLT placement. No assays for HPV, another important potential participant in the oral SCC cascade, were completed on the dysplastic tissue sample.

In a 1989 study, Kaugars and colleagues[62] evaluated 108 patients with histologically confirmed diagnoses of epithelial dysplasia of the oral cavity and a prior history of SLT use and found 44 instances of dysplasia in the location where the patients had reportedly placed SLT. The most common lesional locations were the buccal mucosa/vestibule and alveolar ridge/gingiva. No difference was found in various dysplastic histologic grades for lesions with the use of either snuff or chewing tobacco. The study by Kaugar and colleagues, however, failed to fully take into account the confounding variables of smoking, the use of alcohol, or oral infection with HPV.

An investigation in 1993 by Wray and McGuirt[63] involved the review of medical records from 128 elderly white female patients with oral carcinoma, all of whom were reported to have used SLT exclusive of other carcinogens. The average age of the patients in the study was 78 years, and just more than two-thirds of the patients had used SLT for 40 years or more. About 26% of patients had multiple oral lesions, suggesting that the lesions in fact represented what is now recognized as part of the proliferative verrucous leukoplakia continuum, a multifocal form of oral leukoplakia known to favor women and documented to be HPV associated.[64] No lesions in the study by Wray and McGuirt were accessed for the presence of HPV. Nonetheless, the study is one of the most compelling in the literature to suggest a possible cause-and-effect relationship between SLT and oral SCC because of the exclusion of the confounding variables of smoking and alcohol in the population studied, even in the face of a lack of molecular assessment of any tissue for HPV.

Two large and important prospective studies of mortality among men who used snuff or chewing tobacco in the United States showed no specific link between the use of SLT and oral cancer,[65] but men in the 2 studies who used SLT had higher death rates from all causes and it is reasonable, as the investigators suggest, that SLT, like other tobacco products, increases mortality from heart disease and stroke.

Meta-analysis of the relationship between the European and American SLT users and oral cancer was performed by Weitkunat and colleagues[66] in an investigation in 2007. These investigators reviewed the literature and completed a meta-analysis of 32 epidemiologic studies published between 1920 and 2005, which discussed a link between oral cancer and SLT use. The study included tests for homogeneity and publication bias. The investigators concluded that SLT as used in the United States and Europe carries at most a minor increased risk of oral cancer but that elevated risks in specific populations or from a specific product could not be definitely excluded on the basis of their review. The increased risk for oral cancer, the investigators determined, was primarily evident in studies that were conducted before 1980. No increased risk for oral cancer was seen in studies in Scandinavia. Oral cancer risk was found to be higher in case control studies with hospital controls and in women. The risk significantly decreased in 7 studies that adjusted for smoking and alcohol elimination.

In a study in 2004, Waterbor and colleagues[67] investigated disparities between public health educational materials and the scientific evidence suggesting that SLT causes cancer. These investigators reviewed 4-dozen health education brochures that reported the dangers of SLT use, all printed between 1981 and 2001 and available to the public in 2002. The brochures stated that SLT use causes oral leukoplakia, other oral conditions, and cancers of the oral cavity, larynx, pharynx, esophagus, stomach, pancreas, lung, breast, prostate, bladder, and kidney. However, a review of the scientific literature to determine whether these claims were substantiated showed that there is evidence for cancer causation by SLT only for oral leukoplakia and several other oral conditions. The evidence that SLT causes oral cancer was clearly suggestive, whereas the evidence for causation of other cancers was either absent or contradictory.

Rodu[6] has also reported that SLT use has a low potential for initiating oral cancer but that STK rarely develops into oral cancer, largely because there are marked differences between STK and standard oral leukoplakia, especially in regard to the frequency of dysplastic development in the 2 types of lesions. This investigator further reports that dysplasia is seen very infrequently in STK and that even when dysplasia is found in STK, it is usually found in an earlier stage than in standard oral leukoplakias. Rodu's finding is supported by the fact that typical non-SLT–associated oral leukoplakia, as described by Waldron and Shafer[68] in a study in 1975 of 3256 cases, showed a transition rate to dysplasia of approximately 20%, much higher than the 3% seen with STK.

Rodu reports that no distinctions in the literature related to the risk for oral cancer have been made between dry snuff and moist snuff, even though these products are quite different in relation to their tobacco content, method of processing, and ability to initiate dysplastic mucosal changes. In a follow-up study to the site-specific cancer comparative cause studies of 1977 by Wynder and Stellman,[69] Rodu and Cole[70] reported relative risk estimates for developing oral cancer from the use of SLT. This study again documented that SLT use was associated with low cancer risk and all RR estimates reported were less than 2. Dry snuff especially showed very little risk for oral cancer initiation according to the investigators. Nonetheless, the scientific literature supports the fact that there is a risk for oral cancer associated with SLT use and, whether minimal or not, the risk is real.[71–74]

One significant problem, however, with most studies that have been performed concerning SLT use and the risk for oral cancer relates to the fact that most epidemiologic studies that have been done do not control for the 3 most important oral cancer determinants, cigarette smoking, alcohol, and HPV infection. Important research in this arena is therefore a must.

Boffetta and colleagues[75] reported in a study in 2008 that in India and Sudan, more than 50% of oral cancers can be attributed to the use of SLT and that as many as 4% of the oral cancers in men in the United States are attributable to the use of SLT. These investigators concluded that the cancer risk in SLT users is probably lower than that in smokers but higher than that in nontobacco users. Although the earlier studies of Volger and colleagues,[76] Winn and colleagues,[77] Blot and colleagues,[78] and Kabat and colleagues[79] suggest that SLT results in a RR for oral cancer, the investigations by Wydner and colleagues,[71] Peacock and colleagues,[80] Vincent and Marchetta,[81] Martinez,[82] Mashberg,[72] and Schwartz[83] all indicate that the risk is low. In support of this concept, a 1975 study by Smith and colleagues[84] found no cases of oral cancer in 1550 individuals with STKs who were followed up for 10 years. A 1991 study by Christen and colleagues[85] found no cases of oral cancer among 550 regular SLT users who were followed up for 6 years, and a retrospective study of 200,000 snuff users by Axéll and colleagues[86] in Sweden found only 1 case of oral cancer developing in that population per year.

If the incidence of STK developing into oral cancer is an uncommon finding, the question that must be answered is whether there are predictable clinical, histopathologic, or molecular findings in tissue samples from SLT users that can identify high-risk STKs at their earliest precancerous transformational stage. Few studies have addressed this issue, and not until the STK clinical classification studies of Axéll and colleagues[20] and similar clinical and molecular studies of Greer and colleagues,[87] Shroyer and Greer,[88] and Palefsky and colleagues[54] did researchers begin to access which clinical grades of STK represented the highest risk potential to patients, what specific clinical patterns in those lesions put patients at increased risk for developing oral cancer, and what molecular events associated with STK development might be harbingers of neoplasia.

RISK-ASSOCIATED CLINICAL AND MOLECULAR FINDINGS IN STK

Because most STKs are generally reversible when SLT is discontinued,[22] defining which specific clinical lesions carry neoplastic risk is of extreme importance. Studies

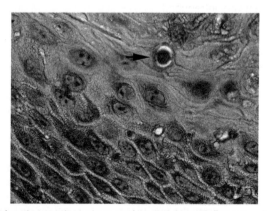

Fig. 13. HPV capsid antigen staining in a grade II STK (*arrow*) (hematoxylin and eosin stain, original magnification × 400).

in the author's laboratory have shown that those clinical grades of STKs described by either Axéll[20] or Greer and Poulson,[8] which demonstrate a markedly papillary or velvety surface, appear to have the highest risk for possible neoplastic transition. Shroyer and Greer[88] and Greer and colleagues[19] have reported that such STKs show a higher degree of cytologic atypia than lesions that have a typical grade I homogeneous leukoplakic appearance or even an undulating grade II or III surface. These investigators have also reported that more than 40% of the high-risk STKs they

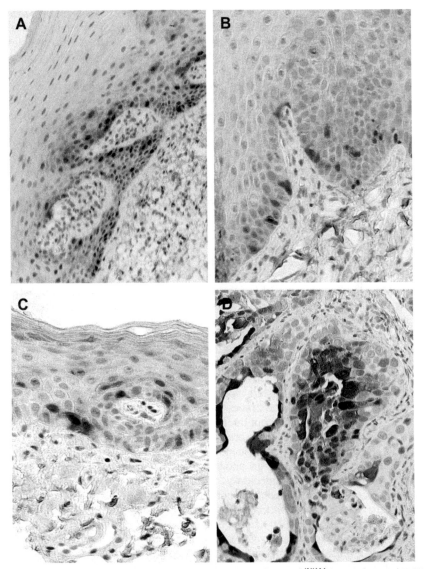

Fig. 14. (A–C) Immunohistochemical (ISH) localization of HPV-16^{INK4A} in grade I and II STKs (hematoxylin and eosin stain, original magnification A, × 100; B, × 200; C, × 200). (D) ISH p16^{INK4A} staining for SLT-associated SCC in the patient shown in **Fig. 11B**. The tissue sample was β-globin positive and PCR informative for HPV-16 (hematoxylin and eosin stain, original magnification × 300).

studied harbored HPV-specific antigens (**Fig. 13**).[48,49] Overexpression of the enzyme telomerase, a key marker of cellular immortalization, has also been documented in precancerous verrucous hyperplasia and in STK.[87]

Because a significant proportion of oral SCC, perhaps as high as 30% of cases, are now thought to be related to infection with HPV and because investigators have identified high-risk HPV DNA[87–89] as well as other abhorrent regulatory genes in 15% to 40% of STKs or STK-associated oral SCC, it seems logical that HPV may play a synergistic developmental role in certain STKs that go on to develop into cancer.

Greer and colleagues[19] recently examined the role of p16[INK4A] protein as a possible surrogate marker of HPV-mediated carcinogenesis in a series of 140 tissue samples, including 81 STK samples of various grades, 29 oral SCC samples, and 30 samples of control cases of benign alveolar ridge keratoses, to determine if p16[INK4A] expression might be a reliable marker for precancer and cancer in those lesions. Although HPV DNA was detected in biopsy samples from grade I, II, and III STK and oral SCC (**Fig. 14**), its presence did not fully correlate with p16[INK4A] expression. The study did, however, demonstrate an apparent relationship between the grade of STK and presence of HPV. HPV was not detected in grade III STK, perhaps because just as with high-grade cervical dysplasias, high-grade STKs are driven by HPV viral integration and support only a low copy number of HPV DNA. Those cases of STKs in the study that harbored HPV were all grades I and II clinically, and 15 of the 21 of those lesions were described clinically by the submitting dentist or oral surgeon as having a bumpy velvetlike surface, a clinical feature that should be considered high risk.

SUMMARY

Epidemiologic studies throughout the literature suggest that the use of moist snuff, as is typically used in the United States, is associated with a real but minimal risk for oral cancer. Most investigations involving the use of moist snuff in Sweden suggest that there is little demonstrable risk for oral cancer with the use of that product. Thus, the risk for oral cancer development with SLT use seems to be real but limited.

What is known for certain is that the use of SLT products puts patients at risk for a host of oral lesions aside from dysplasia or cancer, including the 3 grades of STK, periodontitis, gingival and alveolar bone damage, and possible delayed wound healing. There is a risk of tooth structure abrasion associated with the use of SLT, but chemical erosion of tooth structure appears not to be a risk. Because more than one-fifth of the content of some brands of SLT can be sugar, SLT users can be at risk for increased dental caries, but because the tobacco washes away the bacteria that frequently causes caries, there are but a few definitive reports in the literature that detail a cause-and-effect relationship between the use of SLT and dental caries.

Use of SLT products has been shown to result in histologically degenerative changes to salivary glands, principally glandular fibrous[11] at the site where the tobacco is placed, but the impact of such change seems to be clinically negligible. Altered taste has been reported in association with the use of SLT, as it has been with smoking, but this alteration has not been extensively studied.

Tooth staining and staining of prosthetic devices such as dentures, can occur when SLT products are used. The intensity of the staining appears to be dependent on the amount of available plaque and calculus present in a patient's mouth as well as on the amount of SLT that is used.

It seems that among the standard 3 grades of STK, the lesions that have the greatest risk for transition to dysplasia or oral cancer are those that have a velvety or papillary surface texture, regardless of the grade. The molecular mechanisms that detail exactly how HPV infection or a host of other molecular aberrations might be related to the induction of oral cancer in SLT users has not been fully elucidated, but HPV clearly plays a role in oral SCC development and investigations in that arena remain ongoing.

Perhaps the most appropriate statement concerning the risk of developing head and neck cancer from not just SLT but tobacco in all forms was spelled out in a summary statement of the International Head and Neck Cancer Epidemiology Consortium in 2009. This group examined pooled data from 17 European and American case control studies (11, 221 cases and 16, 168 controls) in an attempt to access the risk of head and neck cancer from the interaction between tobacco and alcohol,[90] and concluded that "a substantial proportion of head and neck cancers cannot be attributed to tobacco or alcohol use, particularly for the oral cavity and for head and neck cancer among women and among young-onset cases." It is important in the future to determine if a large percentage of oral cancers (SCC) in patients with a documented history of SLT use fall into this category.

REFERENCES

1. Christen AG, Swanson BZ, Glover ED, et al. Smokeless tobacco: the folklore and social history of snuffing, sneezing, dipping and chewing. J Am Dent Assoc 1982; 105(5):821–9.
2. Christen AG. The case against smokeless tobacco: five facts for the health professional to consider. J Am Dent Assoc 1980;101(3):464–9.
3. Glover ED, Schroeder KL, Henningfield JE, et al. An interpretative review of smokeless tobacco research in the United States. Part II. J Drug Educ 1989; 19(1):1–19.
4. U.S. Department of Health and Human Services. The health consequences of using smokeless tobacco: a report of the Advisory Committee of the Surgeon General. DHHS Publication, No. 86–2874. Bethesda (MD): U.S. Department of Health and Human Services, Public Health Service, National Institutes of Health, National Cancer Institute; 1986.
5. Wahlberg I, Ringberger T. Smokeless tobacco. In: Davis DL, Nielsen MT, editors. Tobacco: production, chemistry and technology. Oxford (United Kingdom): Blackwell Science; 1999. p. 452–60.
6. Rodu B. Smokeless tobacco and oral cancer: a review of the risks and determinants. Crit Rev Oral Biol Med 2004;15(5):252–63.
7. Federal Trade Commission. Report to Congress for the years 1998 and 1999. Available at: http://www.ftc.gov/reports/tobacco/smokeless98_99.htm. Accessed September 25, 2010.
8. Greer RO, Poulson TC. Oral tissue alterations associated with the use of smokeless tobacco by teenagers. Part I. Clinical findings. Oral Surg Oral Med Oral Pathol 1983;56(3):275–84.
9. Albert HR, Koh G, Connolly GN. Free nicotine content and strategic marketing of moist snuff tobacco products in the United States. Tob Control 2008;17(5):332–8.
10. Christen AG, Armstrong WR, McDaniel RK. Intraoral leukoplakia, abrasion, periodontal breakdown and tooth loss in a snuff dipper. J Am Dent Assoc 1979;98(4): 584–6.
11. Greer RO, Poulson TC, Boone ME. Smokeless tobacco associated oral changes in juvenile, adult and geriatric patients: clinical and histomorphologic features. Gerodontics 1986;2(1):87–98.
12. Squier CA. Smokeless tobacco and oral cancer: a cause for concern? CA Cancer J Clin 1984;34(5):242–7.

13. Murti PR, Gupta PC, Bhonsle DK. Smokeless tobacco use in India: effects on oral mucosa. In: National Institutes of Health Monograph 2. Smokeless tobacco or health: an international perspective. Bethesda (MD): NIH Publication No. 93-3461; 1993. p. 51–7. Chapter 2.

14. Bergström JJ. The use of smokeless tobacco in Sweden. In: National Institutes of Health Monograph 2. Smokeless tobacco or health: an international perspective. Bethesda (MD): NIH Publication No. 93-3461; 1993. p. 74–77. Chapter 2.

15. Pindborg JJ, Renstrup G. Studies in oral leukoplakia II. Effect of snuff on oral epithelium. Acta Derm Venereol Suppl 1963;43(4):271–6.

16. Grady D, Greene J, Daniels TE, et al. Oral mucosal lesions found in smokeless tobacco users. J Am Dent Assoc 1990;121(1):117–23.

17. Sinusas K, Coroso JG, Sopher MD, et al. Smokeless tobacco use and oral pathology in a professional baseball organization. J Fam Pract 1992;34(6): 713–8.

18. Greene TC, Ernster VL, Grady DG, et al. Oral mucosal lesions: clinical findings in relation to smokeless tobacco use among US baseball players. Monograph 2. Smokeless tobacco or health: an international perspective. Bethesda (MD): NIH Publication No. 93-3461; 1993. p. 41–50. Chapter 2.

19. Greer RO, Meyers A, Said M, et al. Is p16^{INK4A} protein expression in oral smokeless tobacco lesions a reliable precancerous marker? Int J Oral Maxillofac Surg 2008;37(9):840–6.

20. Axéll T, Mörnstad H, Sundström B. The relation of clinical picture to histopathology of snuff dippers lesions in a Swedish population. J Oral Pathol 1976; 5(4):229–36.

21. Hirsch JM, Heyden G, Thilander H. A clinical, histomorphological and histochemical study of snuff-induced lesions on varying severity. J Oral Pathol 1982;11(5):387–98.

22. Larsson Å, Axéll T, Andersson G. Reversibility of snuff dippers, lesion in Swedish moist snuff users: a clinical and histologic follow-up study. J Oral Pathol Med 1991;20(6):258–64.

23. Andersson G, Axéll T, Curvall M. Reduction in nicotine intake and oral mucosal changes among users of Swedish oral moist snuff after switching to a low-nicotine product. J Oral Pathol Med 1995;24(6):244–50.

24. Roosaar A, Johansson AL, Sandborgh-Englund G, et al. A long-term follow-up study on the natural course of snus-induced lesions among Swedish snus users. Int J Cancer 2006;119(2):392–7.

25. Rosenquist K, Wennerberg J, Schildt EB. Use of Swedish moist snuff, smoking and alcohol consumption in the aetiology of oral and oropharyngeal squamous cell carcinoma. A population-based case-control study in Southern Sweden. Acta Otolaryngol 2005;125(9):991–8.

26. Modéer T, Lavstedt S, Xhlund C. Relation between tobacco consumption and oral health in Swedish schoolchildren. Acta Odontol Scand 1980;38(4):223–7.

27. Jungell P, Malmström M. Snuff-induced lesions in Finnish recruits. Scand J Dent Res 1985;93(5):442–7.

28. Salonen L, Axéll T, Helldén L. Occurrence of oral mucosal lesions, the influence of tobacco habits and an estimate of treatment time in an adult Swedish population. J Oral Pathol Med 1990;19(4):170–6.

29. Frithiof L, Anneroth G, Lasson U, et al. The snuff-induced lesion. A clinical and morphological study of a Swedish material. Acta Odontol Scand 1983;41(1):53–64.

30. Andersson G, Axéll T. Clinical appearance of lesions associated with the use of loose and portion-bag packed Swedish moist snuff: a comparative study. J Oral Pathol Med 1989;18(1):2–7.

31. Andersson G, Bjornberg G, Curvall M. Oral mucosal changes and nicotine disposition in users of Swedish smokeless tobacco products: a comparative study. J Oral Pathol Med 1994;23(4):161–7.

32. Rolandsson M, Hellqvist L, Lindqvist L, et al. Effects of snuff on the oral health status of adolescent males: a comparative study. Oral Health Prev Dent 2005; 3(2):77–85.

33. Beck JD, Koch GG, Offenbacher S. Incidence of attachment loss over 3 years in older adults—new and progressing lesions. Community Dent Oral Epidmiol 1995; 23(5):291–6.

34. Kallischnigg G, Weitkunat R, Lee P. Systemic review of the relation between smokeless tobacco and non-neoplastic oral disease in Europe and the United States. BMC Oral Health 2008;8:13. Available at: http://www.biomedcentrol. com, 1472-6831/8/13. Accessed May 1, 2008.

35. Martin GC, Brown JP, Elfler CW, et al. Oral leukoplakia status six weeks after cessation of smokeless tobacco use. J Am Dent Assoc 1999;130(7):945–54.

36. Creath C, Shelton WO, Wright JT, et al. The prevalence of smokeless tobacco use among adolescent male athletes. J Am Dent Assoc 1988;116(1):43–8.

37. Poulson TC, Lindenmuth JE, Greer RO. A comparison of the use of smokeless tobacco in rural and urban teenagers. CA Cancer J Clin 1985;34(5):248–61.

38. Grasser JA, Childers E. Prevalence of smokeless tobacco use and clinical leukoplakia in a military population. Mil Med 1997;162(2):401–4.

39. Payne JB, Johnson GK, Reinhardt RA, et al. Histological alterations following short-term smokeless tobacco exposure in humans. J Periodont Res 1998; 33(5):274–9.

40. Offenbacker S, Weathers DR. Effects of smokeless tobacco on the periodontal mucosal and caries status of adolescent males. J Oral Pathol 1985;14(2): 169–81.

41. Wolfe MD, Carlos JP. Oral health effects of smokeless tobacco use in Navajo Indian adolescents. Community Dent Oral Epidemiol 1987;15(4):230–5.

42. Cummings KM, Michalek AM, Carl W, et al. Use of smokeless tobacco in a group of professional baseball players. J Behav Med 1989;12(6):559–67.

43. Stewart CM, Baughman RA, Bates RE. Smokeless tobacco use among Florida teenagers: prevalence, attitudes and oral changes. Fla Dent J 1989;60(1):38–42.

44. Ernster VL, Grady DG, Greene JC, et al. Smokeless tobacco use and health effects among baseball players. JAMA 1990;264(2):218–24.

45. Tomar SL, Winn DM, Swango PA, et al. Oral mucosal smokeless tobacco lesions among adolescents in the United States. J Dent Res 1997;76(6):1277–86.

46. Smith JF, Mincer HA, Hopkins KP, et al. Snuff-dippers lesion: a cytological and pathological study in a large population. Arch Otolaryngol 1970;92(5):450–6.

47. Little SJ, Stevens VJ, LaChance PA, et al. Smokeless tobacco habits and oral mucosal lesions in dental patients. J Public Health Dent 1992;52(2):269–76.

48. Greer RO, Eversole LR, Poulson TC, et al. Identification of human papillomavirus DNA in smokeless tobacco associated keratoses from juveniles, adults, and older patients using immunohistochemical and in situ DNA hybridization techniques. Geriodontics 1987;3(5):201–8.

49. Greer RO, Schroeder KL, Crosby L. Morphologic and immunohistochemical evidence of human papillomavirus capsid antigen in smokeless tobacco keratoses from juveniles and adults. J Oral Maxillofac Surg 1988;46(11):919–29.

50. Daniels TE, Hansen LS, Greenspan JS, et al. Histopathology of smokeless tobacco lesions in professional baseball players. Associations with different types of tobacco. Oral Surg Oral Med Oral Pathol 1992;73(6):720–5.

51. Pindborg JJ, Renstrup G. Studies in oral leukoplakia. I. The influence of snuff on the connective tissue of the oral mucosa. Preliminary report. Acta Pathol Microbiol Scand 1962;55(5):412–4.

52. Archard HO, Tarpley TM Jr. Clinicopathologic and histochemical characterization of submucosal deposits in snuff dipper's keratosis. J Oral Pathol 1972;1(1):3–11.

53. Greer RO, Douglas JM, Breeze P, et al. Evaluation of oral and laryngeal specimens for human papillomavirus (HPV) DNA by dot blot hybridization. J Oral Pathol Med 1990;19(1):35–8.

54. Palefsky JM, Greenspan JS, Daniels TE. Interaction between smokeless tobacco-related carcinogens and human papillomaviruses in the pathogenesis of oral cancer and dysplasia. In: National Institutes of Health Monograph 2. Smokeless tobacco or health: an International Perspective. Bethesda (MD): NIH Publication No. 93-3461; 1993. p. 175–82. Chapter 3.

55. Robertson PB, Walsh NM, Greene JC. Oral effects of smokeless tobacco use by professional baseball players. Adv Dent Res 1997;11(3):307–12.

56. Bastiaan KJ. The effects of tobacco smoking on periodontal tissues. J West Soc Periodont 1979;27(4):120–5.

57. Sinusas K, Coroso JG. A 10 year study of smokeless tobacco use in a professional baseball organization. Med Sci Sports Exerc 2006;38(2):1204–7.

58. Tomar SL, Winn DM. Chewing tobacco use and dental caries among US men. J Am Dent Assoc 1999;130(11):1601–10.

59. Hirsh JM, Livian G, Edwards S, et al. Tobacco habits among teenagers in the city of Göteborg, Sweden, and possible association with dental caries. Swed Dent J 1991;15(3):117–23.

60. Bergström J, Keilani H, Lundholm L, et al. Smokeless tobacco (snuff) use and periodontal bone loss. J Clin Periodontal 2006;33(8):549–54.

61. Mecklenberg R, Stotts C. Recommendations for the control of smokeless tobacco. In: National Institutes of Health Monograph 2. Smokeless tobacco or health: an international perspective. Bethesda (MD): NIH Publication No. 93-3461; 1993. p. 337–49. Chapter 8.

62. Kaugars GE, Mehailescu WL, Gunsolley JC, et al. Smokeless tobacco use and oral epithelial dysplasia. Cancer 1989;64(7):1527–30.

63. Wray A, McGuirt WF. Smokeless tobacco usage associated with oral carcinoma. Incidence, treatment, outcome. Arch Otolaryngol Head Neck Surg 1993;119(9):929–33.

64. Greer RO, Shroyer K, Crosby L. Identification of human papillomavirus DNA in smokeless tobacco keratoses and premalignant and malignant oral lesions, by PCR amplification with consensus sequence primers. In: National Institutes of Health Monograph 2. Smokeless tobacco or health: an international perspective. Bethesda (MD): NIH Publication, No. 93-3461; 1993. p. 183–9. Chapter 3.

65. Henly SJ, Thun JJ, Connell C, et al. Two large prospective studies of mortality among men who use snuff or chewing tobacco (United States). Cancer Causes Control 2005;16(4):347–58.

66. Weitkunat R, Sanders E, Lee PN, et al. Meta-analysis of the relation between European and American smokeless tobacco and oral cancer. BMC Public Health 2007;15(7):334–54.

67. Waterbor JW, Adams RM, Robinson JM, et al. Disparities between public health educational materials and the scientific evidence that smokeless tobacco causes cancer. J Cancer Educ 2004;19(1):17–28.

68. Waldron CA, Shafer WG. Leukoplakia revisited. A clinico-pathologic study of 3256 oral leukoplakias. Cancer 1975;36(4):1386–92.

69. Wynder EL, Stellman SD. Comparative epidemiology of tobacco-related cancers. Cancer Res 1977;37(12):4608–22.
70. Rodu B, Cole P. Smokeless tobacco use and cancer of the upper respiratory tract. Oral Surg Oral Med Oral Pathol Oral Radiol Endod 2002;93(5):511–5.
71. Wynder EL, Bross IJ, Feldman RM, et al. A study of etiological factors in cancer of the mouth. Cancer 1957;10(6):1300–23.
72. Mashberg A, Bofetta P, Winkelman R, et al. Tobacco smoking, alcohol drinking and cancer of the oral cavity and oropharynx among US veterans. Cancer 1993;72(4):1369–75.
73. Mattson ME, Winn DM. Smokeless tobacco: association with increased cancer risk. NCI Monogr 1989;8:13–6.
74. McGuirt WF, Wray A. Oral carcinoma and smokeless tobacco use: a clinical profile. In: National Institutes of Health Monograph 2. Smokeless tobacco or health: an international perspective. Bethesda (MD): NIH Publication No. 93-3461; 1993. p. 91–5. Chapter 3.
75. Boffetta P, Hecht S, Gray P, et al. Smokeless tobacco and cancer. Lancet Oncol 2008;9(7):667–75.
76. Volger WR, Lloyd JW, Milmore B. A retrospective study of etiological factors in cancer of the mouth. Cancer 1962;15(2):246–58.
77. Winn DM, Blot WJ, Shy CM, et al. Snuff dipping and oral cancer among women in the Southern United States. N Engl J Med 1981;304(13):745–9.
78. Blot WJ, McLaughlin JK, Winn D, et al. Smoking and drinking in relation to oral and pharyngeal cancer. Cancer Res 1988;48(6):3282–7.
79. Kabat GC, Chang CJ, Wynder EL. The role of tobacco, alcohol use, and body mass index in oral and pharyngeal cancer. Int J Epidemiol 1994;23(3):1137–44.
80. Peacock EE, Greenberg BG, Brawley BW. The effect of snuff and tobacco on the production of oral carcinoma: an experimental and epidemiological study. Ann Surg 1960;151(4):542–50.
81. Vincent RG, Marchetta F. The relationship of the use of tobacco and alcohol to cancer of the oral cavity, pharynx or larynx. Am J Surg 1963;106(4):501–5.
82. Martinez I. Factors associated with cancer of the esophagus, mouth and pharynx in Puerto Rico. J Natl Cancer Inst 1969;42(6):1069–94.
83. Schwartz SM, Daling JR, Doody DR, et al. Oral cancer risk in relation to sexual history and evidence of human papillomavirus infection. J Natl Cancer Inst 1998;90(11):1626–36.
84. Smith JF. Snuff-dippers lesion. A ten-year follow-up. Arch Otolaryngol 1975; 101(5):276–7.
85. Christen AG, McDonald JL, Christen JA. The impact of tobacco use and cessation on non-malignant and precancerous oral and dental diseases and conditions: a comprehensive review. Indianapolis (IN): Indiana University School of Dentistry Teaching Monograph; 1991. p. 7–13.
86. Axéll T, Mornstad H, Sundström B. Snuff and cancer of the oral cavity. A retrospective study. Läkartidningen 1978;75(5):1224–6.
87. Greer RO, Hoernig G, Shroyer KR. Telomerase expression in precancerous oral verrucous leukoplakia. Int J Oral Biol 1999;24(2):1–5.
88. Shroyer KR, Greer RO. Detection of human papillomavirus DNA by in situ DNA hybridization and polymerase chain reaction in premalignant and malignant oral lesions. Oral Surg Oral Med Oral Pathol 1991;71(6):708–13.
89. Kulkarni V, Saranath D. Concurrent hypermethylation of multiple regulatory genes in chewing tobacco associated oral squamous cell carcinomas and adjacent normal tissues. Oral Oncol 2004;40(2):145–53.

90. Hashibe M, Brenan P, Shu-chun C, et al. Interaction between tobacco and alcohol use and the risk of head and neck cancer: pooled analysis in the international head and neck cancer epidemiology consortium. Cancer Epidemiol Biomarkers Prev 2009;18(2):541–50.

Oral Infections and Antibiotic Therapy

Marilyn E. Levi, MD[a],*, Vincent D. Eusterman, MD, DDS[b]

KEYWORDS

• Oral infection • Odontogenic infection • Antibiotics
• Neck infection

Oral infections commonly originate from an odontogenic source in adults and from tonsil and lymphatic sources in children. Bacterial contamination of adjacent sterile tissue with normal oral flora result in infections the microbiology of which is usually predictable, and together with implementation of appropriate antibiotic options, can lead to successful treatment. Odontogenic infections arise as a result of advanced dental caries or from periodontal disease. Dental disease produces pulpitis, which may progress to periapical abscesses and can spread through bone, soft tissue, and into deeper structures. Periodontal infections from gingivitis, periodontitis, or periodontal abscess may be severe and also spread to deeper structures. Serious oral infections that go untreated may spread superiorly to the orbits and brain, to the retropharyngeal space or pleural space resulting in an empyema. Hematogenous spread may result in endocarditis, seeding of prosthetic material and other metastatic foci. Oral trauma, radiation injury, chemotherapy mucositis, salivary gland infection, lymph node abscess, and postoperative infection are potential nonodontogenic sources of infections that could potentially be life threatening. This article reviews the serious nature and potential danger that exists from oral infection and the antibiotics available to treat them. Successful treatment requires an understanding of the microflora, the regional anatomy, the disease process, the treatment methods available, and interdisciplinary team collaboration.

ANATOMY

Oral infections spread in a pathway of least resistance often into the oral cavity or into the deep spaces of the neck, which may become life threatening. Deep-space infections originate most commonly from odontogenic sources in adults and from tonsil

---

Financial disclosure: the authors have nothing to disclose.
[a] Department of Medicine, Division of Infectious Diseases, University of Colorado Denver, 1635 Aurora Court, Mail Stop B-163, Aurora, CO 80045, USA
[b] Department of Otolaryngology-Head and Neck Surgery, University of Colorado School of Medicine, Denver Health Medical Center, 777 Bannock, Denver, CO 80204, USA
* Corresponding author. University of Colorado Denver, 1635 Aurora Court, Mail Stop B-163, Aurora, CO 80045.
E-mail address: Marilyn.Levi@ucdenver.edu

Otolaryngol Clin N Am 44 (2011) 57–78
doi:10.1016/j.otc.2010.10.003
0030-6665/11/$ – see front matter © 2011 Elsevier Inc. All rights reserved.

and other lymphatic sources in children. Spaces in the neck are created between the superficial, middle and deep layers of the deep cervical fascia. These spaces are inter-connected (**Fig. 1**). Three posterior pharyngeal spaces, the retropharyngeal space (RPS), the danger space (DS), and the prevertebral space (PVS), and a lateral pharyn-geal space, the visceral vascular space (VVS), extend from the skull base to the medi-astinum and beyond. The RPS extends to the upper mediastinum and contains the nodes of Rouviere, which involute by age 6 years; the RPS can rupture posteriorly into the DS. The DS extends to the inferior mediastinum; it lies just behind the RPS, between the alar anteriorly and the prevertebral fascia posteriorly. The PVS lies behind the DS and may extend to the coccyx as it has the vertebral body as the posterior wall and prevertebral fascia as the anterior boundary. Laterally, the VVS, which contains all 3 layers of the deep cervical fascia, extends from the skull base behind the parapharyng-eal space to the mediastinum. The VVS contains the carotid artery, jugular vein, and vagus nerve. Smaller lateral suprahyoid spaces (temporal, masticator, submandibular, peritonsillar, and parotid) empty into the parapharyngeal space (PPS), which has access to mediastinum by way of the the RPS and VVS. The PPS is also known as the pharyngomaxillary space or lateral pharyngeal space. The PPS is divided into ante-rior and posterior portions. The anterior component contains parapharyngeal fat and the tonsillar fossa. It has no boundaries and may access other spaces; infections here are considered surgical emergencies.[1] The posterior component of the PPS is

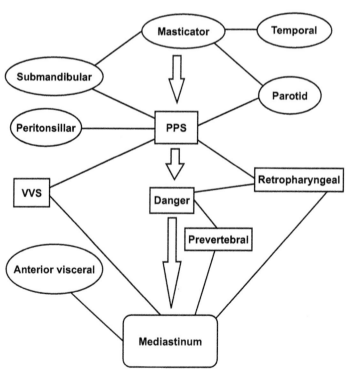

Fig. 1. Deep neck-space communications identify the parapharyngeal space (PPS) as a major communication link for odontogenic infections to reach the mediastinum by way of the ret-ropharyngeal (RPS), danger (DS), prevertebral (PVS), and the visceral vascular (VVS) spaces.

a neurovascular space and infections here are generally limited to the capsule of the lymph node.[1] The anterior infrahyoid neck has 2 additional spaces: the anterior visceral space (AVS) or pretracheal space extending from the thyroid cartilage to the superior mediastinum and the suprasternal space of Burns.

Lateral neck radiographs are a useful screening tool, with a sensitivity of 84% and specificity of 100%. An RPS abscess can be identified here by measuring the distance from the vertebra to the pharyngeal air space. An abscess is considered present when the distance at C2 greater than 7 mm, at C6 greater than 14 mm (in children), and C6 greater than 22 mm (in adults). The computed tomography (CT) scan is the workhorse for deep and superficial oral-facial infections. CT scans evaluating deep neck-space infections must include the mediastinum to rule out mediastinitis. Early recognition and treatment of mediastinitis can prevent the progressive sequela of respiratory failure requiring prolonged intensive care treatment (**Figs. 2** and **3**).

ORAL MICROBIOLOGY
Odontogenic Infections

The type of bacteria found within odontogenic infections are part of the microbiota of the oral cavity. These infections are frequently polymicrobial and their invasiveness may be determined by the specific combinations present[2,3] as specific bacteria vary in their pathogenicity. More than 700 bacterial species have been identified in the oral cavity,[4] although less than 1% are cultured routinely in the clinical laboratory.[5] In addition, eradication of all oral flora is not required for treatment of odontogenic infections, as most are nonpathogenic commensals. Ecologic niches exist within the oral cavity, whereby normal colonizing bacteria reside within biofilms. These biofilms are comprised of polysaccharides that have 2 functions: allowing bacteria to live in a protected milieu and forming a barrier against potential pathogens.

In the oral cavity, more than 80% of the cultured bacteria include *streptococci, Peptostreptococcus, Veillonella, Lactobacillus, Actinomyces* and *Corynebacterium*. Quantitative measurements of the oral flora indicate that most bacteria are anaerobes in specific locations.[6] Although specific organisms are located in most areas of the oral cavity, it is not a homogeneous environment. Certain bacteria colonize different parts of the mouth. *Streptococcus salivarius* and *Veillonella* colonize the tongue, buccal mucosa, and saliva. *Streptococcus sanguinis, Streptococcus mutans, Streptococcus mitis* and *Actinomyces viscosus* are found on tooth surfaces. The gingival crevice contains the anaerobes *Fusobacterium, Porphyromonas, Prevotella*, and anaerobic spirochetes.[7,8]

The normal oral flora may be altered with tobacco use, pregnancy, diet, nutrition, age, oral hygiene, deciduous teeth eruption, dental caries, periodontal disease, antibiotics, hospitalization, and by genetic or racial factors. In these situations, commensal flora may become pathogenic and cause tissue inflammation and destruction. Plaque is a supragingival biofilm that is located on the tooth surface above the gingival margin and can produce dental caries from bacterial byproducts. These plaques are composed of gram-positive facultative (grows with or without oxygen) and microaerophilic (requires low oxygen) cocci and rods. Bacteria found within caries may cause pulpitis or endodontic infection, and potentially extend down the root canal to produce a periapical abscess. This abscess can perforate the alveolar bone and extend into the adjacent soft tissue of the face, or deep neck and lead to serious sequelae (see **Fig. 2**). Subgingival plaques and tartar are found below the gingival margin, and may lead to periodontal disease such as gingivitis,

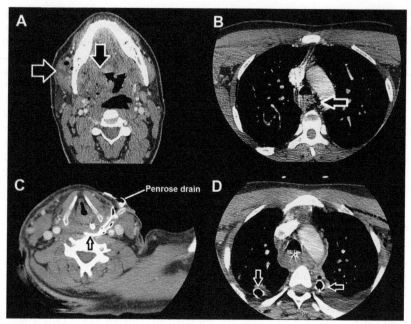

Fig. 2. Patient RF is a 35-year-old man who presented with progressive dysphagia and airway obstruction from a #31 dental abscess. CT scans (*A*) showed a large odontogenic abscess (*arrows*) with air extending into the parapharyngeal space. CT of the mediastinum (*B*) shows mediastinum air (*arrow*) consistent with early mediastinitis. The patient underwent tooth extraction and bilateral neck exploration. (*C*) Penrose drain placement in front of the sterno-cleidomastoid and carotid sheath into the DS (*arrow*). (*D*) Bilateral drainage of an empyema with chest tubes (*arrows*). Wound cultures showed normal oral flora with Gram stain showing many gram-positive and -negative bacilli and gram-positive cocci. Anaerobic cultures showed mixed aerobic and anaerobic flora with few pigmented *Provotella* and *Porphyromanas* groups. The patient was started on clindamycin and metronidazole (Flagyl) while awaiting cultures. On day 2, Flagyl was stopped and piperacillin sodium/tazobactam sodium (Zosyn) added. On day 4 clindamycin was stopped and vancomycin was added for fever spikes believed to be caused by MRSA. Following fever spikes and increased white count, a bronchioalveolar lavage showed *Pseudomonas* and *Enterobacter* sensitive to cephapine. Zosyn was intermediately sensitive and was stopped; cephapine was started in combination with clindamycin. The patient required 38 days of hospitalization.

periodontitis, and periodontal abscess (see **Fig. 3**). These plaques comprise mainly gram-negative anaerobic (grows without oxygen) rods and motile forms, such as spirochetes.[9] Necrotizing periodontal disease (acute necrotizing ulcerative gingivitis) is common in patients with very poor oral hygiene. It is caused by bacterial infection that includes anaerobes (*Prevotella intermedia* and *Fusobacterium*) as well as spirochetes such as *Borellia* and *Treponema*. This condition can progress to gangrenous stomatitis or noma in patients with weak immune systems or in the malnourished, leading to severe facial disfigurement.

The bacterial milieu within dental caries, gingivitis, and periodontitis differ from each other. *Streptococcus mutans* is clearly associated with dental caries,[10] and is the only organism that has been isolated consistently from decayed dental fissures and carious teeth, compared with noncarious teeth.[9] Conversely, the normal oral

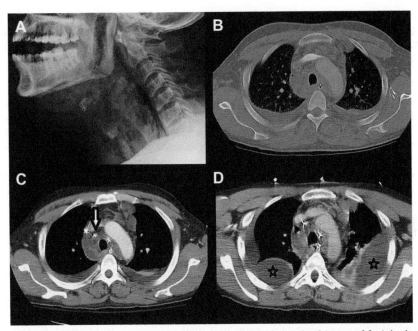

Fig. 3. Patient TM is a 32-year-old man who presented with a 4-day history of facial edema, fever, and dysphagia. The source of infection was a lateral periodontal abscess at tooth #18. A lateral neck radiograph (*A*) identified air in the retropharyngeal space, a Ludwig angina, and left neck phlegmon. CT scan (*B*) showed soft tissue extending into the superior and middle mediastinum with punctate air suspicious for a diffuse mediastinitis. The patient underwent tracheotomy and drainage of the neck and mediastinum through a very purulent pretracheal space. The transcervical mediastinal drains shown in (*C; arrow*) failed to prevent the progression of the infection into the pleural cavity. (*D*) The patient required thoracotomy to drain the empyema (*stars*) of the right chest and mediastinum. The patient's aerobic wound cultures showed moderate *Streptococcus milleri* group, Gram stains revealed many gram-positive and -negative bacilli, many gram-positive cocci, and many gram-negative diplococci. Anaerobic cultures showed mixed bacterial flora without additional identification. The patient was started on clindamycin and then changed to ampicillin/sulbactam (Unasyn) per infectious disease recommendations for *S milleri*, then changed to Zosyn for slow resolution of the Ludwig angina. The patient required 27 days of hospitalization.

flora within subgingival plaques includes *Streptococcus oralis, Streptococcus sanguinis,* and *Actinomyces.*[11] However, in the presence of gingivitis, the flora shifts to anaerobic gram-negative rods such as *Prevotella intermedia, Capnocytophaga,* and *Peptostreptococcus.* Adults with chronic periodontitis have oral flora that evolve to include anaerobic gram-negatives, motile organisms, and spirochetes,[4] including *Porphyromonas gingivalis, Prevotella intermedia, Actinobacillus actinomycetemcomitans, Tannerella forsythensis* (formerly *Bacteroides forsythensis*), and *Treponema denticola.*[12] In contrast, early or juvenile periodontitis seen predominantly in adolescents is most commonly made up of *Capnocytophaga* and *Actinobacillus actinomycetemcomitans.*[13]

Suppurative odontogenic infections such as deep neck-space infections from periapical abscesses is polymicrobial, commonly including both aerobic bacteria (*Streptococcus*) and anaerobes, specifically *Peptostreptococcus, Actinomyces,* pigmented *Bacteroides*, and *Fusobacterium nucleatum*.[13,14] Patients with severe underlying illnesses may become colonized with pathogens such as methicillin-resistant *Staphylococcus aureus* (MRSA) and facultative gram-negative bacilli.[15] These pathogens should be considered during selection of empiric antibiotic treatment.

Nonodontogenic Infections

Nonodontogenic oral infections are related to chemical, thermal, or trauma injury and may be associated with almost any microorganism. Sexually transmitted pathogens such as herpes simplex, *Neisseria gonorrhea*, and *Treponema pallidum* may be considered. Childhood viruses may be identified in the oral cavity. In chemotherapy-associated mucositis or in patients with human immunodeficiency virus (HIV) infection, opportunistic oral infections should be considered and may include *Candida, Aspergillus, Mucormycosis*, mixed gram-negatives, herpetic gingivostomatitis,[15] and *Histoplasma capsulatum*.

ANTIBACTERIALS

The proper selection of antibacterials has a twofold benefit: (1) the rapid eradication of infection, which decreases the degree of tissue destruction; and (2) decreasing the use of inappropriate antibiotics to prevent the development of antibiotic resistance. In addition to becoming familiar with the indigenous microbiota of the oral cavity, the patient's immune status, community-acquired versus nosocomial exposures, allergy profile, and previous antibiotic usage that may predispose to resistant organisms need to be considered. For example, if a patient has been treated with penicillin in the past and presents with a relapsed infection, it is likely that the offending pathogen is resistant to penicillin and will require an alternate antibiotic choice. In addition, antibiotics containing the narrowest spectrum based on results of culture and susceptibility testing should be selected.

β-Lactam Antibiotics

All β-lactams exert the same basic mechanism of action, the inhibition of bacterial cell wall synthesis by binding to penicillin-binding proteins.[16,17] Although the exact pathway is unknown, it is thought that bactericidal antibiotics such as the penicillins irreversibly destroy cell walls through the production of hydroxyl radicals.[17] Resistance to β-lactam antibiotics has been increasing through the production of a variety β-lactamases. These are bacteria-derived enzymes that promote resistance to β-lactam agents that are selected through antibiotic pressure. This phenomenon proves the importance of controlled antibiotic use and has resulted in government mandates to hospitals to form antibiotic stewardship programs.

Penicillins

Penicillin is the primary class of β-lactams and is divided into 5 groups:

1. Natural penicillins
2. First generation penicillin
3. Second generation penicillin
4. Third generation penicillin
5. Fourth generation penicillin.

Natural penicillins Penicillin G and penicillin V are natural penicillins and are most useful for non–β-lactamase producing gram-positive bacteria, such as streptococci, staphylococci, enterococci, gram-positive rods such as *Listeria monocytogenes* and most anaerobes (an important exception is *Bacteroides*). Bacteria that are sensitive to natural penicillins tend to be more effectively inhibited by this group compared to the semi-synthetic penicillins.[18–20] Penicillin penetrates the normal blood-brain barrier poorly but achieves therapeutic levels in the presence of inflamed meninges when administered in high intravenous doses. Oral penicillin V and intravenous/intramuscular penicillin G are interchangeable except against gram-negative organisms, as oral penicillin V is less active against *Neisseria* and *Haemophilus*. Penicillin G is bactericidal with the notable exception of *Enterococcus* for which it is bacteriostatic and in some cases, resistant because of production of penicillinase.[16] Therefore, serious enterococcal infections require synergistic combination therapy of a cell wall active agent (such as the penicillins or vancomycin) with gentamicin, which decreases protein synthesis. Gentamicin synergy is commonly reported as part of *Staphylococcus* and *Enterococcus* susceptibility testing. Penicillin and the semi-synthetic penicillins are cleared by the kidneys and require dose adjustment if the patient has abnormal renal function.

First generation penicillin Nafcillin, oxacillin, cloxacillin, and dicloxacillin are antistaphylococcal penicillins resistant to hydrolysis by penicillinase. They are the drugs of choice for penicillin-resistant *Staphylococcus aureus* and *Staphylococcus epidermidis* but are not active against oxacillin-resistant staphylococci. They also cover streptococci including *Streptococcus pneumoniae*, *Streptococcus viridans*, *Streptococcus pyogenes*, and other hemolytic streptococci and anaerobic gram-positive bacilli such as *Clostridium*. This group is not superior to penicillin for the treatment of penicillin-susceptible streptococci, and if susceptibilities allow, penicillin should be used for infections with these organisms. Conversely, in the case of oxacillin-susceptible staphylococcal infections, this group is more active than vancomycin based on clinical and in vitro studies.[18] These agents are not active against enterococci, *Listeria monocytogenes*, and gram-negative pathogens such as *Neisseria*.

This group of antibiotics is classically associated with acute kidney injury, specifically acute tubulointerstitial nephritis (TIN) that can be diagnosed by the presence of eosinophils in the urine or renal biopsy. If TIN is suspected, discontinuation of the antibiotic is often adequate for renal recovery. Nafcillin is metabolized primarily through the liver and to a lesser extent, through the kidneys. If nafcillin is to be used in patients with liver disease, close monitoring of liver functions is recommended. Nafcillin is stable in solution and may be used in the homecare setting as a continuous infusion for a 24-hour period. Complete blood count monitoring is recommended in addition to renal and liver functions, as neutropenia is reported if used for more than 3 weeks. The original penicillinase-resistant penicillin, methicillin, is no longer used because of a high incidence of TIN.

Second generation penicillin Ampicillin and amoxicillin are aminopenicillins that have identical coverage as penicillin against the same non–β-lactamase containing gram-positive pathogens. This group has additional coverage against non–β-lactamase producing strains of *Haemophilus influenzae*, *Escherichia coli*, *Proteus mirabilis*, *Salmonella*, and *Shigella* but lacks coverage against *Pseudomonas aeruginosa*. The overall prevalence of ampicillin-resistant, β-lactamase producing nontypeable *Haemophilus influenzae* strains is 30%, but geographic variability exists. In addition to *Haemophilus influenzae*, other pathogens important in the pathogenesis of otitis media and sinusitis such as *Moraxella catarrhalis* may produce β-lactamases, resulting in resistance to the aminopenicillins. Therefore, knowledge of the local susceptibilities is recommended.[21,22]

Aminopenicillins have an increased incidence of drug hypersensitivity reactions with rashes compared with other penicillins. This is most evident when these agents are used for the treatment of exudative tonsillitis in the face of infectious mononucleosis. Nonaminopenicillins should be considered for empiric therapy of exudative tonsillitis pending culture and monospot results. Comparing these 2 agents, amoxicillin has enhanced intestinal absorption (particularly at mealtime) and is preferable to oral ampicillin, which is destroyed by low gastric pH. Both middle ear fluid and serum levels are higher with the use of amoxicillin.[21]

Third generation penicillin Ticarcillin, the only third generation penicillin available, is less active than ampicillin against penicillin-resistant streptococci and relatively inactive against enterococci. Ticarcillin has a broader spectrum of activity against β-lactamases of organisms like *Pseudomonas aeruginosa*, *Enterobacter*, and *Proteus*. Ticarcillin is no longer available as a single drug because of potential hydrolysis by β-lactamases, and is used in combination with the β-lactamase inhibitor clavulanate. This addition has further expanded the coverage of ticarcillin-clavulanate to include *Staphylococcus aureus* (except for MRSA) and anaerobes. Ticarcillin-clavulanate is a disodium salt, which may result in volume overload and may cause a bleeding diathesis by prolonging the bleeding time and interfering with platelet function,[23] particularly in the presence of renal failure.

Fourth generation penicillin Piperacillin is an acyl ureidopenicillin (extended spectrum β-lactam), which is a derivative of ampicillin with activity against gram-positive species, *Neisseria*, *Haemophilus* and many members of Enterobacteriaceae. It has excellent activity against anaerobes and is more active than ticarcillin against *Pseudomonas aeruginosa*. As opposed to ticarcillin, pipercillin may be used as a single agent. However, because of β-lactamase production by *Pseudomonas aeruginosa* and *Enterobacter*, a combination of pipercillin with the β-lactamase inhibitor tazobactam is commonly used.

β-Lactamase Inhibitors

β-Lactamase inhibitors such as clavulanate and sulbactam are weak β-lactam compounds, but when coadministered with β-lactam antibiotics, bind and inactivate β-lactamase enzymes. The commonly used combination agents include ampicillin-sulbactam, ampicillin-clavulanate, pipercillin-tazobactam, and ticarcillin-clavulanate. The net result is successful eradication of β-lactamase producing bacteria, particularly *Haemophilus influenzae*, *Moraxella catarrhalis*, *Staphylococcus aureus*, *Bacteroides*, and Enterobacteriaceae. Clinically, the oral combination of amoxicillin-clavulanate and intravenous combination of ampicillin-sulbactam are commonly used in the treatment of head and neck infections.

Cephalosporins

Cephalosporins represent a popular group of β-lactam agents that cover a broad spectrum of organisms and are easy to administer with low toxicity issues. They can often be used in place of penicillins when patients have a history of mild rashes associated with penicillin use. Conversely, cephalosporins should not be used in patients who describe anaphylaxis, angioedema, urticaria, or asthma when using penicillin.[24] The half-lives of these agents vary, resulting in dosing ranges between once daily and four times daily depending on renal function. The pharmacokinetics allow for therapeutic levels in peritoneal, pleural, synovial fluid, and pericardial tissues with biliary concentrations that exceed serum levels.[25] In terms of pneumococcal susceptibility, resistance or reduced susceptibility to any cephalosporin infers alteration in the bacterial penicillin-binding proteins and resistance to the entire group.[26] They are considered active against most gram-positive pathogens and are divided into generations based on their spectrum of activity against aerobic and facultative gram-negative bacteria.

First-generation cephalosporins Cefazolin, the most commonly used intravenous first-generation cephalosporin available is recommended for patients who are allergic to penicillin. It has similar activity against most gram-positive cocci including *Staphylococcus aureus*, group A β-hemolytic *Streptococcus* (*Streptococcus pyogenes*), and penicillin-susceptible *Streptococcus pneumonia*. It is used for surgical prophylaxis for head and neck surgery that requires crossing the oropharyngeal mucosal barrier.[27] Cefazolin lacks activity against oxacillin-resistant staphylococci, penicillin-resistant pneumococci, *Listeria monocytogenes*, and enterococci. In terms of gram-negative bacteria, coverage is more limited to enteric pathogens, such as most strains of *Escherichia coli*, *Klebsiella pneumoniae*, and *Proteus mirabilis*. Cefazolin is inactive against nonenteric gram-negatives such as *Pseudomonas aeruginosa* and *Acinetobacter*, indole-positive *Proteus*, *Enterobacter*, *Serratia*, and gram-negative cocci such as *Neisseria meningococcus* and *Haemophilus influenzae*. In terms of anaerobes, cefazolin lacks coverage of *Bacteroides* and should not be used if this pathogen is suspected.

The first-generation oral cephalosporins include cephalexin, cefadroxil, and cephadrine (not available in the United States). These agents are similar in antibacterial spectrum, but differ in dosing schedules. These agents have high oral bioavailability and are active against *Streptococcus pyogenes*. They are not useful against penicillinase-producing *Streptococcus pneumoniae*, *Haemophilus Influenzae*, and *Moraxella catarrhalis*, and are therefore not recommended for sinusitis, otitis media, or lower respiratory tract infections.

Second-generation cephalosporins In the United States, second-generation cephalosporins include cefaclor, cefprozil, cefuroxime, and cefoxitin. This group has broader gram-negative coverage than the first-generation cephalosporins but less gram-positive activity. There are 2 basic subgroups. The first subgroup with activity against *Haemophilus influenzae* includes cefuroxime, the only intravenous formulation in this subgroup, which also covers strains of *Enterobacter* and indole-positive *Proteus*, compared with cefazolin. Intravenous and oral cefuroxime is stable against ampicillin-resistant, β-lactamase producing *Haemophilus influenzae*. It is the only second-generation cephalosporin to cross the blood-brain barrier and is approved for the treatment of *Haemophilus influenzae* meningitis.[28] However, because of reports of treatment failures and delayed responses, third-generation cephalosporins are now the preferred treatment of *Haemophilus influenzae*.[27] They are less active than amoxicillin against *Streptococcus pneumoniae*, specifically strains with intermediate susceptibility to penicillin and should not be used with strains that are fully resistant. Cefuroxime also covers β-lactamase producing *Moraxella catarrhalis*. In comparison, cefprozil is less active against *Haemophilus influenzae* and *Streptococcus pneumoniae*, and is inactive against *Moraxella catarrhalis*. Cefaclor is the least active of this group, with poor coverage of *Moraxella catarrhalis* and *Haemophilus* strains. This agent is also associated with serum sickness. The second subgroup is the cephamycins, which also covers anaerobes such as *Bacteroides* and includes agents such as cefoxitin, cefmetazole, and cefotetan. The spectrum of activity of cephamycins includes common aerobic and facultative gram-negatives and anaerobes and is optimal for gastrointestinal and pelvic infections,[27] with no clear advantage in the prophylaxis or treatment of oral infections.

Third-generation cephalosporins Ceftriaxone and cefotaxime cover many important infections because of their broad coverage, high potency, low toxicity issues and favorable pharmacokinetics, such as high levels in the cerebrospinal fluid. These compounds have less activity against gram-positive pathogens compared with the first-generation cephalosporins, although they are usually useful for pneumococci that have intermediate susceptibility to penicillin. Pneumococcal strains that are completely resistant to penicillin are commonly resistant to the third-generation cephalosporins as well.[24,26,29] Agents such as cefixime and ceftibuten may be used for acute otitis media or sinusitis only when resistant pneumococci have been previously treated. Oral cefpodoxime, cefdinir, and cefditoren are technically third-generation cephalosporins but exert the same antibacterial activity as the second-generation agents. Cefpodoxime is considered the most active of the oral cephalosporins for the treatment of acute otitis media and sinusitis.

Third-generation cephalosporins have the advantage of being resistant to the common β-lactamases of gram-negative bacilli with enhanced activity against Enterobacteriaceae such as *Escherichia coli*, *Serratia* spp, *Proteus mirabilis*, indole-positive *Proteus*, *Klebsiella*, *Citrobacter*, and *Enterobacter*. Some Enterobacteriaceae have recently developed β-lactamase enzymes such as extended spectrum β-lactamases (ESBLs), carbapenemases and AmpC β-lactamases. These enzymes pose a growing threat to the continued usefulness of these agents.

There are 2 basic subgroups of third-generation cephalosporins based on coverage of *Pseudomonas aeruginosa*. One subgroup will lack pseudomonal coverage, including ceftriaxone, cefotaxime, cefdinir, cefditoren, cefotetan (a cephamycin), cefixime, ceftibuten, cefpodoxime and ceftizoxime. A second subgroup will cover *Pseudomonas aeruginosa*, the most commonly being ceftazidime. Ceftazidime has poor activity against gram-positives and should be reserved for *Pseudomonas aeruginosa* infections.[27]

Ceftriaxone and cefotaxime are the only third-generation cephalosporins that maintain excellent activity against *Streptococcus pneumoniae*, including those isolates reported as intermediate or high-level resistance to penicillin. Conversely, third-generation agents such as ceftriaxone, cefotaxime, and ceftazidime[30] achieve higher cerebrospinal fluid levels in the presence of inflamed meninges and are approved for the treatment of bacterial meningitis. If multidrug resistant pneumococcus is suspected, intravenous vancomycin can be added to ceftriaxone or cefotaxime. Ceftriaxone is considered more potent than cefotaxime against gram-positive pathogens and requires only single daily dosing. It can be used in intramuscular form for persistent otitis media and gonococcal infections.

Fourth-generation cephalosporins Cefepime is the only fourth-generation cephalosporin available in the United States. It has enhanced penetration through the outer membrane of gram-negative bacteria and is less susceptible to inactivation by certain β-lactamases of gram-negative bacilli. As a result, 75% to 80% of Enterobacteriaceae that are resistant to ceftazidime are susceptible to cefepime. Cefepime is also active against gram-positive cocci such as *Streptococcus pneumoniae* and staphylococci compared with ceftazidime.[31,32] However, both ceftazidime and cefepime usually have excellent activity against *Pseudomonas aeruginosa*, depending on susceptibility testing of the individual isolates and provide nonnephrotoxic and nonototoxic alternatives to aminoglycosides.

Fifth-generation cephalosporins Cetobiprole is the only fifth-generation cephalosporin produced thus far, and is available in Europe. The fifth-generation cephalosporins are active against MRSA, ampicillin-resistant enterococci, *Streptococcus pneumoniae*, and *Pseudomonas aeruginosa*. They also share similar activity with many third- and fourth-generation cephalosporins against gram-negative bacilli.[33–35]

Carbapenems
Carbapenems are a class of β-lactam antibiotics with the widest spectrum of antibacterial coverage because they are commonly resistant to β-lactamases.[36–38] The 4 approved agents in the United States include ertapenem, imipenem-cilastatin, meropenem, and doripenem. Their general coverage includes (1) gram-positive organisms including *Listeria* and *Enterococcus faecalis* (but not against MRSA and vancomycin-resistant *Enterococcus faecium*), (2) gram-negative organisms, including beta-lactamase producing *Haemophilus influenzae*, *Neisseria gonorrheae*, the Enterobacteriaceae, *Pseudomonas aeruginosa*, *Acinetobacter*, and ESBLs. Carbapenems other than ertapenem are the drugs of choice for the treatment of carbapenem-susceptible, multiresistant *Acinetobacter baumannii* infections, although carbapenem resistance is a growing problem[39–41] and (3) anaerobes including *Bacteroides fragilis*, anaerobic gram-positive cocci, *Fusobacterium, Prevotella,* and *Porphyromonas*.

There are variations in the susceptibility of carbapenems. Ertapenem is the only carbapenem that has poor activity against *Pseudomonas aeruginosa* compared with doripenem, which is most effective, including strains resistant to antipseudomonal penicillins and cephalosporins. Although imipenem-cilastatin, meropenem, and doripenem may exhibit activity against *Pseudomonas aeruginosa* initially, resistance may occur when these agents are used as monotherapy[37] and coadministration with aminoglycosides should be considered.

Imipenem-cilastatin, meropenem, and doripenem are useful for the treatment of a wide variety of infections including bacteremias, bone and soft tissue infections, pneumonia, and serious hospital-acquired or mixed infections. They may be used as single agents for the empiric treatment of unidentified infections pending culture results or when treatment with cephalosporins or penicillin has been unsuccessful.[36,37]

Ertapenem has a narrower spectrum of activity compared with the other carbapenems. It is active against most Enterobacteriaceae and anaerobes but less useful for *Pseudomonas aeruginosa*, *Acinetobacter*, and gram-positive pathogens, such as penicillin-resistant pneumococci and enterococci. Unlike meropenem, it is not approved for meningitis although it penetrates the blood-brain barrier. It has the advantage of single daily dosing and is used in skin and soft tissue, pelvic, gastrointestinal infections, community-acquired pneumonia and urinary tract infections.

Imipenem is coadministered with cilastatin, an inhibitor of dehydropeptidase I, an enzyme that cleaves imipenem. Imipenem is more active against highly resistant pneumococci and has some activity against *Enterococcus faecalis*. Both imipenem and meropenem have excellent penetration into the cerebrospinal fluid in the presence of inflamed meninges.[42,43] The main toxicity of imipenem is central nervous system (CNS) involvement with myoclonus, altered mental status and seizures,[44] and should be used with caution in patients with underlying CNS or renal disease.

Meropenem has less central nervous system toxicity[43] and may be used in patients with underlying CNS or renal disease. It has a spectrum of activity similar to imipenem,[36] but is more active against *Haemophilus influenzae*. It is the only carbapenem approved for the treatment of bacterial meningitis.[45]

Doripenem is the most recently approved carbapenem and, together with merope-nem, has enhanced activity against gram-negative bacilli. Doripenem is the most active carbapenem against *Pseudomonas aeruginosa* and is approved for complicated intra-abdominal infections and urinary tract infections.[46,47] Data suggest that doripenem may be used for nosocomial pneumonia[47] and oral and dental surgical infections.[46]

Monobactams

Aztreonam is the only monobactam available. Monobactams are β-lactams that have the β-lactam ring alone, and not fused to another ring. They are used exclusively for gram-negative aerobic bacterial infections[48,49] and have no activity against gram-positive or anaerobic bacteria. They are very active against *Haemophilus influenzae* and *Neisseria gonorrheae* infections as well as *Escherichia coli, Klebsiella, Serratia* and *Proteus* but less activity against *Pseudomonas aeruginosa* compared with imipe-nem or ceftazidime. For patients who are allergic to penicillin, ertapenem can be added to clindamycin or vancomycin for the treatment of oral infections.

Aminoglycosides

Aminoglycosides including gentamicin, tobramycin, streptomycin and amikacin have bactericidal activity against susceptible gram-negative bacilli and may be additive or synergistic with penicillins or cephalosporins against gram-positive cocci or gram-negative bacilli. Aminoglycosides block protein synthesis and resistance has remained relatively low. Despite these properties, the toxicity issues with aminoglycosides often limit their use. Renal toxicity results in acute kidney injury ranging from 0% to 50%.[50] Ototoxicity can produce irreversible cochlear and vestibular damage. Although few patients complain of hearing loss, damage is noted in up to 62% of asymptomatic high-frequency audiograms.[51] Overall, the incidence is reported to be between 3% and 14%.[52] A commonly used definition of drug-induced ototoxicity is an increased auditory threshold of 15 dB or greater at any of 2 or more frequencies.[51,52] Toxicity is identified initially in the outer hair cells of the organ of Corti, although the exact interac-tions are unknown.[52,53] Vestibular toxicity occurs in the type 1 hair cell of the ampullary cristae and is symptomatic with nausea, vomiting, and true vertigo.[54] Neuromuscular blockade can result in weakness of respiratory muscles, dilated pupils, and flaccid paralysis, and can be rapidly reversed with intravenous calcium gluconate.[55]

Macrolides

Macrolides activity to block bacterial protein synthesis comes from the presence of the macrolide ring. The commonly used macrolide antibiotics include erythromycin, azithromycin, and clarithromycin. Erythromycin has activity against streptococci and pneumococci compared with penicillin but has become less popular than azithromy-cin and clarithromycin because of gastrointestinal intolerance, more limited spectrum of activity, decreased oral absorption and a longer half-life.[56] Specifically, most strains of *Haemophilus influenzae* are resistant to erythromycin, so that its use as monother-apy in otitis media is limited. Erythromycin may be an effective agent against *Moraxella catarrhalis* and respiratory pathogens such as *Mycoplasma pneumoniae, Chlamydia pneumoniae, Legionella pneumophilia*, and *Bordatella pertussis*.[57] Erythromycin is also useful for *Mycoplasma* or pharyngitis caused by Chlamydiae. There are several issues that may limit the use of erythromycin. Resistance to erythromycin may develop early in treatment, including *Haemophilus influenzae* and *Streptococcus pneumoniae*. There is no activity against MRSA. Gastrointestinal distress is common but is improved with use of enteric-coated preparations. There is risk of inadequate absorp-tion if taken with food. Reversible hearing loss can occur with high doses of intravenous erythromycin. Prolongation of QT interval is found with all macrolides. Significant drug interactions exist with statins, antiarrythmics, sildenafil citrate (Viagra), theophylline, cyclosporine, warfarin, carbamezapine, benzodiazepines, digoxin, methylprednisolone, alfentanil, and dopamine agonists.[58] Compared with erythromycin and clarithromycin, azithromycin has more activity against gram-negative bacteria, particularly *Haemophilus influenzae* and *Moraxella catarrhalis*.[59] Azithromycin also has the benefit of lacking the drug interactions listed earlier.

Clindamycin

Clindamycin is a semisynthetic derivative of lincomycin, a natural antibiotic produced by the actinobacterium *Streptomyces lincolnensis*. It is bacteriostatic by inhibiting protein synthesis. Clindamycin is an excellent agent for the treatment of infections of the oral cavity and surpasses penicillin in the eradication of streptococci in tonsillo-pharyngitis, likely because of the β-lactamase production of some of the polymicrobial flora, resulting in resistance to penicillin. It is effective against most pneumococci and streptococci and most penicillin-resistant staphylococci including some MRSA isolates. It also shows enhanced activity against most clinically important anaerobes, especially *Bacteroides fragilis*, although resistance is now being reported.[60–62] It concentrates well in saliva, mucus, respiratory tissues, and bone, and is the drug of choice for the treatment of osteomyelitis with susceptible pathogens. From a head and neck standpoint, clindamycin is particularly useful in the treatment of the polymicrobial oral infections, including *Bacteroides* and other anaerobes common in chronic tonsillitis and deep neck abscesses of oral and dental origin. The main concerns with regard to clindamycin are gastrointestinal distress with nausea and vomiting and a risk of esophagitis. This risk can be minimized with ingestion during meals, and yogurt or acidophilus. *Clostridium difficile* pseudomembranous colitis is a complication that may occur after all antibacterial agents but has been classically associated with clindamycin. Treatment includes discontinuation of the antibiotic and treatment with oral metronidazole, vancomycin, or nitazoxanide. Clindamycin has poor penetration of the blood-brain barrier, and therefore not useful for the treatment of intracranial infections. Penicillin-resistant pneumococci are becoming increasingly resistant to clindamycin.

Metronidazole

Metronidazole is useful in the treatment of oral infections by virtue of its activity against clinically important anaerobes including *Bacteroides*, *Prevotella*, *Fusobacterium*, *Peptostreptococcus* (anaerobic *Streptococcus*), and *Clostridium*. One study of metronidazole showed inhibition of periodontal pathogens, irrespective of its β-lactamase production, except for *Actinomyces*.[63] Specifically, metronidazole relieves the pain of pharyngeal and tonsillar ulcers associated with Vincent angina and may improve the tonsillitis of infectious mononucleosis, inferring a significant role of anaerobic bacteria in these conditions. In addition, it is used in the treatment of perioral dermatitis, acute necrotizing gingivitis, and childhood granulomatous periorificial dermatitis.

Metronidazole lacks activity against all aerobic bacteria, an issue in the treatment of oral infections, which are often polymicrobial. Therefore, combination of metronidazole with other agents such as the penicillins, cephalosporins, and quinolones is required for the treatment of mixed infections such as tonsillitis, sinusitis, odontogenic disease, infected cholesteatoma, or deep neck abscesses.[63,64] Patients treated with metronidazole need to be reminded to avoid alcohol consumption because of the risk of a disulfuram-like reaction.

Vancomycin

Given the increasing incidence of MRSA and penicillin-resistant pneumococcal infections, vancomycin use has become more prevalent. A glycopeptide antibiotic, it is of particular importance to otolaryngology-head and neck surgeons because of its use in combination with gram-negative and anaerobic antibiotics for head and neck infections, and because of its potential for vancomycin-associated ototoxicity.[62] It is bactericidal against almost all *Staphylococcus*, *Streptococcus*, *Pneumococcus*, *Enterococcus*, and *Clostridium* species. One of the first reports of vancomycin usage included 6 cases of severe ototoxicity[65] with high-frequency sensorineural hearing loss described in up to 12% and higher in the elderly.[66] Concomitant use of aminoglycosides is believed to potentiate the toxicity of vancomycin. In rare cases, tinnitus and vertigo may develop and precede the hearing loss.[67] The ototoxicity is reversible with discontinuation of the drug. If vancomycin dosing exceeds 2 g/d, monitoring for renal function and vancomycin trough levels between 15 and 20 µg/mL is recommended. Vancomycin is known to produce red man or red neck syndrome with rapid infusions in 3.4% to 11.2% of cases.[68,69] Classically, patients experience a rapid onset of an erythematous rash and/or pruritis involving the head, neck, and upper trunk that may or may not be associated with angioedema and hypotension anaphylactoid reaction. This reaction resolves with discontinuation of vancomycin without other measures in most cases. The risk of this adverse reaction can be reduced by decreasing the rate of the infusion, and if necessary, the use of antihistamines. Reversible neutropenia occurs in 1% to 2%[70,71] with a more recent report of thrombocytopenia with severe bleeding.[72] There are reports of nephrotoxicity ranging from 0% to 12%,[70,73] which increases with combined use of other nephrotoxic agents such as aminoglycosides.

Linezolid

Linezolid is a synthetic antibiotic that has activity against MRSA and vancomycin-resistant *Enterococcus* (VRE) and can be used for patients with penicillin allergies. Although this agent also has activity against pneumococcus, it lacks activity against penicillin-resistant strains. It has been used for the treatment of parotitis. The major concerns regarding linezolid include thrombocytopenia and pancytopenia (particularly with more than a 2-week course), high cost, serotonin syndrome when used in conjunction with monoamine oxidase inhibitor antidepressants, hypertension when used together with decongestants containing pseudoephedrine, ephedrine, or phenylephrine, and increasing reports of peripheral neuropathy and lactic acidosis.

Daptomycin

Daptomycin has rapid bactericidal activity against staphylococci, pneumococci, and enterococci[74,75] including MRSA, vancomycin-intermediate *Staphylococcus aureus* and vancomycin-resistant *Enterococcus* isolates. In addition to aerobic gram-positive activity, it has in vitro activity against gram-positive anaerobes such as *Peptostreptococcus* and *Clostridium perfringens* although established guidelines for susceptibility testing are not available. It has the advantage of once daily intravenous dosing and is approved for skin and soft tissue infections, bacteremia, and right-sided endocarditis. The 2 caveats with daptomycin use are the lack of lung penetration, and therefore it is not indicated for the treatment of pneumonia, and increase in creatine phosphokinase (CPK) level and associated muscle toxicity.

Sulfonamides

Sulfonamides have been in existence since the 1930s and exert antimicrobial activity against many *Haemophilus influenzae* isolates. However, trimethoprim (TMP)-sulfamethoxazole (SMZ) should not be used as a first-line agent against otitis media, particularly when resistant respiratory pathogens are present.[76] This class of bacteriostatic antibiotics has only variable activity against pneumococci, streptococci, anaerobes, and *Moraxella catarrhalis*. Therefore, it is common to use sulfa in combination with other agents such as SMZ with TMP, which is believed to potentiate the action of sulfonamides by the inhibition of folic acid synthesis and ultimately protein synthesis.[77] Classically, TMP-SMZ has been used together with erythromycin for the treatment of acute otitis media and purulent rhinosinusitis against *Haemophilus influenzae* and pneumococci in the pediatric population. More recently, TMP-SMZ has been useful for the treatment of MRSA, although susceptibility testing needs to be done. TMP-SMZ has an effective role in the treatment and prevention of relapse of Wegener granulomatosis, as an adjuvant to immunosuppressive agents.[78] It is the most common agent for the prophylaxis and treatment of *Pneumocystis carinii*, a cause of otitis media and mastoiditis in individuals infected with HIV with CD4 counts less than 200/mm^3. Sulfonamides have several adverse reactions that require monitoring. These include rashes (ranging from mild morbilliform rashes to urticaria and Stevens Johnson syndrome), blood dyscrasias (ranging from aplastic anemia, agranulocytosis, and thrombocytopenia), nephrotoxicity, type 4 renal tubular acidosis, and drug interactions with phenytoin, rifampin, warfarin, oral hypoglycemics, methotrexate, and cyclosporine.

ANTIFUNGALS

There are 3 basic classes of antifungal agents: azoles, echinocandins, and polyenes. In the event of a serious fungal infection, an infectious diseases consultation should be considered to assist with antifungal selection and management of potential drug interactions and toxicities.

Azoles include fluconazole, itraconazole, voriconazole, and posaconazole. Fluconazole covers *Candida albicans* and many nonalbicans *Candida*. It is the primary antifungal agent used to treat oropharyngeal and esophageal candidiasis. It is also used for the treatment of cryptococcal meningitis. It has excellent penetration of the cerebrospinal fluid, eye, and saliva. Some *Candida* isolates such as *Candida glabrata* may be resistant to fluconazole. Therefore, susceptibility testing is indicated in cases of severe fungal infections.

Itraconazole is active against aspergillosis, molds such as dematiaceous fungi (dark pigmented molds, eg, *Curvularia*, *Alternaria*, and *Bipolaris*) as well as *Candida*. It is recommended for the treatment of allergic fungal sinusitis dosed at 200 mg twice daily followed by 100 mg daily for 3 months.[50] There are 2 formulations; the oral suspension is combined with cyclodextrin and has superior bioavailability compared with the tablet form.

Voriconazole has excellent activity against *Aspergillus* spp and is recommended as first-line therapy for invasive aspergillosis including invasive fungal sinusitis. It also has activity against *Scedosporium* and *Fusarium* and enhanced activity against nonalbicans *Candida*. In 30% of patients, voriconazole has been associated with mild, reversible visual alteration developing 30 minutes after dosing and persisting for 30 minutes. The visual changes are described as blurry vision, color vision change, and/or photophobia and is reversible. Prolongation of the QT interval has also been reported and should be taken into account in patients with underlying conduction abnormalities.[79]

Posaconazole has the additional benefit of excellent activity against zygomycetes such as mucormycosis compared with amphotericin, although it is not approved by the US Food and Drug Administration for this indication. It also has activity against *Candida*, including fluconazole-resistant isolates, *Aspergillus*, dermatophytes, *Blastomyces*, and dimorphic fungi such as coccidiomycosis, histoplasmosis, and cryptococcosis. It is available only in oral suspension and should be taken with a full meal or liquid nutritional supplements to enhance absorption.

The azoles share some similar adverse reactions including abnormal liver function tests with dose adjustment or discontinuation in patients who develop liver disease, and drug interactions resulting in increased levels of cyclosporine and tacrolimus.

Echinocandins are a class of antifungal agents that include caspofungin, micafungin, and anidulafungin. Their mechanism of action differs from azoles and the amphotericin preparations and covers *Candida*, including fluconazole-resistant strains, and *Aspergillus*. They are well tolerated with some specific differences. Caspofungin decreases the metabolism of cyclosporine and tacrolimus, resulting in increased levels and hepatotoxicity. Dosing may be decreased from 50 mg to 35 mg in the presence of liver disease. Micafungin increases levels of nifedipine and rapamycin, and anidulafungin has less issues with hepatotoxicity.

Polyenes involve the amphotericin preparations with broad antifungal coverage that includes *Candida*, *Aspergillus* and *Zygomyces*. The most common preparation is intravenous, although amphotericin has been used as a nasal rinse for the treatment of fungal sinusitis. The dosing as a nasal rinse is amphotericin B 250 μg/mL of sterile water, with 20 mL irrigated into each nostril twice daily.[80] The main side effects are nephrotoxicity, infusion related fevers, rigors, hypotension, nausea/vomiting and tachypnea, anemia, and electrolyte abnormalities. Ambisome, Abelcet and Amphotec are lipid formulations of amphotericin that have been developed to decrease the nephrotoxicity of amphotericin.

ANTIVIRALS

Acyclovir, valacyclovir, and famciclovir are active against herpes simplex and herpes zoster. Acyclovir is available in topical ointment, oral and intravenous formulations. The topical ointment is useful for the treatment of mucocutaneous herpes simplex infections in immunocompromised patients, although oral or intravenous acyclovir is also used in this population. The oral and intravenous formulations are also used for the treatment of local and disseminated herpes infections such as herpes zoster oticus.[81] Patients who experience frequent reactivations of herpes infections may benefit from chronic suppressive therapy, for example, with acyclovir 400 mg twice daily.

Patients who present with rash or vesicles along the ear canal and pinna may have Ramsey-Hunt syndrome (herpes zoster) and benefit from antivirals. Bell's palsy is possibly related to herpetic viral infections or idiopathic causes; clinicians are electing to treat a possible viral cause with antivirals.

ANTIBIOTIC CONSIDERATIONS FOR SPECIFIC INFECTIONS
Oral Infections of Odontogenic Sources

These infections are related to dental caries, pulpitis, periapical abscess, gingivitis, gingival abscess, and periodontal disease. Significant complications can include intracranial, retropharyngeal, or pleuropulmonary extension, and hematogenous extension to heart valves and prosthetic devices. Antibiotic considerations are based on knowledge of the most prevalent oral flora as described previously.

Antibiotic choice is ampicillin-sulbactam, amoxicillin-clavulanate, or penicillin plus metronidazole. If the patient is allergic to penicillin, clindamycin is appropriate. Cefoxitin or moxifloxacin can be considered, however, anaerobic coverage may be inadequate. Avoid erythromycin and tetracyclines because of increasing resistance among some strains of streptococci and limited anaerobic activity.

Radiation and Chemotherapy Resulting in Ulcerative Mucositis

The treatment of head and neck malignancies with surgery, chemotherapy, and radiation therapy is commonly associated with infectious complications.[82] Patients may develop osteonecrosis of the mandible, radionecrosis of the laryngeal cartilage, or pharyngocutaneous fistulas. The most common pathogens involved include *Staphylococcus aureus* and *Pseudomonas aeruginosa*.[83] Because of the chronicity of these infections, multiple debridements with deep intraoperative cultures and sensitivities can help guide the choice of antibiotics. A broad-spectrum antibiotic is appropriate in this setting, such as pipercillin-tazobactam, ticarcillin-clavulanate, or a carbapenem (excluding ertapenem because of the lack of adequate *Pseudomonas aeruginosa* activity). If patients are known to be carriers of MRSA, the addition of vancomycin would be prudent. Osteomyelitis of the jaw is complicated by the presence of teeth and exposure to the oral environment. Both clindamycin and moxifloxacin have excellent bone penetration and are recommended, often for weeks or months.[84]

Deep Neck Infections of Odontogenic Sources

These infections occur from direct extension from the teeth or hematogenous spread from transient bacteremias, which commonly occur during or after dental procedures, particularly with the extraction of infected teeth.[85] Complications include spread to the mediastinum[86,87] and intracranial suppuration such as cavernous sinus thrombosis, which can be avoided with antibiotic therapy. Antibiotic choices can be made based on the predictable oral flora, such as *Streptococcus viridans* and other streptococci and anaerobes such as *Bacteroides* and *Peptostreptococcus*. These pathogens are associated with suppurative orofacial and odontogenic infections such as Ludwig's angina and can be treated with intravenous penicillin G plus metronidazole, ampicillin-sulbactam, clindamycin, or cefoxitin. Lateral pharyngeal or retropharyngeal space infections can be treated with penicillin plus metronidazole, ampicillin-sulbactam, or clindamycin. Although antibiotic therapy is important in this setting, the most important treatment of odontogenic and nonodontogenic orofacial infections is surgical drainage and debridement of necrotic tissue.[8,9]

Invasive Fungal Sinusitis

The causal agents are commonly the filamentous fungi such as *Aspergillus, Mucorales*, and *Rhizopus*, and dematiaceous (black mold) fungi such as *Alternaria, ipolaris*, and *Curvularia*. These infections may become fulminant and disseminate, often associated with an immunocompromised state such as diabetes mellitus, malignancy with neutropenia, or high-dose corticosteroid use. The treatment includes wide debridement with clean margins and antifungal therapy, such as intravenous liposomal amphotericin B 3 to 5 mg/kg daily plus/minus posaconazole 400 mg by mouth three times a day (no oral formulation). Echinocandins (caspofungin, anidulafungin, micafungin) are used for *Aspergillus* only because this class of antifungals has no coverage for additional molds such as the dematiaceous fungi or mucorales and may be considered suboptimal therapy unless combined with posaconazole or amphotericin preparations.

REFERENCES

1. Sichel JY, Attal P, Hocwald E, et al. Redefining parapharyngeal space infections. Ann Otol Rhinol Laryngol 2006;115(2):117–23.
2. Dahlen G. Microbiology and treatment of dental abscesses and periodontal endodontic lesions. Periodontol 2000 2002;28:206–39.
3. Preshaw PM, Serymour RA, Heasman PA. Current concepts in periodontal pathogenesis. Dent bacterial diversity within the human subgingival crevice. Proc Natl Acad Sci U S A 1999;96:14547–52.
4. Brinig MM, Lepp PW, Ouverney CC, et al. Prevalence of bacteria of division TM7 in human subgingival plaque and their association with disease. Appl Environ Microbiol 2003;69:1678–94.
5. Sutter VL. Anaerobes as normal oral flora. Rev Infect Dis 1984;6:S62.
6. Costello EK, Lauber CL, Hamady M, et al. Bacterial community variation in human body habitats over space and time. Science 2009;326:1694.
7. Jousimies-Somer H, Summanen P. Recent taxonomic changes and terminology update of clinically significant anaerobic gram-negative bacteria (excluding spirochetes). Clin Infect Dis 2002;35(Suppl 1):517–21.
8. Chow AW. Infections of the oral cavity, neck and head. In: Mandell GL, Bennett JE, Douglas RG, editors. Principles and practice of infectious diseases. 7th edition. Philadelphia: Churchill Livingstone Elsevier; 2010. p. 855–71.
9. Chow AW. Odontogenic infections. In: Schlossberg D, editor. Infections of the head and neck. New York: Springer-Verlag; 1987. p. 148–60.
10. Selwitz RH, Ismail AI, Pitts NB. Dental caries. Lancet 2007;369:51–9.
11. Haffajee AD, Cugini MA, Tanner A, et al. Subgingival microbiota in healthy, well-maintained elder and periodontitis subjects. J Clin Periodontol 1998;25: 346–53.
12. Matto J, Asikainen S, Vaisanen ML, et al. Role of *Porphyromonas gingivalis*, *Prevotella intermedia*, and *Prevotella nigrescens* in extraoral and some odontogenic infections. Clin Infect Dis 1997;25(Suppl 2):S194–8.
13. Brook I. Microbiology and management of endodontic infections in children. J Clin Pediatr Dent 2003;28:13–7.
14. Hull MW, Chow AW. An approach to oral infections and their management. Curr Infect Dis Rep 2005;7:17–27.
15. Epstein JB. Mucositis in the cancer patient and immunosuppressed host. Infect Dis Clin North Am 2007;21:503–22.
16. Ghuysen JM. Molecular structure of penicillin-binding proteins and beta-lactamases. Trends Microbiol 1994;2:372–80.
17. Kohanski MA, Dwyer DJ, Hayete B, et al. A common mechanism of cellular death induced by bactericidal antibiotics. Cell 2007;130:797–810.
18. Marcy SM, Klein JO. The isoxazolyl penicillins: oxacillin, cloxacillin, and dicloxacillin. Med Clin North Am 1970;54:1127–43.
19. Herman DJ, Gerding DN. Antimicrobial resistance among enterococci. Antimicrob Agents Chemother 1991;35:1–4.
20. Mulligan ME, Murray-Leisure KA, Ribner BS, et al. Methicillin-resistant *Staphylococcus aureus*: a consensus review of the microbiology, pathogenesis and epidemiology with implications for prevention and management. Am J Med 1993;94:313.
21. Klimek J, Nightingale C, Lehmann W, et al. Comparisons of concentrations of amoxicillin in serum and middle ear fluid of children with chronic otitis media. J Infect Dis 1977;155(6):999–1002.

22. Murphy TF. *Haemophilus* species (including *H. influenzae* and chancroid). In: Mandell GL, Bennett JE, Dolin R, editors. Principles and practice of infectious diseases. 7th edition. Philadelphia (PA): Churchill, Livingstone Elsevier; 2010. p. 2911–9.
23. Johnson GJ, White JG. Proceedings: platelet dysfunction induced by parenteral administration of carbenicillin and ticarcillin. Thromb Diath Haemorrh 1975;34(1): 341–2.
24. Pichichero ME. A review of evidence supporting the American Academy of Pediatrics recommendation for prescribing cephalosporin antibiotics for penicillin-allergic patients. Pediatrics 2005;115:1048–57.
25. Bohnen JM, Solomkin JS, Dellinger EP, et al. Guidelines for clinical care: anti-infective agents for intra-abdominal infections. Arch Surg 1992;127:83.
26. Reichmann P, Konig A, Linares J, et al. A global gene pool for high-level cephalosporin resistance in commensal *Streptococcus* species and *Streptococcus pneumoniae*. J Infect Dis 1997;176:1001.
27. Andes DR, Craig WA. Cephalosporins. In: Mandell GL, Douglas RG, Bennett JE, editors. Principles and practice of infectious diseases. 7th edition. Philadelphia (PA): Churchill, Livingstone Elsevier; 2010. p. 323–39.
28. Schaad UB, Suter S, Gianella-Borradori A, et al. A comparison of ceftriaxone and cefuroxime for the treatment of bacterial meningitis in children. N Engl J Med 1990;322:141.
29. Tomasz A. Antibiotic resistance in *Streptococcus pneumoniae*. Clin Infect Dis 1997;24:S85.
30. Quagliarello VJ, Scheld WM. Treatment of bacterial meningitis. N Engl J Med 1997;336:708.
31. Barckow D, Schwigon CD. Cefepime versus cefotaxime in the treatment of lower respiratory tract infection. J Antimicrob Chemother 1993;32(Suppl B):187–93.
32. Zervos M, Nelson M, Cefepime Study Group. Cefepime versus ceftriaxone for empiric treatment of hospitalized patients with community-acquired pneumonia. Antimicrob Agents Chemother 1998;42:729–33.
33. Yun HC, Ellis MW, Jorgensen JH. Activity of ceftobiprole against community-associated methicillin-resistant *Staphylococcus aureus* isolates recently recovered from US military trainees. Diagn Microbiol Infect Dis 2007;59(4):463.
34. Widmer A. Ceftobiprole: a new option for treatment of skin and soft-tissue infections due to methicillin-resistant *Staphylococcus aureus*. Clin Infect Dis 2008; 46(5):656–8.
35. Noel GJ, Bush K, Bagchi P, et al. A randomized, double-blind trial comparing ceftobiprole medocaril with vancomycin plus ceftazidime plus ceftazidime for the treatment of patients with complicated skin and skin-structure infections. Clin Infect Dis 2008;46(5):647–55.
36. Condon RE, Walker AP, Sirinek KR, et al. Meropenem versus tobramycin plus clindamycin for treatment of intraabdominal infections: results of a prospective, randomized double-blind clinical trial. Clin Infect Dis 1995;21:544.
37. Chang DC, Wilson SE. Meta-analysis of the clinical outcome of carbapenem monotherapy in the adjunctive treatment of intra-abdominal infections. Am J Surg 1997;174:284.
38. Available at: http://www.fda.gov/bbs/topics/NEWS/2007/NEW01728.html. Accessed October 14, 2010.
39. Kumarasamy KK, Toleman MA, Walsh TR, et al. Emergence of a new antibiotic resistance mechanism in India, Pakistan, and the UK: a molecular, biological and epidemiological study. Lancet Infect Dis 2010;10:597–602.

40. Dauner DG, May JR, Steele JC. Assessing antibiotic therapy for *Acinetobacter baumannii* infections in an academic medical center. Eur J Clin Microbiol Infect Dis 2008;27:1021–4.

41. Maragakis IL, Perl TM. *Acinetobacter baumannii*: epidemiology, antimicrobial resistance, and treatment options. Clin Infect Dis 2008;46:1254–63.

42. Jacobs RF, Kearns GI, Brown AL, et al. Cerebrospinal fluid penetration of imipenem and cilastatin (primaxin) in children with central nervous system infections. Antimicrob Agents Chemother 1986;29:670–4.

43. Nicolau DP. Pharmacokinetic and pharmacodynamic properties of meropenem. Clin Infect Dis 2008;47:532–40.

44. Calandra G, Lydick E, Carrigan J, et al. Factors predisposing to seizures in seriously ill patients receiving antibiotics: experience with imipenem/cilastatin. Am J Med 1988;84:911.

45. Mohr JF 3rd. Update on the efficacy and tolerability of meropenem in the treatment of serious bacterial infections. Clin Infect Dis 2008;47:S41–51.

46. Keam SJ. Doripenem: a review of its use in the treatment of bacterial infections. Drugs 2008;68(14):2021–57.

47. Chastre J, Wunderink R, Prokocimer P, et al. Efficacy and safety of intravenous infusion of doripenem versus imipenem in ventilator-associated pneumonia: a multicenter, randomized study. Crit Care Med 2008;36(4):1089–96.

48. Barry AL, Thornsberry C, Jones RN, et al. Aztreonam: antibacterial activity, beta-lactamase stability, and interpretive standards and quality control guidelines for disk-diffusion susceptibility tests. Rev Infect Dis 1985;7:S594–604.

49. Brummett RE, Fox KE. Aminoglycoside induced hearing loss in humans. Antimicrob Agents Chemother 1989;33:797–800.

50. Ferguson BJ. What role do systemic corticosteroids, immunotherapy, and antifungal drugs play in the therapy of allergic fungal rhinosinusitis? Otolaryngol Head Neck Surg 1998;124(10):1174–8.

51. Fausti SA, Henry JA, Schaffer HI, et al. High frequency audiometric monitoring for early detection of aminoglycoside ototoxicity. J Infect Dis 1992;165:1026–32.

52. Hutchin T, Cortopassi G. Proposed molecular and cellular mechanism of aminoglycoside ototoxicity. Antimicrob Agents Chemother 1994;38:2517–20.

53. Amiko M, Bagger-Sjoback D, et al. Gentamicin binding to the isolated crista ampullaris of the guinea pig. Res Commun Chem Pathol Pharmacol 1982;37:333–42.

54. Minor LB. Gentamicin-induced bilateral vestibular hypofunction. JAMA 1998;279: 541–4.

55. Singh YN, Harvey AL, Marshall IG. Antibiotic-induced paralysis of the mouse phrenic nerve-hemidiaphragm preparation, and reversibility by calcium and by neostigmine. Anesthesiology 1978;48:418–42.

56. Fairbanks DNF. Pocket guide to antimicrobial therapy in otolaryngology-head and neck surgery. 13th edition. Alexandria (VA): American Academy of Otolaryngology-Head and Neck Surgery Foundation, Inc; 2007. p. 10–11.

57. Sivapalasingam S, Steigbigel NH. Macrolides, clindamycin and ketolides. In: Mandell GL, Douglas RG, Bennett JE. Principles and practice of infectious diseases. 7th edition. Philadelphia (PA): Churchill, Livingstone Elsevier; 2010. p. 427–48.

58. Bahal N, Nahata MC. The new macrolide antibiotics: azithromycin, clarithromycin, dirithromycin, roxithromycin. Ann Pharmacother 1992;26:46–55.

59. Credito KL, Lin G, Pankuch GA, et al. Susceptibilities of *Haemophilus influenzae* and *Moraxella catarrhalis* to ABT-773 compared to their susceptibilities to 11 other agents. Antimicrob Agents Chemother 2001;45:67–72.

60. Ednie LM, Spangler SK, Jacobs MR, et al. Antianaerobic activity of the ketolide RU 64004 compared to activities of four macrolides, five beta-lactams, clindamycin and metronidazole. Antimicrob Agents Chemother 1997;41:1037–41.

61. Snydman DR, Jacobus NV, McDermott LA, et al. National survey on the susceptibility of the *Bacteroides fragilis* group: report and analysis of trends in the United States from 1997 to 2004. Antimicrob Agents Chemother 2008;51:1649–55.

62. Dalmau D, Cayouette M, Lamothe F, et al. Clindamycin resistance in the *Bacteroides fragilis* group: association with hospital acquired infections. Clin Infect Dis 1997;24:874–7.

63. Milazzo I, Blandino G, Caccamo F, et al. Faropenem, a new penem: antibacterial activity against selected anaerobic and fastidious periodontal isolates. J Antimicrob Chemother 2003;51:721–5.

64. Salvatore M, Meyers BR. Metronidazole. In: Mandell GL, Douglas RG, Bennett JE. Principles and practice of infectious diseases. 7th edition. Philadelphia (PA): Churchill, Livingstone Elsevier; 2010. p. 419–26.

65. Geraci JE, Heilman FR, Nichols DR, et al. Antibiotic therapy of bacterial endocarditis. VII. Vancomycin for acute micrococcal endocarditis. Proc Staff Meet Mayo Clin 1958;33:172–91.

66. Forouzesh AA, Moise PA, Sakoulas G. Vancomycin ototoxicity: a re-evaluation in an era of increasing doses. Antimicrob Agents Chemother 2009;53(2):483–6.

67. Murray BE, Nannini EC. Glycopeptides (vancomycin and teicoplanin), streptogramins (quinipristin-dalfopristin), and lipopeptides (daptomycin). In: Mandell GL, Douglas RG, Bennett JE. Principles and practice of infectious diseases. 7th edition. Philadelphia (PA): Churchill, Livingstone Elsevier; 2010. p. 449–67.

68. Matzke GR, Zhanel GG, Guay DR. Clinical pharmacokinetics of vancomycin. Clin Pharmacokinet 1986;11:257–82.

69. O'Sullivan TL, Ruffling MJ, Lamp KC, et al. Prospective evaluation of red man syndrome in patients receiving vancomycin. J Infect Dis 1993;168:773–6.

70. Downs NJ, Neihart RE, Dolezal JM, et al. Mild nephrotoxicity associated with vancomycin use. Arch Intern Med 1989;149:1777–81.

71. Rybak MJ, Albrecht LM, Boike SC, et al. Nephrotoxicity of vancomycin, alone or with an aminoglycoside. J Antimicrob Chemother 1990;25:679–87.

72. Von Drygalski A, Curtis BR, Bougie DW, et al. Vancomycin-induced immune thrombocytopenia. N Engl J Med 2007;356:904–10.

73. Farber BF, Moellering RC. Retrospective study of the toxicity of preparations of vancomycin from 1974 to 1981. Antimicrob Agents Chemother 1983;23: 138–41.

74. Hanberger H, Nilsson LE, Maller R, et al. Pharmacodynamics of daptomycin and vancomycin on *Enterococcus faecalis* and *Staphylococcus aureus* demonstrated by studies of initial killing and postantibiotic effect and influence of Ca^{2+} and albumin on these drugs. Antimicrob Agents Chemother 2001;45:454–9.

75. Akins RL, Rybak MJ. Bactericidal activities of two daptomycin regimens against clinical strains of glycopeptide intermediate-resistant *Staphylococcus aureus*, vancomycin-resistant *Enterococcus faecium* and methicillin-resistant *Staphylococcus aureus* isolates in an in vitro pharmacokinetic model with simulated endocardial vegetations. Antimicrobial Agents Chemother 2001;45:454–9.

76. Yelland MJ. The efficacy of oral cotrimoxazole in the treatment of otitis externa in general practice. Med J Aust 1993;158:697–9.

77. Leiberman A, Leibovitz E, Piglansky L, et al. Bacteriologic and clinical efficacy of trimethoprim-sulfamethoxazole for treatment of acute otitis media. Pediatr Infect Dis J 2001;20:260–4.

78. McRae D, Buchanan G. Longterm sulfamethoxazole-trimethoprim in Wegener's granulomatosis. Arch Otolaryngol 1993;119(1):103–5.

79. Rex JH, Stevens DA. Systemic antifungal agents. In: Mandell GL, Bennett JE, Douglas RG. Principles and practice of infectious diseases. 7th edition. Philadelphia (PA): Churchill, Livingstone Elsevier; 2010. p. 549–63.

80. Ponikau JU, Sherris DA, Weaver A, et al. Treatment of chronic rhinosinusitis with intranasal amphotericin B: a randomized, placebo-controlled, double-blind pilot trial. J Allergy Clin Immunol 2005;115(1):125–31.

81. Uscategui T, Doree C, Chamberlain IJ, et al. Antiviral therapy for Ramsay Hunt syndrome (herpes zoster oticus with facial palsy) in adults. Cochrane Database Syst Rev 2008;4:CD006851.

82. Lofti CJ, Cavalcanti RC, Costa e Silva AM, et al. Risk factors for surgical site infections in head and neck cancer surgery. Otolaryngol Head Neck Surg 2008;138: 74–80.

83. Brook I, Hirokawa R. Microbiology of wound infection after head and neck cancer surgery. Ann Otol Rhinol Laryngol 1989;98:323–5.

84. Sharkawy AA. Cervicofacial actinomycosis and mandibular osteomyelitis. Infect Dis Clin North Am 2007;21:543–56.

85. Lockhart PB, Durack DT. Oral microflora as a cause of endocarditis and other distant site infections. Infect Dis Clin North Am 1999;13:833–50.

86. Furst IM, Ersil P, Caminiti M. A rare complication of tooth abscess-Ludwig's angina and mediastinitis. J Can Dent Assoc 2001;67:324–7.

87. Garatea-Crelgo J, Gay-Escoda C. Mediastinitis from odontogenic infection. Report of three cases and review of the literature. Int J Oral Maxillofac Surg 1991;20:65–8.

Recurrent Aphthous Stomatitis

Amit Chattopadhyay, BDS, MDS, FFPH, MPH, CPH,
PGDHHM, PGDMLS, PhD[a],*, Kishore V. Shetty, BDS, DDS, MS, MRCS[b]

KEYWORDS

• Recurrent • Oral • Aphthous • Stomatitis • Diagnosis
• Management

Recurrent aphthous stomatitis (RAS) in the oral cavity a painful ulcer that causes causing substantial morbidity in the United States and elsewhere. RAS is one of the most common oral ailments. These ulcers have been generally described to typically appear first in childhood and tend to abate around the third decade of life.[1] Patients often report a family history of RAS. However, contrary to general belief, the burden of RAS among adults is high. RAS often is confused with intraoral ulcers associated with several systemic diseases or conditions. However, experts have suggested reserving the term *recurrent aphthous stomatitis* for recurrent ulcers confined to the mouth and seen in the absence of systemic disease.[1] Recurrent ulcers that do not have all the typical clinical characteristics or a childhood onset may perhaps be termed *aphthous-like ulcers* and not labeled as RAS.

CLINICAL PRESENTATION

RAS anywhere in the oral cavity is painful, and is one of the most common oral ailments. The disease is characterized by recurring painful ulcers of the mouth that are round or ovoid and are surrounded by inflammatory halos. These ulcers typically appear first in childhood. RAS may present as small ulcers 2 to 8 mm in diameter, called *minor aphthous ulcers*, and may heal spontaneously in 10 to 14 days. Larger ulcers, often 1 cm or more in diameter, are called *major recurrent aphthous ulcers*. *Herpetiform ulcers* are a bunch of small pinpoint ulcers occurring close together that may later coalesce.

Severe RAS is a rare but extremely disabling disorder. The lower vestibule is the most commonly involved site.[2] Most recurrent aphthous ulcers develop on freely movable nonkeratinized oral mucosa, including the buccal mucosa, vestibules, inner lips, under surface of the tongue, and soft palate. Although sometimes prodromal

Financial disclosures/conflicts of interest: The authors have nothing to disclose.
[a] ARCAB, 8603 Watershed Court, Gaithersburg, MD 20877, USA
[b] Private Dental Practice, Denver, CO 80238, USA
* Corresponding author.
E-mail address: amit.arcab@hotmail.com

Otolaryngol Clin N Am 44 (2011) 79–88
doi:10.1016/j.otc.2010.09.003
0030-6665/11/$ – see front matter © 2011 Published by Elsevier Inc.

oto.theclinics.com

symptoms such as altered sensation or focal erythema or slight swelling may be present, these are usually ignored by most patients until the painful ulcers develop.

EPIDEMIOLOGY

Among the most commonly cited studies for RAS prevalence,[3–11] only three are population-based,[3,4,7] of which the only one performed in the United States[7] involved school children and was based on the National Institute of Dental Research (renamed the National Institute of Dental Research and Craniofacial Research [NIDCR]) National Survey of Oral Health in US School Children (1986–1987). Although various factors have been reported to be associated with RAS, independent risk or causative factors of RAS have not been clearly established in population-based studies, and most evidence comes from convenience samples and clinic-based studies.[2]

Historically, reports have provided varying estimates for prevalence of RAS, ranging from 1% to 66% among adults[8,10,12–14] and 1% to 40% among children.[7,8,15] Most of these estimates were derived from hospital-based studies that could be subject to several selection biases. Most of these reports likely overestimated RAS prevalence because of improper sampling design for the purpose of estimating true disease burden. Sampling design and selection of study populations seriously impact the conclusion of studies, and convenience samples can provide estimates that may not reflect reality. Results based on data from the Third National Health and Nutrition Examination Survey (NHANES III), analyzed with appropriate nesting and weighting statements to adjust the variance for the complex sampling design of the survey, can be generalized to the United States population. Such a study found a substantially lower prevalence of RAS (1.03% overall), which, when stratified by age, suggests a 0.85% prevalence among adults and 1.5% prevalence among children and adolescents.[2]

This population-based study in the United States found that overall the prevalence of recurrent aphthous ulcers was 1030 per 100,000 persons (95% CI, 830–1220).[2] The prevalence of RAS among children was 1500 per 100,000 (95% CI, 1090–1910), which was greater than that among adults, at 850 per 100,000 (95% CI, 630–1070). It is estimated that in the United States, at least 3 million people have RAS, of which approximately 2 million are aged 17 years or older and 1 million are younger than 17 years.[2]

Multivariable analyses to determine independent risk indicators and risk factors in adults suggested that adjusted odds of RAS were greatest for persons aged 17 to 29 years (adjusted odds ratio [OR], 2.7; 95% CI, 1.4–5.5), men (adjusted OR, 1.7; 95% CI, 0.9–2.8), and persons with low serum insulin levels (OR, 2.0; 95% CI, 0.9–4.4). Never-smokers had greater risk for recurrent aphthous ulcers (OR, 9.2; 95% CI, 2.8–30.1) than people who smoked more than 10 cigarettes per day.[2] Results from a separate analysis based on NHANES III data show RAS-associated age distribution and sex differences (**Figs. 1** and **2**).

ASSOCIATIONS AND ETIOLOGY

Box 1 lists various causative and predictive factors suggested to be associated with RAS, none of which has been proven conclusively to be independently associated with RAS.[9–11,15–23]

Oral streptococci were suggested as important determinants of RAS, either as direct pathogens or as an antigenic stimulus culminating in the genesis of antibodies that may cross-react with keratinocyte antigenic determinants.[24] However, this was later refuted.[25] Similarly, *Mycobacterium tuberculosis*,[26] *Helicobacter pylori*,[27,28] herpes viruses,[29–31] varicella zoster virus,[32] and cytomegalovirus[33–35] have been

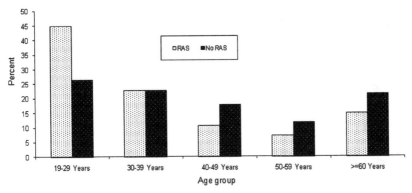

Fig. 1. Association of RAS with age: case-control analysis, NHANES-II.

implicated in RAS. Low insulin levels might be independently associated with greater odds of RAS.[2] A recent study also reported that RAS was associated with Behçet's disease, with 63 of 4000 registered subjects having RAS (5.8%).[33]

One study showed that phagocytic functions of salivary and peripheral blood neutrophils were reduced in patients with RAS compared with healthy subjects.[36] The ingestion ability of salivary neutrophils was also decreased with that of peripheral blood neutrophils in patients with RAS. These findings suggested that RAS may be characterized by consistent changes in salivary and peripheral blood neutrophil functions, and that the pathophysiology of RAS may be associated with reduction in phagocytic functions of neutrophils.[36]

Among other potentially etiologic associations, "a genetic predisposition is present, as shown by an increased frequency of certain human leucocyte antigen (HLA) types, and a positive family history in some patients with RAS. Attempts to implicate a variety of bacteria or viruses in the etiology have failed. Reactions to heat shock proteins (hsp) are one possibility: patients with RAS have circulating lymphocytes reactive with peptide 91–105 of hsp 65–60."[37]

Poor understanding of the cause of RAS has also spawned various possible treatment regimens proposed through clinical case series and clinical trials, with no strong evidence supporting or refuting efficacy or effectiveness of any of the treatments.

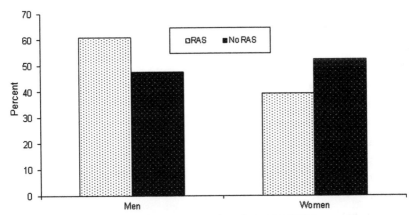

Fig. 2. Association of RAS with sex: case-control analysis, NHANES-II.

Box 1
Conditions and causative factors possibly associated with RAS

Trauma

Variety of physical and chemical trauma

Foods and nutrients

Chocolates

Dairy products

Nuts

Tomatoes

Wheat

Deficiency

Vitamins B_1, B_2, and B_6

Folate

Zinc

Iron

Chemokines, biological body products

TNF-α

Interleukins

Heat shock proteins

Systemic conditions

Endocrinologic

    Menstruation

    Low insulin levels

Gastroenterologic

    Crohn's disease

    Malabsorption syndrome

    Celiac disease

    Ulcerative colitis

    Gluten enteropathy

Hematologic

    Anemia

    Cyclical neutropenia

    Hematologic malignancies

Immunologic

    Immunodeficiencies (T-cell responses and defects, HIV)

Microbiologic

    Streptococci

    M tuberculosis

    H pylori

    Herpes viruses

Varicella zoster

Cytomegalovirus

Multiorgan diseases

Behçet's disease

MAGIC (mouth and genital ulcers with inflamed cartilage) syndrome

Marshall's syndrome

Reactive arthritis

Erythema multiforme

Genetic

HLA B51

Others

Keratinocyte maturity deficiency

Defective mucosal epithelial turnover

Behavioral factors

Smoking

Oral contraceptives

Psychological

Physiologic stress

Medications

Nonsteroidal anti-inflammatory drugs

β-blockers

Nicorandil

Alendronate

MANAGEMENT

RAS may sometimes be resistant to treatment (**Table 1**). Topical or intralesional corticosteroids and local anesthetics are used for palliative therapy. Suggested treatment modalities have aimed at either providing symptomatic relief or affecting a biologic cure, with no clear indication of superiority of either. No specific treatment for RAS is yet available.[15,38,39] The goals of RAS treatment have been to control pain, promote healing, and decrease numbers of future ulcers.[39] The treatments that have been attempted are listed in **Box 2**.

Few adequately powered clinical trials have tested the efficacy of therapeutic agents for RAS. Most current evidence is assembled from small studies. However, some recent developments show encouraging signs in RAS treatment that may help generate hypotheses that could potentially lead to strong clinical trials. One multicenter retrospective cohort study followed up on 92 patients (76 with oral or bipolar RAS, and 16 with Behçet's disease) at 14 centers for 40 months and assessed for effect of thalidomide on RAS. Groups were treated with either intermittent or regular therapy. Overall, "Thalidomide was rapidly effective: 85% (78/92) entered complete remission (CR) within a median of 14 days"; however, adverse events were reported by 84% of patients (mild, 78%; severe, 22%).[41]

Table 1 Commonly used topical and systemic agents for treatment of recurrent aphthous stomatitis	
Topical Agents for Recurrent Aphthous Ulcers	
Amlexanos	Most effective for minor ulcers
Antibiotics	May be used as a rinse for patients with multiple ulcers
Chlorhexidine gluconate	Effectiveness is unpredictable
Corticosteroids	Superpotent strength formulations are most effective
Systemic Agents for Recurrent Aphthous Ulcers	
Colchicine	Suppressive therapy limited by gastrointestinal toxicity
Dapsone	Suppressive therapy requires careful laboratory testing
Pentoxifylline	Least toxic suppressive therapy controlled efficacy studies are needed
Thalidomide	Acute treatment for patients with ulcerations unresponsive to topical therapy

Recently, much interest has focused on the use of irsogladine maleate for treatment of RAS, because it is viewed as a promising potential therapy. Irsogladine maleate (6-(2,5-Dichlorophenyl)-1,3,5-triazine-2,4-diamine maleate) is a type 4 phosphodiesterase (PDE4) and works as a mucosa protector that inhibits gastric mucosal injury induced by monochloramine and ischemia-reperfusion.[42] Moreover, irsogladine maleate activates gap junctional intercellular communication in mucosa, which is thought to contribute to improving gastric mucosal barrier function.[43] It further inhibits superoxide production in human neutrophils[44] and has been shown to inhibit in vitro and in vivo angiogenesis.[45]

A recent study suggested that the recovery of gap junctional intercellular communication by irsogladine maleate in the gingival epithelium may be a normal process in gingival epithelial homeostasis. Irsogladine maleate counters gap junctional intercellular communication reduction induced by interleukin-8 or Actinobacillus actinomycetemcomitans in cultured human gingival epithelial cells.[46] In another open-label, single-center study study, Nanke and colleagues[47] administered irsogladine, 2 to 4 mg/d, orally to 10 patients with Behçet's disease and recurrent oral aphthous ulcers. They reported that irsogladine was effective in all 10 patients and that the mean ulcer count decreased in all patients 3 months after administration. More recently, Inui and colleagues[48] reported some success with irsogladine maleate in a pilot study involving 16 patients. These studies seem to suggest that thalidomide and irsogladine maleate may be candidates for well-conducted clinical trials in the treatment of RAS.

The role of irsogladine maleate in healing of gastric ulcers lends credibility to successes in RAS management. In a pilot study of irsogladine maleate given after H pylori eradication treatment, the rate of healing of gastric ulcers was high, at 79.2%.[49] A recently reported multicenter, double-blind, randomized clinical trial[50] assessed 321 patients with a single H pylori-positive gastric ulcer. The trial participants were given eradication treatment and then assigned randomly to a treatment group (4 mg/d irsogladine maleate; n = 150) or a control group (placebo; n = 161). The results showed that irsogladine maleate was effective for treating gastric ulcers after H pylori eradication. The high healing rates observed in patients with or without successful eradication show the usefulness of irsogladine maleate treatment regardless of the outcome of eradication,[45] indicating efficacious mucosal healing after therapy. Irsogladine maleate is an enhancer of gastric mucosal protective factors. It increases the production of intracellular cyclic adenosine monophosphate (cAMP)

Box 2
Attempted treatments for RAS

Topical applications

Anesthetics

Protective bioadhesives

Corticosteroids

Antimicrobial mouth rinses

Aphthasol

Local cauterization

Sucralfate

Amyloglucosidase

Glucose oxidase

Systemic agents[40]

Colchicine

Dapsone

Pentoxifylline

Levamisole

Systemic corticosteroids

Azathioprine

Methotrexate

Cyclosporine A

Chlorambucil

Cyclophosphamide

Infliximab

Etanercept

Interferon α

Thalidomide

---

through inhibiting phosphodiesterase activity, and thus activates intracellular communication, prevents a reduction in gastric mucosal blood flow, increases anti-inflammatory activity, and prevents the reduction of mucosal hydrophobicity. Its efficacy has been shown in various models of gastric mucosal injury.[50]

RAS remains a common disorder, for which the precise cause, long-term behavior, preventive factors, and precise etiopathology are not well understood. Clear definitive treatments are not yet available. The management paradigm for RAS continues to be essentially palliative and has the goal of reducing pain and inflammation, and minimizing physical damage to the affected mucosa.

REFERENCES

1. Scully C. Aphthous ulceration. N Engl J Med 2006;355:165–72.
2. Chattopadhyay A, Chatterjee S. Risk indicators for recurrent aphthous ulcers among adults in the US. Community Dent Oral Epidemiol 2007;35:152–9.

3. Axéll T, Henricsson V. The occurrence of recurrent aphthous ulcers in an adult Swedish population. Acta Odontol Scand 1985;43:121–5.
4. Axéll T, Henricsson V. Association between recurrent aphthous ulcers and tobacco habits. J Dent Res 1985;43:121–5.
5. Rennie JS, Reade PC, Hay KD, et al. Recurrent aphthous stomatitis. Braz Dent J 1985;159:361–7.
6. Rogers RS III. Recurrent aphthous stomatitis. Clinical characteristics and associated systemic disorders. Semin Cutan Med Surg 1997;16:278–83.
7. Kleinman DV, Swango PA, Pindborg JJ. Epidemiology of oral mucosal lesions in United States Schoolchildren: 1986–87. Community Dent Oral Epidemiol 1994; 22:243–53.
8. Field EA, Allan RB. Oral ulceration—aetiopathogenesis, clinical diagnosis and management in the gastrointestinal clinic. Aliment Pharmacol Ther 2003;18: 949–62.
9. Porter SR, Scully C, Pedersen A. Recurrent aphthous stomatitis. Crit Rev Oral Biol Med 1998;9:306–12.
10. Rivera-Hidalgo F, Shulman JD, Beach MM. The association of tobacco and other factors with recurrent aphthous stomatitis in an US adult population. Oral Dis 2004;10:335–45.
11. Ferguson MM, Carter J, Boyle P. An epidemiological study of factors associated with recurrent aphthae in women. J Oral Med 1984;39:212–7.
12. Zunt SL. Recurrent aphthous stomatitis. Dermatol Clin 2003;21:33–9.
13. Sohat-Zabarski R, Kalderon S, Klein T, et al. Close association of HLA B-51 in persons with recurrent aphthous stomatitis. Oral Surg Oral Med Oral Pathol 1992;74:455–8.
14. Dorsey C. More observations on relief of aphthous stomatitis on resumption of cigarette smoking. Calif Med 1964;101:377–8.
15. Ferguson MM, McKay HD, Lindsay R, et al. Progeston therapy for menstrually related aphthae. Int J Oral Surg 1978;7:463–70.
16. Bittoun R. Recurrent aphthous ulcers and nicotine. Med J Aust 1991;154:471–2.
17. Ferguson MM, Wray D, Carmichael HA, et al. Coeliac disease associated with recurrent aphthae. Gut 1980;21:223–36.
18. Soames JV, Southam JC. Oral pathology. 3rd edition. Oxford (UK): Oxford University Press; 1998.
19. Freysdottir J, Lau S, Fortune F. Gammadelta T cells in Behçet's disease (BD) and recurrent aphthous stomatitis(RAS). Clin Exp Immunol 1999;118:451–7.
20. Natah SS, Hayrinen-Immonen R, Hietanen J, et al. Immunolocalisation of tumor necrosis factor-alpha expressing cells in recurrent aphthous ulcer lesions (RAU). J Oral Pathol Med 2000;29:19–25.
21. Sun A, Chu CT, Liu BY, et al. Expression of interleukin-2 receptor by activated peripheral blood lymphocytes upregulated by the plasma level of interleukin-2 in patients with recurrent aphthous ulcers. Proc Natl Sci Counc Repub China B 2000;24:116–22.
22. Lehner T, Lavery E, Smith R, et al. Association between the 65-kilodalton heat shock protein, Streptococcus sanguis, and the corresponding antibodies in Behcets syndrome. Infect Immun 1991;59:1434–41.
23. Ferguson R, Basu MK, Asquith P, et al. Jejunal mucosal abnormalities in patients with recurrent aphthous ulceration. Br Med J 1976;1:11–3.
24. Endre L. Recurrent aphthous ulceration with zinc deficiency and cellular immune deficiency. Oral Surg Oral Med Oral Pathol 1991;72:559–61.

25. Lindemann RA, Riviere GR, Sapp JP. Serum antibody responses to indigenous oral mucosal antigens and selected laboratory-maintained bacteria in recurrent aphthous ulceration. Oral Surg Oral Med Oral Pathol 1985;59:585.

26. Greenspan JS, Gadol N, Olson JA, et al. Lymphocyte function in recurrent aphthous ulceration. J Oral Pathol 1985;14:495–502.

27. Pervin K, Childersrton A, Shinnick T, et al. T cell epitope expression of mycobacterial and homologous human 65-kilodalton heat shock protein peptides in short term lines from patients with Behçet's disease. J Immunol 1983;154:174–7.

28. Porter SR, Barker G, Scully C, et al. Serum IgG antibodies to helicobacter pylori in patients with recurrent aphthous stomatitis and other oral disorders. Oral Surg Oral Med Oral Pathol Oral Radiol Endod 1997;83:325–8.

29. Shimoyama T, Horie N, kato T, et al. Helicobacter pylori in oral ulcerations. J Oral Sci 2000;42:225–9.

30. Pedersen A. Recurrent aphthous ulceration: virological and immunological aspects. APMIS 1993;37(Suppl):1–37.

31. Di Alberti L, Ngui SL, Porter SR, et al. Presence of human herpesvirus-8 variants in the oral tissue of human immunodeficiency virus-infected individuals. J Infect Dis 1997a;175:703–7.

32. Di Alberti L, Porter SR, Speight P, et al. Detection of human herpesvirus-8 DNA in oral ulcer tissues of HIV infected individuals. Oral Dis 1997;3(Suppl 1):S133–4.

33. Klein P, Weinberger A, Altmann VJ, et al. Prevalence of Behçet's disease among adult patients consulting three major clinics in a Druze town in Israel. Clin Rheumatol 2010;29(10):1163–6.

34. Leimola-Virtanen R, Happonen RP, Syrjanen S. Cytomegalovirus (CMV) and Helicobacter pylori (HP) found in oral mucosal ulcers. J Oral Pathol Med 1995;24:14–7.

35. Pedersen A, Hornsleth A. Recurrent aphthous ulceration: a possible clinical manifestation of reaction of varicella zoster of cytomegalovirus infection. J Oral Pathol Med 1993;22:64–8.

36. Kumar BP, Keluskar V, Bagewadi AS, et al. Evaluating and comparing phagocytic functions of salivary and blood neutrophils in patients with recurrent aphthous ulcers and controls. Quintessence Int 2010;41(5):411–6.

37. Jurge S, Kuffer R, Scully C, et al. Mucosal disease series. Number VI. Recurrent aphthous stomatitis. Oral Dis 2006;12(1):1–21.

38. Ship J. Recurrent aphthous stomatitis—an update. Oral Surg Oral Med Oral Pathol Oral Radiol Endod 1996;81:141–7.

39. Barrons RW. Treatment strategies for recurrent aphthous ulcers. Am J Health Syst Pharm 2001;58:41–53.

40. Altenburg A, Abdel-Naser MB, Seeber H, et al. Practical aspects of management of recurrent aphthous stomatitis. J Eur Acad Dermatol Venereol 2007;21(8):1019–26.

41. Hello M, Barbarot S, Bastuji-Garin S, et al. Use of thalidomide for severe recurrent aphthous stomatitis: a multicenter cohort analysis. Medicine (Baltimore) 2010;89(3):176–82.

42. Kyoi T, Kitazawa S, Tajima K, et al. Phosphodiesterase type IV inhibitors prevent ischemia-reperfusion-induced gastric injury in rats. J Polyn Soc 2004;95:321–8.

43. Ueda F, Ban K, Ishima T. Irsogladine activates gap-junctional intercellular communication through M1 muscarinic acetylcholine receptor. J Pharmacol Exp Ther 1995;274:815–9.

44. Kyoi T, Noda K, Oka M, et al. Irsogladine, an anti-ulcer drug, suppresses super-oxide production by inhibiting phosphodiesterase type 4 in human neutrophils. Life Sci 2004;76:71–83.
45. Nozaki S, Maeda M, Tsuda H, et al. Inhibition of breast cancer regrowth and pulmonary metastasis in nude mice by anti-gastric ulcer agent, irsogladine. Breast Cancer Res Treat 2004;83:195–9.
46. Fujita T, Ashikaga A, Shiba H, et al. Irsogladine maleate counters the interleukin-1 beta-induced suppression in gap-junctional intercellular communication but does not affect the interleukin-1 beta-induced zonula occludens protein-1 levels in human gingival epithelial cells. J Periodont Res 2008;43:96–102.
47. Nanke Y, Kamatani N, Okamoto T, et al. Irsogladine is effective for recurrent oral ulcers in patients with Behçet's disease: an open-label, single-centre study. Drugs R D 2008;9(6):455–9.
48. Inui M, Nakase M, Okumura K, et al. Irsogladine Maleate in the management of recurrent aphthous stomatitis: a pilot study. Spec Care Dentist 2010;30(2):33–4.
49. Masuyama H, Ishida M, Morita K, et al. An open-label, multi-center study of irso-gladine maleate for gastric ulcer healing after eradication of Helicobacter pylori. Ther Res 2008;29:415–22.
50. Hiraishi H, Haruma k, Miwa H, Goto H, et al. Clinical trial: irsogladine maleate, a mucosal protective drug, accelerates gastric ulcer healing after treatment for eradication of helicobacter pylori infection - the results of a multicentre, double-blind, randomized clinical trial (IMPACT Study). Aliment Pharmacol Ther 2010; 31(8):824–33.

Oral Lichen Planus

Pallavi Parashar, BDS, DDS

KEYWORDS

- Lichen planus • Oral • Lichenoid
- Potentially malignant oral disorders • Therapy • Causes
- Diagnostic criteria

Lichen planus (LP) is derived from the Greek *leichen* meaning tree moss and the Latin *planus* meaning flat. Erasmus Wilson first described LP in 1869,[1] as a chronic disease affecting the skin, scalp, nails, and mucosa, with possible rare malignant degeneration.[2] Francois Henri Hallopeau reported the first oral lichen planus (OLP)–related carcinoma in 1910.[1]

The true cause of LP remains obscure. Treatment is generally geared to alleviating symptoms.[3] Cutaneous lesions of LP are self-limiting and pruritic; however, oral lesions are chronic, rarely remissive, and are frequently the source of morbidity. Cutaneous lesions are characteristically erythematous to violaceous, flat-topped, pruritic, polygonal papules with the surface showing a network of fine lines (Wickham striae) affecting the flexor surfaces of arms, wrists, ankles, and genitalia.[3,4] Apart from cutaneous LP in patients with OLP, there is a high prevalence of other skin diseases such as eczema and psoriasis in patients with OLP.[5]

OLP constitutes 9% of all white lesions affecting the oral cavity.[6] Most patients with OLP have no associated cutaneous LP or LP at any other mucosal site, so the process is often referred to as isolated OLP. Less often, a subset of patients can have simultaneous involvement of the oral mucosa and cutaneous or other mucosal sites, such as in the vulvovaginal-gingival syndrome,[7] or penogingival syndrome.[4] Genital LP is associated with approximately 20% of OLP, whereas cutaneous LP is associated with approximately 15% of OLP. However, some studies suggest that the association between cutaneous LP and OLP is closer to 70% to 77%.[1] OLP has been well documented in patients with esophageal LP.[4]

The diagnosis of OLP is made based on a strict combination of clinical criteria as well as histopathologic evaluation.[8]

FREQUENCY

LP has a varied prevalence based on different geographic regions, but it generally affects approximately 1% to 2% of the world's population.[3] Many large-scale studies of OLP have been conducted in India. The prevalence of OLP ranges between 0.5%

Department of Diagnostic and Biological Sciences, University of Colorado Denver School of Dental Medicine, 13065 East 17th Avenue, Mail Stop 844, Aurora, CO 80045, USA
E-mail address: pallavi.parashar@ucdenver.edu

Otolaryngol Clin N Am 44 (2011) 89–107
doi:10.1016/j.otc.2010.09.004　　　　　　　　　　　　　oto.theclinics.com
0030-6665/11/$ – see front matter © 2011 Elsevier Inc. All rights reserved.

and 3% and may occur in 70% to 77% of patients with cutaneous LP.[1] However, some studies report that isolated OLP (without cutaneous involvement) occurs more commonly.[5]

RACE

OLP affects people of all ethnic groups.[6] In general, the prevalence of OLP is 0.5% in certain Japanese populations, 1.9% in Swedish populations, 0.38% in Malaysian populations, and 2.6% in Indian populations.[9]

SEX

Women are affected more commonly than men. In a study from Japan, the incidence of OLP in men was 59.7 per 100,000 versus 188.0 per 100,000 for women.[10]

AGE

Typically, LP affects individuals between the ages of 30 and 60 years.[1] It is rare in children, with the youngest case documented in a child aged 3 months.[11] Of the cases of OLP reported in children, there is a higher prevalence in the Indian population, suggesting probable differences in the genetic background and/or environmental triggers.[12]

CAUSES

Numerous reports have tried to clarify the role viruses may play in the development of OLP, including Varicella zoster virus, Epstein-Barr virus, cytomegalovirus, human herpes virus, human papilloma virus, and hepatitis C virus (HCV).[13] The association between OLP and liver disease has been investigated since 1978.[14] The pathogenic role of HCV in the development of OLP is still undecided. It is believed that the immune reaction mediated by HCV replication may cause damage to the basal layer cells and result in OLP lesions, resulting in an extrahepatic manifestation of HCV.[15] Some studies suggest that the hepatitis C virus exerts an indirect effect, possibly mediated by the modulation of cytokines and lymphokines in the pathogenesis of oral erosive LP.[16] In a recent review and meta-analysis, it was concluded that patients with LP have a higher risk of being HCV seropositive and, similarly, HCV-infected patients had a higher probability of developing LP.[17]

Although controversial, psychological disorders and stress are believed to represent possible causal factors in OLP.[18,19] A few investigators have found that patients with OLP have significantly higher stress, anxiety, and depression levels compared with healthy individuals.[2]

PATHOPHYSIOLOGY

Although many possible causes explaining the pathogenesis of LP have been proposed, the exact cause remains unclear.[4] OLP is classified as an inflammatory disease of the stratified squamous epithelium, and it is still unclear what antigen, whether endogenous or exogenous in origin, triggers the inflammatory immune response in OLP lesions.

Most data suggest that OLP is a CD8+ T cell–mediated autoimmune disease. However, the triggering factors and pathogenic mechanism are still not conclusively identified.[1] There seems to be no definite role of B cells, plasma cells, immunoglobulins, or complements in the mediation of LP.[20] In a study comparing the T cell clone response of lesional LP and normal mucosa, the T cell lines in patients with LP were significantly more cytotoxic and were identified as CD8+.[21] These CD8+ T cells are believed to induce keratinocyte apoptosis and cause epithelial basal cell layer damage via several possible suggested mechanisms: (1) secretion of tumor necrosis factor-α (TNF-α), which binds the TNF-α receptor 1 on the keratinocyte surface; (2) the binding of CD95 (Fas) on the keratinocyte surface with CD95L, which is expressed on the T cell surface; and (3) entry and assimilation of granzyme B secreted by T cells into the keratinocytes by perforin-induced membrane pores.[22] A variety of factors are believed to trigger the cytotoxicity of CD8+ T cells. One is the expression of major histocompatibility complex class (MHC) II presented by the langerhans cells and keratinocytes, which secrete interleukin-12 (IL-12) thus activating the CD4+ T cells. This activation of CD4+ T cells and subsequent expression of interleukin-2 (IL-2) and interferon-γ (INF-γ), in association with the MHC class I, which are associated with basal keratinocytes, promotes cytotoxic CD8+ T cell induction of keratinocytes apoptosis.[4,23] The immunologic abnormality leads to a delay in the growth of mucosal epithelium that is responsible for hyperkeratosis.[24]

Polymorphisms and genetic variations in the expression of cytokines have been linked with the risk of developing lesions of OLP and governs whether lesions are limited to the oral cavity (INF-γ), or skin (TNF-α).[25]

Another nonspecific mechanism in the development of LP is believed to be the degranulation of mastocytes and a posterior activation of matrix metalloproteinases, which degrades components of the extracellular matrix and basal membrane and also participates in the migration of lymphocytes through the epithelium. OLP lesions have more than 60% of degranulated mastocytes in comparison with normal mucosa.[26]

Genetics, familial clustering, and human leukocyte antigen association, although initially implicated to play a role in the pathogenesis of OLP, are no longer considered critical factors.[20]

CLINICAL FINDINGS

LP may affect the hair follicles, nails, esophagus, and, less frequently, the eyes, urinary tract, genitals, nasal mucosa, and larynx.[1] Scalp involvement causes pruritic, follicular and perifollicular, scaly, violaceous papules, referred to as lichen planopilaris, and can also lead to permanent patchy hair loss. When LP affects nails, it causes pitting, subungual hyperkeratosis, permanent nail loss, and so forth.[20]

The clinical presentation orally is nearly always in a bilateral, symmetric pattern.[27] The buccal mucosa (bilaterally) is the most typical site of involvement, but other panoral mucosal sites and the lips can also be involved.[9] After the buccal mucosa and tongue, the gingiva seems to be commonly involved. If only the erosive subtype of OLP affects the gingival tissue, the descriptive clinical term desquamative gingivitis (DG) is often used. OLP is confined to the gingiva in about 10% of patients.[4,28] Lesions of OLP affecting the palate, floor of the mouth, and upper lip are not common.[4]

Most patients with OLP show no increased prevalence of cigarette smoking or alcohol consumption.[3] Although OLP patients do not seem to have an increased risk of diabetes, diabetics who develop OLP have an increased frequency of atrophic-erosive lesions, especially affecting the tongue.[29] A correlation between OLP and hypertension has also been proposed.[30] An association between OLP, diabetes mellitus, and hypertension has been described, the triad being termed the Grinspan syndrome.[31]

CLINICAL FEATURES

To better define the criteria for diagnosis of OLP, the World Health Organization (WHO) devised a set of clinicopathologic criteria in 1978 (**Box 1**).[32] Because these criteria lacked consensus regarding a clinical and histologic diagnosis of OLP, modifications were proposed to the WHO criteria in 2003 (**Box 2**), which resulted in a substantial increase in consensus and clinicopathologic correlation.[33,34] In addition, knowledge about history of systemic diseases, history of drug use, and cutaneous lesions can be helpful in arriving at a definite diagnosis.[8]

The oral manifestations of OLP have been described in many large studies. Clinically, there are 6 clinical subtypes of OLP that can be seen individually or in combination: papular, reticular, plaquelike, atrophic, erosive, and bullous.[1] The most common of these are the reticular, erosive, and plaquelike subtypes, and these variants can coexist within the same patient.[7] Mucosal lesions are usually bilateral and involve multiple sites within the oral cavity. The most common presentation is that of pinpoint white papules that gradually enlarge and come together to form the reticular or plaquelike pattern.[27] In the absence of the classic reticular pattern on oral mucosal surfaces, which appears as multiple papules with a network of small, raised, whitish-gray, lacy lesions referred to as Wickham striae (**Fig. 1**), it is challenging to clinically diagnose nonreticular types.[4,7] Histologic confirmation of the diagnosis is thus required.[27]

The erosive form of OLP may present with erythema caused by inflammation or epithelial thinning, or both, and ulceration/pseudomembrane formation with periphery of the lesion surrounded by reticular keratotic striae (**Figs. 2** and **3**).[9] Gingival lesions frequently present with erythema and ulceration affecting the marginal and attached gingiva, as a manifestation of erosive LP (**Fig. 4**). The plaque form of OLP mimics leukoplakia in that it appears as a white, homogeneous, slightly elevated, multifocal, smooth lesion (**Fig. 5**).[9] The plaque form of OLP commonly affects the dorsum of

---

Box 1
WHO diagnostic criteria (1978) of OLP

Clinical criteria

- Presence of white papule, reticular, annular, plaque-type lesions, gray-white lines radiating from the papules
- Presence of lacelike network of slightly raised gray-white lines (reticular pattern)
- Presence of atrophic lesions with or without erosion, and possibly also bullae

Histopathologic criteria

- Presence of thickened ortho- or parakeratinized layer in sites that are normally keratinized, and, if site is normally nonkeratinized, this layer may be thin
- Presence of Civatte bodies in basal layer, epithelium, and superficial part of connective tissue
- Presence of a well-defined bandlike zone of cellular infiltration that is confined to the superficial part of the connective tissue, consisting mainly of lymphocytes
- Signs of liquefaction degeneration in the basal cell layer

Data from Kramer IR, Lucas RB, Pindborg JJ, et al. Definition of leukoplakia and related lesions: an aid to studies on oral precancer. Oral Surg Oral Med Oral Pathol 1978;46:518–39.

Box 2
Modified WHO diagnostic criteria of OLP and oral lichenoid lesions

Clinical criteria

- Presence of bilateral, more or less symmetric lesions
- Presence of a lacelike network of slightly raised gray-white lines (reticular pattern)
- Erosive, atrophic, bullous, and plaque-type lesions are only accepted as a subtype in the presence of reticular lesions elsewhere in the oral mucosa

In all other lesions that resemble OLP but do not complete the aforementioned criteria, the term "clinically compatible with" should be used.

Histopathologic criteria

- Presence of a well-defined, bandlike zone of cellular infiltration that is confined to the superficial part of the connective tissue, consisting mainly of lymphocytes
- Signs of liquefaction degeneration in the basal cell layer
- Absence of epithelial dysplasia

When the histopathologic features are less obvious, the term "histopathologically compatible with" should be used.

Final diagnosis of OLP or oral lichenoid lesions (OLL)

To achieve a final diagnosis, clinical as well as histopathologic criteria should be included

OLP

A diagnosis of OLP requires fulfillment of clinical and histopathologic criteria

OLL

The term OLL will be used in the following conditions:

1. Clinically typical of OLP but histopathologically only compatible with OLP
2. Histopathologically typical of OLP but clinically only compatible with OLP
3. Clinically compatible with OLP and histopathologically compatible with OLP

From van der Meij EH, van der Waal I. Lack of clinicopathologic correlation in the diagnosis of oral lichen planus based on the presently available diagnostic criteria and suggestions for modifications. J Oral Pathol Med 2003;32(9):510.

---

the tongue and buccal mucosa. Bullous LP may present with bullae ranging from a few millimeters to a few centimeters in diameter. Typically, bullae ulcerate and become covered by whitish pseudomembrane.[34] Bullous LP is uncommon in the oral cavity, as is the papular type of OLP.

Lichenoid reactions (OLL/oral lichenoid reactions [OLR]) have similar features, clinically and histologically, to LP, but have a less characteristic morphology or have a distinct cause, unlike OLP (**Fig. 6**). OLL therefore needs to be distinguished because treatment modalities are different from those for OLP.[7]

SYMPTOMS AND SIGNS

Symptoms and signs can range from patients being unaware of the disease, with lesions that are completely asymptomatic as in reticular OLP, to those experiencing mucosal sensitivity and burning and debilitating pain. Approximately two-thirds of the patients affected with OLP experience oral discomfort. Because OLP has periods

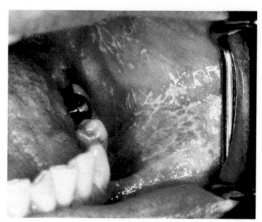

Fig. 1. Diffuse reticular lichen planus characterized by multiple interlacing white keratotic lines or striae, referred to as Wickham striae, affecting the left labial mucosa and buccal mucosa. (*Courtesy of* Robert O. Greer, DDS, ScD, CO, USA.)

of relapses and remissions, during a period of exacerbation there may be an increase in symptoms and clinical signs. During periods of quiescence, symptoms and signs of OLP are diminished.[20] Factors such as stress may aggravate the clinical presentation of the disease. Precipitating factors similar to the Koebner phenomenon, which is characteristic of cutaneous LP whereby lesions develop in response to trauma, can also affect the oral cavity. Sharp cusps and ill-fitting dental prosthesis may be the triggers. Chronic accumulation of plaque and calculus can also exacerbate OLP, perhaps because of the Koebner phenomenon.[9,28] Gingival OLP can eventually lead to gingival recession, advanced periodontal disease, and so forth, and therapeutic periodontal procedures may aggravate these conditions.[35] An association between OLP and xerostomia has been established.[36]

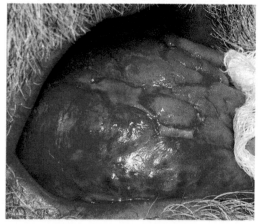

Fig. 2. The right dorsolateral surface of the tongue exhibiting extensive ulceration covered by pseudomembrane resulting from erosive lichen planus.

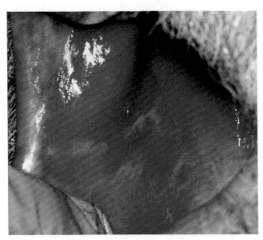

Fig. 3. Right buccal mucosa depicting a central area of ulceration with peripheral erythema and radiating white keratotic striae, a feature of erosive lichen planus.

HISTOLOGIC FINDINGS

The histologic features of OLP were first described by Dubreuill in 1906 and later revised by Shklar[37] in 1972. The WHO developed a set of histopathological criteria for OLP in 1978,[32] which was most recently modified in 2003 (see **Box 2**).

Definite diagnostic histologic findings include liquefactive degeneration of the basal cells, colloid bodies (Civatte, hyaline, cytoid), homogeneous infiltrate of lymphocytes in a dense, bandlike pattern along the epithelium-connective tissue interface in the superficial dermis, cytologically normal maturation of the epithelium, sawtooth rete ridges, and hyperkeratosis (orthokeratosis or parakeratosis) (**Fig. 7**). In addition, the surface epithelium may show signs of ulceration, typically seen in erosive LP.[6] If the erosive component is severe, bullae may form in the area of the epithelial separation, which eventually ulcerate (**Fig. 8**). Several histologic criteria that are considered as exclusionary in diagnosing OLP include the absence of basal cell liquefaction

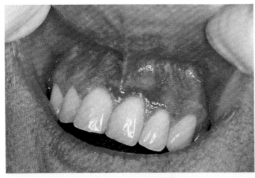

Fig. 4. Erosive lichen planus may affect the gingival tissue, particularly the marginal and attached gingiva. Often, the clinical descriptive term DG is rendered based on this clinical appearance. (*Courtesy of* Robert O. Greer, DDS, ScD, CO, USA.)

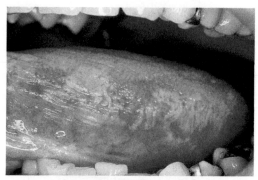

Fig. 5. Smooth, white plaques seen on the dorsolateral surface of tongue. A clinical diagnosis of plaquelike lichen planus was given. Biopsies were taken of the lesion and a histologic diagnosis of lichenoid dysplasia rendered. (*Courtesy of* Robert O. Greer, DDS, ScD, CO, USA.)

degeneration, polyclonal inflammatory infiltrate, abnormal cytology suggestive of dysplasia, abnormal keratinization, flat rete ridges, and absence of colloid bodies.[9]

Krutchkoff and Eisenberg[38] coined the term lichenoid dysplasia (LD) to describe lesions that resemble OLP histologically and also show features of dysplasia. These lesions are considered transitory premalignancies. Histologic features such as atypical cytomorphology, changes in the nuclear/cytoplasmic ratio, nuclear hyperchromatism, increase in mitotic figures, blunted rete ridges, and abnormal keratinization, are all considered to be features suggestive of this type of dysplasia.[9] Genetic studies, such as loss of heterozygosity (LOH), or cytogenetics on OLP with and without dysplasia, suggest that LD is a distinct entity. Also LD is considered a stage of preneoplastic transformation to squamous cell carcinoma (SCC). It is still debated whether OLP can transform to dysplasia, or whether lesions representing LD are early SCC.[39]

DIAGNOSTIC TESTS

Direct immunofluorescence is useful in distinguishing OLP from other lesions, especially vesiculobullous lesions such as pemphigus vulgaris, benign mucous membrane

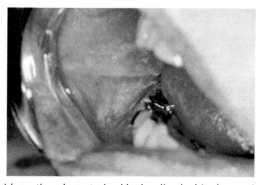

Fig. 6. Oral lichenoid reaction characterized by localized white keratotic striae on the right buccal mucosa in the vicinity of semiprecious metal crowns placed on right lower posterior teeth. (*Courtesy of* Robert O. Greer, DDS, ScD, CO, USA.)

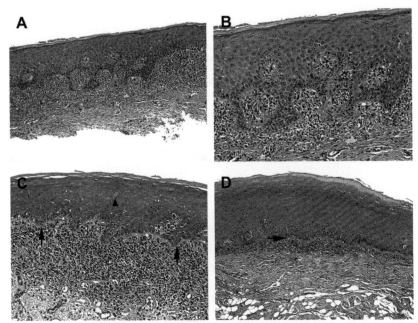

Fig. 7. (*A*) Low-power view of OLP shows hyperkeratosis, sawtooth rete ridges, and a thin bandlike infiltrate of lymphocytes in the superficial connective tissue/lamina propria. (*B*) Higher-power view showing the sawtooth rete ridges and the close approximation of the chronic inflammatory cells to the epithelium. No atypical features are seen in the epithelium. (*C*) High-power view of OLP showing basal cell degeneration (*arrows*) and intact epithelial-connective tissue interface. A colloid body, which is a degenerating keratinocyte, is also seen in the epithelium (*arrowhead*). (*D*) High-power view of OLP showing an acellular, eosinophilic, dense band along the epithelium-connective tissue interface (eosinophilic coagulum) representing byproducts of the liquefaction degeneration of the basal cell layer (*arrow*). (*Courtesy of* Robert O. Greer, DDS, ScD, CO, USA.)

pemphigoid, and linear immunoglobulin A (IgA) bullous dermatitis.[9] Direct immunofluorescence studies of OLP have shown a linear pattern and intense positive fluorescence with antifibrogen outlining the basement membrane zone and cytoidlike bodies with positive immunoglobulin M labeling.

Indirect immunofluorescence studies are not useful in the clinical diagnosis of OLP.

TREATMENT

The primary goal of OLP management is to alleviate symptoms on a long- and short-term basis and to prevent and further screen for malignant transformation.[1] Asymptomatic reticular lesions may require simple observation without any medical intervention. The objective in treating erosive or atrophic lesions of OLP is to relieve symptoms. LP does not have a cure, largely because the cause of OLP remains unknown. Thus treatment is only supportive and palliative.[40]

Multiple treatment modalities have been reported and recommended for OLP. The available options of treatment of OLP are corticosteroids, topical and systemic retinoids, calcineurin inhibitors (cyclosporin, tacrolimus, pimecrolimus), azathioprine, phototherapy, griseofulvin, hydroxyquinone, dapsone, mycophenolate, CO_2 laser,

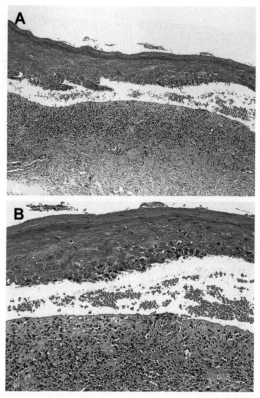

Fig. 8. (*A*) Low-power view of separation of the epithelium from the connective tissue, with the connective tissue showing a thin band of lymphocytes as seen in the deroofing bullous OLP. (*B*) High-power view of the degeneration of the basal cell layer and the sub-basilar separation of the epithelium from the connective tissue. (*Courtesy of* Robert O. Greer, DDS, ScD, CO, USA.)

thalidomide, and low-molecular-weight heparin.[20] The treatment modality for OLP depends on factors such as severity of symptoms, location and extent of the lesions in the oral cavity and the patient's overall health, precipitating psychological factors, possible drug interactions, and compliance of the patient.[41]

The most widely prescribed treatment of OLP involves the use of topical steroids, often required for a prolonged period because of multiple symptomatic episodes. Among topical steroids, the superpotent halogenated steroid clobetasol propionate has been reported to have good efficacy [24,40]; alternatively, triamcinolone and fluocinonide acetonide, which are midpotency and potent fluorinated steroid respectively, are also effective.[4] It is critical to have contact between the mucosal surface and the steroid drug for a few minutes, and therefore formulations such as an oral rinse or adhesive paste are often recommended.[1] Depending on the extent of oral involvement and access to OLP lesions, elixirs such as triamcinalone, dexamethasone, or clobetasol can be used, or topical steroids in adhesive bases, which are more widely used, can be prescribed.[4] Gingival lesions respond better to topical corticosteroids delivered in occlusive custom vinyl carriers because this method of drug delivery increases contact time of the topical agent to the gingiva.[34] Overall, almost a 55% reduction of moderate to severe pain is achieved as a result of topical steroid use.

The prolonged use of topical corticosteroids can result in adverse effects such as candidiasis, bad taste, nausea, dry mouth, sore throat, and, less frequently, moon face, hirsutism, and inhibition of the hypothalamus-pituitary-adrenal axis (HPA), producing adrenal insufficiency and development of features similar to those of Cushing disease.[24,42] Although the use of clobetasol propionate in an adherent vehicle does not cause inhibition of the hypothalamus-pituitary axis, use of the same in doses greater than 100 g/wk on the skin can affect the HPA axis. Management of patients using an aqueous solution of clobetasol propionate can cause transient inhibition of the HPA axis.[42] The patient should be advised to refrain from eating or drinking for 1 hour after use of any formulation of topical steroids.[4]

The use of intralesional steroids has been reported, but their efficacy is not well documented.[1]

Systemic steroids are used only for short-term alleviation of acute or refractory flares of OLP, or for widespread LP when other mucosal sites are also affected.[4] Depending on the severity of the lesion and the patient's weight and response to treatment, short courses of high-dose corticosteroids, such as prednisone 0.5 to 1.0 mg/kg/d, can be prescribed.[24] Prednisone 40 to 80 mg daily is usually effective in bringing about a response, and once a therapeutic response is achieved the steroid should be gradually tapered by reducing the dosage to 5 to 10 mg/d.[4,27] Carbone and colleagues[41] did not find any difference when OLP lesions were treated with systemic prednisone (1 mg/kg/d) and topical steroids versus topical steroids alone.

Treatment of lesions with steroids can lead to the development of secondary candidiasis for which antimycotic treatment is usually effective.[41]

The use of cyclosporine, either in local or systemic form, has been reported, but use of topical steroids seem to be more efficacious.[43]

Tacrolimus has also been used to treat LP.[44] Tacrolimus is available in the form of injections, capsules, and topical preparations.[40] Tacrolimus 0.1% ointment has been reported to show efficacy in the treatment of OLP in cases refractory to topical steroids.[1] Similar reduction in symptoms was found when tacrolimus 0.1% was compared with clobetasol 0.05% in treating OLP.[40] When comparing the efficacy of tacrolimus 0.1% and triamcinolone 0.1% after 6 weeks of treatment of OLP, complete remission was obtained in 30% and 10% of patients receiving tacrolimus and triamcinolone, respectively, and partial improvement was observed in 60% and 35% respectively.[45] Although tacrolimus has proved to have potentially better clinical outcomes, it can cause local irritation, transient taste alterations, possible lesional flare-up after drug withdrawal, and mucosal pigmentation.[44]

Pimecrolimus 1% cream has been suggested to be effective in the management of OLP; however, pimecrolimus has shown comparable efficacy to triamcinolone acetonide 0.1% in several small placebo-controlled trials.[46,47]

Retinoids for treatment of OLP have been used in several clinical trials showing less effectiveness than 0.1% fluocinolone acetonide in orabase when used topically.[48] Unclear results have been reported with systemic use.[49,50]

Extracorporeal photochemotherapy is not commonly prescribed and has been tried for treatment of severe refractory erosive LP. In a study of 12 patients with severe refractory OLP treated by extracorporeal photochemotherapy, complete remission was observed in 9 patients and a partial response in 3 patients.[51] Its use for OLP is questioned because of the oncogenic potential with ultraviolet light.

Surgical removal of OLP, especially isolated plaques or nonhealing erosions, has been performed but limited data exist to advocate this procedure.[4] Cryosurgery and laser surgery have been used to treat OLP, but more studies are needed to prove their efficacy.

Patient education and measures for reducing provoking factors such as mechanical trauma (sharp tooth, ill-fitting prosthesis), chemical irritation (acidic, spicy food or beverages), and the advocating of good oral hygiene to reduce bacterial plaque can help in alleviating symptoms of OLP.[27] Tobacco and alcohol use should also be discouraged.

FOLLOW-UP

Patient follow-up ranging from every 2 months to annually is accepted as part of long-term care for patients with LP largely to screen for changes that may indicate malignant transformation.[52] At a minimum, annual monitoring is recommended.[27] More frequent examinations are recommended for patients with LD/OLP with dysplasia. If changes are noted in a lesion at follow-up visits, then an additional biopsy or biopsies should be performed and the follow-up intervals shortened.[34]

Although the WHO currently regards OLP as a disease that may evolve to cancer, this concept is still controversial. A review of articles published between 1950 and 1976 evaluating the contention that OLP represents a disease with premalignant potential showed that there was insufficient documented evidence to confidently claim that OLP represents a premalignant state.[53] In a recent review by Lodi and colleagues,[13] the published literature was reviewed between 1985 and 2004 and these investigators observed a malignant transformation rate between 0% and 5.3%. Greer and colleagues[6] reviewed 548 cases of OLP, and showed a transition of OLP to SCC in 2.01% of their cases. Three of their patients showed an evolution to LD and SCC from OLP. Eight of their patients showed direct advancement to SCC.[6] Tobacco and alcohol do not seem to be risk factors in OLP-associated SCC,[52] but patients should still be strongly encouraged to avoid or discontinue these habits.[27] Although SCC is exceedingly rare on the dorsum of the tongue, 3 cases of SCC have been reported arising from a long-standing plaque-type OLP on the dorsum of the tongue.[54] The development of squamous cell carcinoma is not restricted to the site of LP involvement. There are no known reliable predictors to evaluate an affected individuals risk of malignant transformation.[7] The highest rate of malignant transformation has been reported in atrophic and erosive lesions.[9] The time interval between the diagnosis of OLP and the identification of cancer varies from 0.5 to 20 years,[4] although the risk is reportedly at a maximum between 3 and 6 years after diagnosis of OLP.[55] Clinically, carcinomas associated with OLP lesions can present as an exophytic or endophytic lesion.[56] Mignogna and colleagues[57] reported an additional risk in OLP-associated SCC because of an increased likelihood to develop a second or third oral malignancy with lymph node metastases. The pathogenesis of the malignant transformation is believed to be the result of accumulation of inducible nitric oxide synthase with 8-nitroguanine and 8-oxo-7,8-dihydro-2'-deoxyguanosine in oral epithelium in OLP, leading to alterations in the DNA and thus promoting malignant transformation.[4] Other theories proposed include the HCV infection status, LOH, and alterations in the p53 system.[58]

LD as an initial diagnosis is more likely to undergo malignant transformation than transformation of LP directly to cancer. Therefore, a diagnosis of OLP with dysplasia should be examined more frequently, that is every 2 to 3 months.[9] Genetic changes documented in SCC have also been proven in OLP with dysplasia, such as LOH at chromosomes 3, 9, and 17, thus suggesting that dysplasia in OLP is a sign of risk of malignant changes.[58] Treatment of LD is directed toward controlling the inflammatory response and treating the dysplastic changes. Surgical or laser excision, topical and systemic therapies including vitamin A and vitamin A analogues, and topical chemotherapy with agents such as bleomycin have been used.[34]

DIAGNOSTIC CONSIDERATIONS

Often clinicians are challenged with oral lesions that have features similar to LP clinically and histologically but also have a less characteristic morphology or have a distinct cause, unlike OLP. Such lesions are referred to as OLL or OLR, terms first coined by Finne and colleagues[59] in 1982. Other names such as contact allergies, or contact lesions have also been given.[60] OLL are classified as (1) lesions arising as a result of allergic contact stomatitis, such as those lesions in direct topographic relation with a dental restorative material; amalgam restorations being the most common; (2) drug-related lichenoid lesions, the most commonly implicated drugs being nonsteroidal antiinflammatory drugs, angiotensin-converting enzyme inhibitors, and β-blockers; (3) lesions in systemic conditions such as in chronic graft versus host disease and lupus erythematosus; and (4) unclassified OLL, those lesions that lack the characteristic features of OLP.[7] OLL related to nonmetallic dental materials are less common. Previously, the widespread use of gold salts and penicillamine were implicated in causing OLL.[27] Overall, OLL may be localized, asymmetric, and affect mucosal sites not commonly affected by OLP. Histologically, the distinction between OLL and OLP is not discriminative. Certain features, such as the presence of a mixed inflammatory infiltrate extending deeper into the lamina propria and superficial submucosa, favor a drug-associated lichenoid oral lesion, as do perivascular inflammation with plasma cells and neutrophils, which are absent in OLP.[61] Drug-related OLL are less common than their cutaneous counterparts.[7] Another useful histologic distinguishing measure between OLP and OLR is the difference in the ratio of degranulated mast cells to the total mast cell population in the reticular zone of the lamina propria.[26] Approximately 60% of mast cells are degranulated in OLP, compared with 20% in the normal mucosa.[13]

Management of OLL depends on the cause of the process, and may require removing the offending amalgam restoration or modifying drugs inducing such lesions. van der Meij and colleagues[62] studied 125 cases OLL for an average follow-up of 53.8 months and found malignant transformation to be 0.71% per year.

Leukoplakia is a clinical diagnosis for white lesions that cannot be rubbed off and that cannot be clinically or pathologically defined as any specific entity (**Fig. 9**). Conversely, erythroplakia is defined as a lesion that cannot be recognized clinically or pathologically as any specific entity and clinically appears as a red velvety lesion.[39] Apart from the reticular subtype of OLP, the other OLP subtypes can be easily confused as leukoplakia or erythroplakia, especially the plaque form.[4]

Proliferative verrucous leukoplakia (PVL) generally appears as irregular white patches or plaques that are multifocal and progress to oral cancer, either verrucous carcinoma or SCC. PVL can be confused with OLP because of its multifocal clinical appearance. The histologic spectrum of PVL is wide, ranging from benign keratosis to invasive SCC.[39]

DG is a clinical descriptive term for gingival lesions showing epithelial desquamation, erythema, erosions, and/or vesiculobullous lesions of the gingival tissue. Although OLP seems to be the most frequent cause of DG, other conditions, such as benign mucous membrane pemphigoid (BMMP) and pemphigus vulgaris (PV), can also have similar manifestations of DG. A variety of other local and systemic conditions, such as erythema multiforme, graft versus host disease, lupus erythematosus (LE), paraneoplastic pemphigus, epidermolysis bullosa acquista, linear IgA

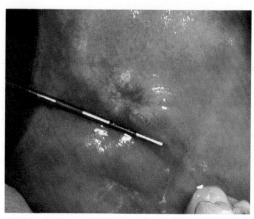

Fig. 9. Localized white plaque involving the right buccal mucosa near the commissure, which was given a clinical diagnosis of leukoplakia and was histologically diagnosed as hyperkeratosis.

disease, chronic ulcerative stomatitis, plasma cell gingivitis, dermatitis herpetiformis, foreign body gingivitis, and psoriasis, can have a similar pattern of presentation.[63]

Pemphigus vulgaris (PV) is an uncommon autoimmune disorder that is important because of its high morbidity and mortality. PV usually involves blistering of the skin and mucous membranes resulting from an abnormal production of autoantibodies that are directed against the epidermal cell surface glycoproteins. PV is almost always found to affect individuals between the fourth and sixth decade. There is no gender predilection. PV normally begins with oral vesicles or bullae that rupture quickly leaving erosions and ulcerations. All oral mucosal surfaces may be affected. More than half of the patients have oral mucosal lesions before the onset of cutaneous lesions. The skin lesions may be found in various stages of ulceration. The histopathology of PV presents as a characteristic intraepithelial separation, which occurs just above the basal cell layer of the epithelium, leaving only the basal cells attached to the connective tissue. The intact basal cells are considered to resemble a row of tombstones.[64]

Cicatricial pemphigoid or BMMP is another autoimmune condition affecting the oral mucosa, skin, and other mucosal surfaces. It affects women more frequently, between the fifth and sixth decade of life. The oral lesions of pemphigoid begin as either vesicles or bullae that may occasionally be identified clinically, which rupture. Histologic examination reveals a separation between the surface epithelium and the underlying connective tissue in the region of the basement membrane, with a mild inflammatory response. Direct immunofluorescence studies are often needed for a definite diagnosis.[64]

LE is difficult to differentiate from LP because of strong similarities in both the clinical and histologic findings. Oral lesions develop in 5% to 25% of patients with LE and affect the palate, buccal mucosa, and gingiva. The clinical appearance of LE can range from being nonspecific to being lichenoid. Histologically, oral lesions of LE show findings similar to those seen in LP. However, the presence of subepithelial edema (sometimes to the point of vesicle formation) and a more diffuse, deep inflammatory infiltrate, often in a perivascular orientation, can favor a diagnosis of LE. Some authorities suggest that direct immunofluorescence studies or histopathologic examination of the cutaneous lesions is best for differentiating LP from LE.[64]

Chronic ulcerative stomatitis (CUS) is a rare mucocutaneous disorder involving the mucosal surfaces and skin. Oral manifestations of patients with CUS may appear as ulcerations and erosions affecting the gingiva, buccal mucosa, and the tongue, thus resembling erosive LP or other vesiculobullous lesions. CUS affects women in the sixth decade of life.[65] Histopathologically, chronic ulcerative stomatitis mimics LP, although the epithelium is atrophic and the inflammatory infiltrate in the connective tissue has a predominance of plasma cells rather than lymphocytes.[64] Direct immunofluorescence studies reveal an immunoglobulin G (IgG) affinity in a perinuclear distribution in the basal and parabasal layers of epithelium.[65]

Lichen planus pemphigoides (LPP) is a rare condition that resembles bullous LP; however, unlike LP, LPP is marked by bullous eruptions on both the LP and normal skin. The histopathology reveals a subepidermal blister, predominantly lymphocytic infiltrate along the basement membrane zone (BMZ), with liquefactive degeneration of the basal keratinocytes and a linear deposition of IgG and/or C3 along the dermal-epidermal interface with direct immunofluorescence. Indirect immunofluorescence often reveals circulating autoantibodies against the BMZ components. The cause of LPP has been linked with treatment with multiple medications including cinnarizine, captopril, ramipril, simvastatin, and antituberculous medications. LPP may also be associated with an internal malignancy, although sometimes these lesions can be idiopathic. LPP affects men and women equally. Acral bullous lesions are more common, with minimal oral involvement. Management of LPP includes topical and systemic steroids, azathioprine, dapsone, or tetracycline plus nicotinamide.[66]

SUMMARY

OLP is a chronic condition that is immune mediated and is characterized by episodic exacerbations and remissions. It is known to be a T cell–mediated condition with predominantly cytotoxic CD8+ T cells. A definite diagnosis of OLP is based on a combination of clinical and histologic findings. The cause of OLP remains elusive, and therefore the treatment goals are directed at alleviating related signs and symptoms. Topical steroids are the first line of treatment of symptomatic OLP. Regular and long-term follow-up of patients with OLP is recommended to evaluate for changes in the lesion and to screen for malignancies.

ACKNOWLEDGMENTS

I would like to express my sincere thanks to Dr Robert O. Greer, Chairman of the Department of Diagnostic and Biologic Sciences, University of Colorado Denver School of Dental Medicine, for his mentorship and continuous support in writing this manuscript. I would also like to thank Dr Henry Barham, Resident in the Department of Otolaryngology, University of Colorado Denver School of Medicine, for his help in writing this article.

REFERENCES

1. Farhi D, Dupin N. Pathophysiology, etiologic factors, and clinical management of oral lichen planus, part I: facts and controversies. Clin Dermatol 2010;28(1): 100–8.
2. Chaudhary S. Psychosocial stressors in oral lichen planus. Aust Dent J 2004; 49(4):192–5.
3. Carbone M, Arduino PG, Carrozzo M, et al. Course of oral lichen planus: a retrospective study of 808 northern Italian patients. Oral Dis 2009;15(3):235–43.

4. Scully C, Carrozzo M. Oral mucosal disease: lichen planus. Br J Oral Maxillofac Surg 2008;46(1):15–21.
5. Bidarra M, Buchanan JA, Scully C, et al. Oral lichen planus: a condition with more persistence and extra-oral involvement than suspected? J Oral Pathol Med 2008; 37(10):582–6.
6. Greer RO, McDowell JD, Hoernig G. Oral lichen planus: a premalignant disease? Pro. Pathol Case Rev 1999;4(1):28–34.
7. van der Waal I. Oral lichen planus and oral lichenoid lesions; a critical appraisal with emphasis on the diagnostic aspects. Med Oral Patol Oral Cir Bucal 2009; 14(7):E310–4.
8. Rad M, Hashemipoor MA, Mojtahedi A, et al. Correlation between clinical and histopathologic diagnoses of oral lichen planus based on modified WHO diagnostic criteria. Oral Surg Oral Med Oral Pathol Oral Radiol Endod 2009;107(6): 796–800.
9. Ismail SB, Kumar SK, Zain RB. Oral lichen planus and lichenoid reactions: etiopathogenesis, diagnosis, management and malignant transformation. J Oral Sci 2007;49(2):89–106.
10. Nagao T, Ikeda N, Fukano H, et al. Incidence rates for oral leukoplakia and lichen planus in a Japanese population. J Oral Pathol Med 2005;34(9):532–9.
11. Pusey WA. Lichen planus in an infant less than 6 months old. Arch Dermatol Syphil 1929;19(4):671–2.
12. Kanwar AJ, De D. Lichen planus in childhood: report of 100 cases. Clin Exp Dermatol 2010;35(3):257–62.
13. Lodi G, Scully C, Carrozzo M, et al. urrent controversies in oral lichen planus: report of an international consensus meeting. Part 1. Viral infections and etiopathogenesis. Oral Surg Oral Med Oral Pathol Oral Radiol Endod 2005;100(1): 40–51.
14. Rebora A, Patri P, Rampini E, et al. Erosive lichen planus and cirrhotic hepatitis. Ital Gen Rev Dermatol 1978;15(2):123–31.
15. Nagao Y, Sata M, Noguchi S, et al. Detection of hepatitis C virus RNA in oral lichen planus and oral cancer tissues. J Oral Pathol Med 2000;29(6):259–66.
16. Femiano F, Scully C. Functions of the cytokines in relation oral lichen planus-hepatitis C. Med Oral Patol Oral Cir Bucal 2005;10(Suppl 1):E40–4.
17. Lodi G, Pellicano R, Carrozzo M. Hepatitis C virus infection and lichen planus: a systematic review with meta-analysis. Oral Dis 2010;16(7):601–12.
18. Rojo-Moreno JL, Bagán JV, Rojo-Moreno J, et al. Psychologic factors and oral lichen planus. A psychometric evaluation of 100 cases. Oral Surg Oral Med Oral Pathol Oral Radiol Endod 1998;86(6):687–91.
19. Allen CM, Beck FM, Rossie KM, et al. Relation of stress and anxiety to oral lichen planus. Oral Surg Oral Med Oral Pathol 1986;61(1):44–6.
20. Sugerman PB, Savage NW. Oral lichen planus: causes, diagnosis and management. Aust Dent J 2002;47(4):290–7.
21. Sugerman PB, Satterwhite K, Bigby M. Autocytotoxic T-cell clones in lichen planus. Br J Dermatol 2000;142(3):449–56.
22. Sugerman PB, Savage NW, Zhou X, et al. Oral lichen planus. Clin Dermatol 2000; 18(5):533–9.
23. Simark Mattsson C, Jontell M, Bergenholtz G, et al. Distribution of interferon-gamma mRNA-positive cells in oral lichen planus lesions. J Oral Pathol Med 1998;27(10):483–8.
24. Thongprasom K, Dhanuthai K. Steroids in the treatment of lichen planus: a review. J Oral Sci 2008;50(4):377–85.

25. Carrozzo M, Uboldi de Capei M, Dametto E, et al. Tumor necrosis factor-alpha and interferon-gamma polymorphisms contribute to susceptibility to oral lichen planus. J Invest Dermatol 2004;122(1):87–94.

26. Jahanshahi G, Aminzadeh A. A histochemical and immunohistochemical study of mast cells in differentiating oral lichen planus from oral lichenoid reactions. Quintessence Int 2010;41(3):221–7.

27. Al-Hashimi I, Schifter M, Lockhart PB, et al. Oral lichen planus and oral lichenoid lesions: diagnostic and therapeutic considerations. Oral Surg Oral Med Oral Pathol Oral Radiol Endod 2007;103(Suppl S25):e1–12.

28. Mignogna MD, Lo Russo L, Fedele S. Gingival involvement of oral lichen planus in a series of 700 patients. J Clin Periodontol 2005;32(10):1029–33.

29. Bagan JV, Donat JS, Penarrocha M, et al. Oral lichen planus and diabetes mellitus. A clinico-pathological study. Bull Group Int Rech Sci Stomatol Odontol 1993; 36(1–2):3–6.

30. Lowe NJ, Cudworth AG, Clough SA, et al. Carbohydrate metabolism in lichen planus. Br J Dermatol 1976;95(1):9–12.

31. Abbate G, Foscolo AM, Gallotti M, et al. Neoplastic transformation of oral lichen: case report and review of the literature. Acta Otorhinolaryngol Ital 2006;26(1): 47–52.

32. Kramer IR, Lucas RB, Pindborg JJ, et al. Definition of leukoplakia and related lesions: an aid to studies on oral precancer. Oral Surg Oral Med Oral Pathol 1978;46(4):518–39.

33. van der Meij EH, van der Waal I. Lack of clinicopathologic correlation in the diagnosis of oral lichen planus based on the presently available diagnostic criteria and suggestions for modifications. J Oral Pathol Med 2003;32(9):507–12.

34. Epstein JB, Wan LS, Gorsky M, et al. Oral lichen planus: progress in understanding its malignant potential and the implications for clinical management. Oral Surg Oral Med Oral Pathol Oral Radiol Endod 2003;96(1):32–7.

35. Eisen D, Carrozzo M, Bagan Sebastian JV, et al. Number V. Oral lichen planus: clinical features and management. Oral Dis 2005;11(6):338–49.

36. Colquhoun AN, Ferguson MM. An association between oral lichen planus and a persistently dry mouth. Oral Surg Oral Med Oral Pathol Oral Radiol Endod 2004;98(1):60–8.

37. Shklar G. Lichen planus as an oral ulcerative disease. Oral Surg Oral Med Oral Pathol 1972;33(3):376–88.

38. Krutchkoff DJ, Eisenberg E. Lichenoid dysplasia: a distinct histopathologic entity. Oral Surg Oral Med Oral Pathol 1985;60(3):308–15.

39. Greer RO. Pathology of malignant and premalignant oral epithelial lesions. Otolaryngol Clin North Am 2006;39(2):249–75.

40. Radfar L, Wild RC, Suresh L. A comparative treatment study of topical tacrolimus and clobetasol in oral lichen planus. Oral Surg Oral Med Oral Pathol Oral Radiol Endod 2008;105(2):187–93.

41. Carbone M, Goss E, Carrozzo M, et al. Systemic and topical corticosteroid treatment of oral lichen planus: a comparative study with long-term follow-up. J Oral Pathol Med 2003;32(6):323–9.

42. Gonzalez-Moles M, Scully C. HPA-suppressive effects of aqueous clobetasol propionate in the treatment of patients with oral lichen planus. J Eur Acad Dermatol Venereol 2010;24(9):1055–9.

43. Yoke PC, Tin GB, Kim MJ, et al. A randomized controlled trial to compare steroid with cyclosporine for the topical treatment of oral lichen planus. Oral Surg Oral Med Oral Pathol Oral Radiol Endod 2006;102(1):47–55.

44. Al Johani KA, Hegarty AM, Porter SR, et al. Calcineurin inhibitors in oral medicine. J Am Acad Dermatol 2009;61(5):829–40.
45. Laeijendecker R, Tank B, Dekker SK, et al. A comparison of treatment of oral lichen planus with topical tacrolimus and triamcinolone acetonide ointment. Acta Derm Venereol 2006;86(3):227–9.
46. Swift JC, Rees TD, Plemons JM, et al. The effectiveness of 1% pimecrolimus cream in the treatment of oral erosive lichen planus. J Periodontol 2005;76(4): 627–35.
47. Passeron T, Lacour JP, Fontas E, et al. Treatment of oral erosive lichen planus with 1% pimecrolimus cream: a double-blind, randomized, prospective trial with measurement of pimecrolimus levels in the blood. Arch Dermatol 2007;143(4):472–6.
48. Buajeeb W, Kraivaphan P, Pobrurksa C. Efficacy of topical retinoic acid compared with topical fluocinolone acetonide in the treatment of oral lichen planus. Oral Surg Oral Med Oral Pathol Oral Radiol Endod 1997;83(1):21–5.
49. Gorsky M, Raviv M. Efficacy of etretinate (Tigason) in symptomatic oral lichen planus. Oral Surg Oral Med Oral Pathol 1992;73(1):52–5.
50. Hersle K, Mobacken H, Sloberg K, et al. Severe oral lichen planus: treatment with an aromatic retinoid (etretinate). Br J Dermatol 1982;106(1):77–80.
51. Guyot AD, Farhi D, Ingen-Housz-Oro S, et al. Treatment of refractory erosive oral lichen planus with extracorporeal photochemotherapy: 12 cases. Br J Dermatol 2007;156(3):553–6.
52. Muñoz AA, Haddad RI, Woo SB, et al. Behavior of oral squamous cell carcinoma in subjects with prior lichen planus. Otolaryngol Head Neck Surg 2007;136(3):401–4.
53. Krutchkoff DJ, Cutler L, Laskowski S. Oral lichen planus: the evidence regarding potential malignant transformation. J Oral Pathol 1978;7(1):1–7.
54. Coombes D, Cascarini L, Booth PW. Carcinoma of the midline dorsum of the tongue. Br J Oral Maxillofac Surg 2008;46(6):485–6.
55. Bermejo-Fenoll A, Sanchez-Siles M, López-Jornet P, et al. Premalignant nature of oral lichen planus. A retrospective study of 550 oral lichen planus patients from south-eastern Spain. Oral Oncol 2009;45(8):e54–6.
56. Lo Muzio L, Mignogna MD, Favia G, et al. The possible association between oral lichen planus and oral squamous cell carcinoma: a clinical evaluation on 14 cases and a review of the literature. Oral Oncol 1998;34(4):239–46.
57. Mignogna MD, Lo Russo L, Fedele S, et al. Clinical behaviour of malignant transforming oral lichen planus. Eur J Surg Oncol 2002;28(8):838–43.
58. Zhang L, Michelsen C, Cheng X, et al. Molecular analysis of oral lichen planus. A premalignant lesion? Am J Pathol 1997;151(2):323–7.
59. Finne K, Göransson K, Winckler L. Oral lichen planus and contact allergy to mercury. Int J Oral Surg 1982;11(4):236–9.
60. Cobos-Fuentes MJ, Martínez-Sahuquillo-Márquez A, Gallardo-Castillo I, et al. Oral lichenoid lesions related to contact with dental materials: a literature review. Med Oral Patol Oral Cir Bucal 2009;14(10):e514–20.
61. Cortés-Ramírez DA, Gainza-Cirauqui ML, Echebarria-Goikouria MA, et al. Oral lichenoid disease as a premalignant condition: the controversies and the unknown. Med Oral Patol Oral Cir Bucal 2009;14(3):E118–22.
62. van der Meij EH, Mast H, van der Waal I. The possible premalignant character of oral lichen planus and oral lichenoid lesions: a prospective five-year follow-up study of 192 patients. Oral Oncol 2007;43(8):742–8.
63. Lo Russo L, Fierro G, Guiglia R, et al. Epidemiology of desquamative gingivitis: evaluation of 125 patients and review of the literature. Int J Dermatol 2009; 48(10):1049–52.

64. Neville BW, Damm DD, Allen CM, et al. Dermatologic diseases. In: Neville BW, Damm DD, Allen CM, editors. Oral and maxillofacial pathology. 3rd edition. Philadelphia: WB Saunders; 2009. p. 741–815.
65. Islam MN, Cohen DM, Ojha J, et al. Chronic ulcerative stomatitis: diagnostic and management challenges–four new cases and review of literature. Oral Surg Oral Med Oral Pathol Oral Radiol Endod 2007;104(2):194–203.
66. Cohen DM, Ben-Amitai D, Feinmesser M, et al. Childhood lichen planus pemphigoides: a case report and review of the literature. Pediatr Dermatol 2009;26(5):569–74.

White Lesions

Indraneel Bhattacharyya, DDS, MSD[a],*, Hardeep K. Chehal, BDS[b]

KEYWORDS

- White lesions • Oral mucosa • Leukoplakia • Hyperkeratosis
- Dysplasia

Increased thickness of the epithelium imparts a white appearance to the oral mucosa by increasing the distance to the underlying blood vessels. Usually this thickening is a result of the increased formation of keratin. Some other less common causes of white lesions are acanthosis or a thickening of the spinous cell layer, edema of the epithelium, or increased fibrosis of the connective tissue thereby reducing blood vessels. Occasionally the surface of an ulcer may appear white, due to collection of fibrin on the surface. In this article the authors discuss white lesions based on putative etiology, that is, hereditary, reactive, inflammation related, immunologic, traumatic, infection related, and idiopathic. Because many other lesions that may appear white have overlapping etiology and/or clinical nature (eg, candidiasis, carcinoma, smokeless tobacco associated lesions), they are discussed in other articles.

DEVELOPMENTAL WHITE LESIONS
Leukoedema

Leukoedema is a common developmental mucosal alteration of unknown cause, rather than a true pathologic change.[1,2] Leukoedema is seen in 90% of all black adults and 50% of black teenagers.[3] This condition has also been reported over a wide range in white adults (10%–90%) but the changes are far less pronounced.[3] Tobacco smoking and chewing are reported to enhance the whiteness and extent of the lesion.[4,5] Similar edematous changes have been seen in the mucosa of the larynx, the vagina, and other mucosal surfaces.[5]

Clinical features
Leukoedema typically presents as a bilateral, diffuse, milky, gray-white asymptomatic area with numerous surface folds, on the buccal mucosa (**Fig. 1**). Rarely it may involve the floor of the mouth and palatopharyngeal tissues.[6] Mucosal changes start as early as age 3 to 5 years and by the end of the teen years, 50% of blacks present with mucosal alterations.[3] An important diagnostic feature of leukoedema stems from its disappearance on stretching.

[a] Department of Oral and Maxillofacial Diagnostic Sciences, Oral & Maxillofacial Pathology, University of Florida College of Dentistry, PO Box 100414, Gainesville, FL 32610, USA
[b] Department of General Dentistry, Oral & Maxillofacial Pathology, Creighton University School of Dentistry, 2802 Webster Street, Omaha, NE 68178, USA
* Corresponding author.
E-mail address: ibhattacharyya@dental.ufl.edu

Otolaryngol Clin N Am 44 (2011) 109–131
doi:10.1016/j.otc.2010.09.009
0030-6665/11/$ – see front matter © 2011 Elsevier Inc. All rights reserved.

oto.theclinics.com

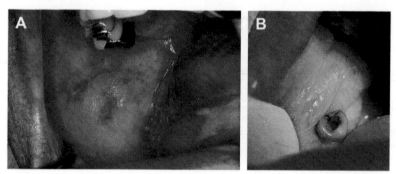

Fig. 1. (A) Diffuse, gray-white appearance of the buccal mucosa in leukoedema. (B) Wrinkled, white appearance in leukoedema may extend throughout the buccal mucosa.

Histopathologic features
Epithelial hyperplasia with significant intracellular edema of the spinous cells, and broad and elongated rete ridges are evident. Keratinization of the surface is also noted.

Differential diagnosis
White sponge nevus, frictional keratosis, smokeless tobacco keratosis, and hereditary benign intraepithelial dyskeratosis.

Treatment
None indicated. No malignant changes have been reported.[3,6]

White Sponge Nevus

White sponge nevus is a rare autosomal dominant disorder resulting from point mutation of either keratin 4 or keratin 13 genes.[6–8] These mutations result in defective keratinization of the oral mucosa, with alterations that may also be seen in the nasal, esophageal, laryngeal, and anogenital mucosa.[6,9,10] A high degree of penetration and variable expression is seen. White sponge nevus typically presents early in life and there is no gender predilection.[9]

Clinical features
White sponge nevus presents as asymptomatic, white, soft and spongy bilateral plaques or macules, typically on the buccal mucosa, but other sites such as the lip, ventral surface of the tongue, and floor of the mouth may also be involved.[11,12] Rare cases of mild discomfort due to secondary infections have been reported.[12]

Histopathologic features
Parakeratosis, marked epithelial thickening, and intracellular edema with perinuclear condensation of keratin is seen. Clear cell changes begin at the parabasalar layer and extend close to the surface.

Differential diagnosis
Leukoplakia, candidiasis, pachyonychia congenita, hereditary benign intraepithelial dyskeratosis, Darier disease, dyskeratosis congenita, lichen planus, lupus erythematosus, chemical burns, and syphilis.

Treatment
None indicated. No malignant changes seen. Treatment of the condition with topical tetracycline has been reported.[12]

Hereditary Benign Intraepithelial Dyskeratosis

Hereditary benign intraepithelial dyskeratosis (HBID) is a rare autosomal dominant disease exhibiting incomplete penetration, characterized by early onset of bulbar conjunctivitis preceded by bilateral gelatinous plaques and asymptomatic oral lesions.[13,14] Also known as Witkop disease, HBID is primarily seen among the descendents of a triracial isolate of whites, Indians, and African Americans in North Carolina.[14–16] HBID usually presents at birth or early childhood.[13–15] Recent studies have linked the gene responsible for HBID to chromosome 4 (4q35).[17]

Clinical features
Oral lesions of HBID are usually asymptomatic and present as white spongy macules or plaques seen on the buccal and labial mucosa, lateral tongue, floor of the mouth, gingiva, and palate, very similar to those seen in white sponge nevus. These lesions usually intensify until the mid-teens, after which they stabilize. The ocular lesions of HBID are particularly interesting; they develop early in life and may vary seasonally. These gelatinous plaques are seen bilaterally on the bulbar conjunctiva. Unlike the oral lesions, ocular lesions are frequently symptomatic.[15] Tearing, redness of the eyes, photophobia, and itching are commonly encountered during the active phase.[14,15] Blindness has also been reported as a result of vascularization of the cornea.[14]

Histopathologic features
Microscopic similarities are seen between oral and ocular lesions. Marked epithelial keratosis and acanthosis are seen. A dyskeratotic process in the form of enlarged hyaline keratinocytes is seen in the upper half of the epithelium. Some of the cells appear to be "engulfed" by surrounding cells forming a "cell within a cell" pattern. The lower half of the epithelium appears normal, with a well-defined epithelium-connective tissue interface.

Differential diagnosis
Leukoedema, dyskeratosis follicularis, focal epithelial hyperplasia, hereditary mucoepithelial dyskeratosis, leukoplakia, and white sponge nevus.

Treatment
None indicated for oral lesions because this is a self-limiting benign condition with no malignant potential. Patients with symptomatic ocular lesions should be referred to an ophthalmologist for surgical removal of the plaques. However, these plaques tend to recur.

Dyskeratosis Congenita

Dyskeratosis congenita is a rare inherited disorder characterized by mucosal leukoplakia, nail dystrophy, and hyperpigmentation of the skin.[18–21] Although it exhibits autosomal dominant, autosomal recessive, or x-linked inheritance patterns, most cases are of the x-linked form.[20,21] Mutation of the DKC1 gene has been determined to be the cause of the x-linked form.[22] The condition manifests itself during the first decade of life. Patients with this disorder are susceptible to developing bone marrow failure as well as malignant transformation of oral and skin lesions.[20,21] Hence identification of the condition is important for early referral and appropriate treatment.[21]

Oral leukoplakic lesions are seen in 80% of cases.[21] These lesions are seen most frequently on the tongue but can also involve the buccal mucosa, lingual mucosa, and palate.[6,18,20,21]

Clinical features

Oral lesions begin with bullae formation on affected surfaces, followed by erosion and finally leukoplakic plaques. Superimposed candidal infection is often seen. Discomfort may be associated with the consumption of spicy and hot foods. The oral lesions are considered to be premalignant and may transform to malignancy over a 10- to 30-year period.[6,18,20,21] Squamous cell carcinoma is the most common malignancy to arise in these lesions.[18] Skin and nail changes increase with age.[21] The most significant clinical manifestation of the disease is bone marrow failure. By the second decade of life patients typically develop anemia, and 94% of patients develop bone marrow failure by the age of 40 years.[21]

Histologic features

Early lesions display hyperkeratosis with epithelial dysplasia, and frank malignant changes are seen eventually as the lesion develops.

Differential diagnosis

Leukoplakia, white sponge nevus, lichen planus, dyskeratosis congenita, candidiasis, hyperkeratosis, epithelial dysplasia, early invasive squamous cell carcinoma, thrombocytopenia, and aplastic anemia.

Treatment

Periodic examination of oral lesions to monitor malignant changes and avoidance of smoking and drinking are of utmost importance. Current treatment for bone marrow failure is allogenic hematopoietic stem cell transplantation. Prognosis is guarded.

Pachyonychia Congenita

Pachyonychia congenita is a rare autosomal dominant disorder mainly characterized by nail dystrophy, subungual and palmoplantar hyperkeratosis, and oral leukoplakic lesions.[23,24] Two major subtypes include pachyonychia congenita type 1 (Jadassohn-Lewandowsky form) and pachyonychia congenita type 2 (Jackson-Lawler form).[25] Oral lesions characterized by leukoplakic lesions of the tongue and buccal mucosa as well as dental abnormalities in the form of neonatal teeth are seen only on pachyonychia congenita type 1.[26] Mutations of keratin 16 gene and keratin 17 gene have been implicated as the cause of pachyonychia congenita type 1 and pachyonychia type 2, respectively.[27,28] The condition manifests itself at birth or very early in life.[24] Cases of late onset, called pachyonychia tarda, have also been reported.[29]

Clinical features

Nail changes are the most outstanding feature, and changes are typically seen at birth.[23,24,26,27] Palmoplantar and follicular keratosis are observed.[23,26] Oral leukoplakic lesions seen on the tongue, buccal mucosa, or rarely the gingiva are not precancerous.[23,24]

Histologic features

Mild to moderate hyperkeratosis and acanthosis of the epithelium are evident.

Differential diagnosis

Leukoplakia and focal palmoplantar keratodermas.

Treatment
None indicated for oral lesions, as there is no malignant potential. General treatment forms are directed at symptom relief, and there is no satisfactory treatment regimen to date.[30]

REACTIVE INFLAMMATORY LESIONS
Physical and Chemical Injuries

Linea alba
Linea alba is a very common oral finding characterized by a white line on the buccal mucosa at the level of the occlusal surface of teeth, and extends from the commissure to as far back as the molar teeth.[31,32] It is often bilateral (**Fig. 2**). This condition is related to pressure or sucking trauma from teeth on the buccal mucosa.[33] According to one study its incidence is seen in up to 13% of the population.[32] Linea alba is typically restricted to teeth-bearing areas of the buccal mucosa.[33]

Clinical features Linea alba usually presents as asymptomatic, bilateral linear white lines, which may be scalloped and may be more intense in the posterior region.[6]

Histologic features Hyperkeratosis overlying normal mucosa is seen.

Differential diagnosis Frictional keratosis and cheek chewing.

Treatment None indicated. Condition may regress spontaneously in some cases.[6]

Frictional, chemical, and thermal keratosis
These lesions are characterized as white plaques that arise as a result of an identifiable source and usually resolve once the causative factor is eliminated. The sources of friction resulting in hyperkeratosis may be an ill-fitting denture, malocclusion, parafunctional habits (**Fig. 3**A), or poor brushing techniques.[6,34] Frictional keratosis is usually seen in young adults. Lips, lateral surface of tongue, and buccal mucosa are common sites.[6,34]

Thermal keratosis can be due to thermal burns in the oral cavity caused by excessively hot (microwaved) foods or heat generated from smoking.[35–37] Lesions are commonly seen on the tongue and palate.[35] Nicotine stomatitis is a tobacco-related form of keratitis causing both chemical and thermal keratosis.[35–37] Heat and carcinogens are the causative factors.[37]

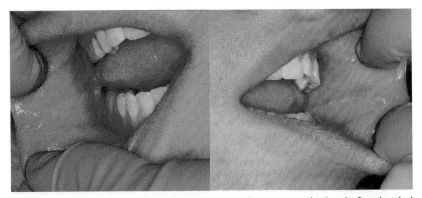

Fig. 2. Linear white line seen bilaterally on the buccal mucosa at the level of occlusal plane of the teeth. The scalloped white line extends from the commissure as far back as the molar teeth.

Chemicals causing burning of the mucosa and resultant hyperkeratosis include aspirin, sodium hypochlorite, hydrogen peroxide, formocresol, paraformaldehyde, cavity varnish, or mouthwashes, to name a few.[38–44] Lesions are typically located on the mucobuccal fold or the gingiva.

Clinical features Frictional keratosis is typically characterized by a poorly demarcated rough area, which can be peeled off occasionally, leaving focal areas of pink mucosa

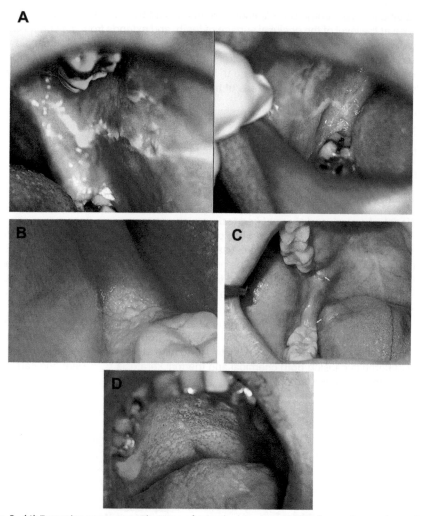

Fig. 3. (A) Extensive asymptomatic areas of raised white frayed and shaggy keratosis on the buccal mucosa bilaterally in a 24-year-old man. Lesions caused by persistent habit of cheek chewing (frictional keratosis). Patient reports that he can "pick off" small fragments of tissue. (B) Thick white corrugated area of leukoplakia distal to the second molar in a 42-year-old man. The area is asymptomatic and corresponds to traumatic biting due to overextended upper molar tooth. (C) Typical areas (arrows) of benign hyperkeratosis associated with masticatory trauma. (D) Nicotine stomatitis with a diffuse white appearance of the hard palate interspersed by red punctate spots representing metaplastically altered and inflamed salivary duct openings.

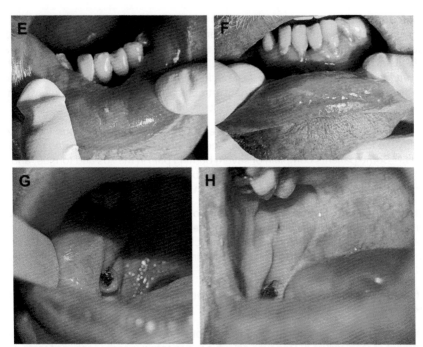

Fig. 3. (*E*) Epithelial necrosis of lower lip mucosa resulting from overuse of alcohol contain-ing mouthwash (chemical burn). (*F*) Same patient as *E*, after 1 week of discontinuation of mouthwash use. Complete resolution is noted without scarring. (*G*) Chemical burn on buccal mucosa resulting from alcohol containing mouthwash. (*H*) Same patient as *G*, 14 days after discontinuation of mouthwash with complete resolution of lesions. (*Courtesy of* Dr Eric Fox, oral surgeon, Coral Springs, FL, USA.)

(see **Fig. 3**A).[6,34] Masticatory trauma often results in thick white corrugated lesions on the retromolar pad areas (see **Fig. 3**B and C). Trauma from mastication or sharp cuspal edges of teeth may also cause similar lesions. Thermal keratosis is characterized by a white lesion with focal areas of ulceration associated with mild to moderate pain. Nicotine keratosis causes opacification of the hard palate with red punctuate spots representing inflamed and metaplastically altered salivary duct openings[36] (see **Fig. 3**D). Chemical keratosis is characterized by a white, irregularly shaped, asymp-tomatic or variably symptomatic lesions (see **Fig. 3**E–H). Thermal and chemically induced lesions are almost always painful.

Histologic features Fractional keratosis lesions simply exhibit hyperkeratosis and acanthosis with fraying and shredding of the keratin layers. These lesions do not show any epithelial dysplasia. Chemical and thermal keratoses display a superficial pseudomembrane composed of necrotic tissue and an inflammatory exudate.

Differential diagnosis Leukoedema, leukoplakia, candidiasis, white sponge nevus, dysplasia, carcinoma in situ, squamous cell carcinoma, oral hairy leukoplakia, and lupus erythematosus.

Treatment Removal of the causative factor leads to resolution of the lesions (see **Fig. 3**G and H). These lesions do not show any malignant potential.

Uremic stomatitis

Uremic stomatitis is a rare oral manifestation of advanced renal failure, typically characterized by an abrupt onset of adherent white plaques on the ventral and dorsal surfaces of the tongue, floor of the mouth, buccal and labial mucosa, as well as the gingiva.[45,46] The etiology is still unclear but it has been suggested that salivary urease hydrolyzes urea in saliva and converts it into ammonia and its compounds, which in turn cause mucosal irritation and burn, resulting in oral lesions.[47,48]

Clinical features Four forms have been described: erythemopultaceous (characterized by the formation of a pseudomembrane), ulcerative, hemorrhagic, and hyperkeratotic.[49] Some patients complain of severe burning pain in the lips and tongue, and an unpleasant taste.[6,45] Patients' breath may be laced with the smell of urea and ammonia.[45] Lesions may be seen anywhere in the oral mucosa (**Fig. 4**).

Histologic features Hyperkeratotic-type lesions demonstrate hyperkeratosis and acanthosis of the epithelial layer. Ballooning keratinocytes are also seen with minimal inflammatory infiltrate in the underlying connective tissue.[46,50] Ulcerative-type lesions demonstrate epithelial necrosis and a dense inflammatory infiltrate in the underlying connective tissue.

Differential diagnosis Frictional keratosis, leukoplakia, carcinoma, and oral hairy leukoplakia.

Treatment Lesions resolve with the lowering of blood urea nitrogen (BUN) levels and treatment of renal failure.[51] Because calculus may contain urease, scaling of teeth may be of help.[52] Hydrogen peroxide mouthwashes have also been shown to resolve the lesions.[45,50,51]

INFECTIOUS WHITE LESIONS
Oral Hairy Leukoplakia

These lesions are typically characterized by unilateral or bilateral white plaques on the lateral border of the tongue as a result of human immunodeficiency virus infections, immunocompromised state, or rarely in immunocompetent patients.[53–55] These

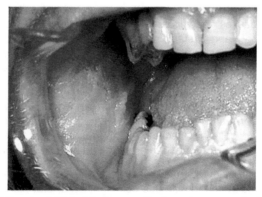

Fig. 4. Multiple white raised "flaky" lesions on the buccal mucosa of a 73-year-old patient with history of renal failure. The lesions were multiple painful and malodorous. The lesions appear very similar to frictional keratosis (cheek chewing). (*Courtesy of* Oral Pathology Department, University of Minnesota School of Dentistry.)

plaques cannot be scraped off. Other sites in the oral cavity include buccal mucosa, floor of the mouth, and soft palate.[53–55] Epstein-Barr virus has been implicated as the causative factor for this lesion.[56,57]

Clinical features
Oral hairy leukoplakia is typically seen on the lateral borders of the tongue (**Fig. 5**). The poorly demarcated white plaques usually have an irregular corrugated surface, and are asymptomatic.[58] Symptomatic lesions causing burning and soreness have also been reported.[59] Size may range from a few millimeters to a few centimeters. Lesions seen on the ventral surface of the tongue may be flat.[54]

Histologic features
Severe hyperkeratosis and acanthosis with an irregular surface is usually seen. Virally effected epithelial cells (koilocytes) with margination of the nuclear chromatin (nuclear beading) is a characteristic feature. Superficial candidal hyphae are also seen frequently.[54,57]

Differential diagnosis
Hyperplastic candidiasis, leukoplakia, tongue chewing, lichen planus, lupus erythematosus, and white sponge nevus.

Treatment
None is required because it is an asymptomatic lesion with no malignant potential.[53] The use of antivirals (acyclovir, gancyclovir, desicyclovir, ziduvudine) usually resolves the condition but the lesions reappear once the medication is discontinued.[60,61] Topical podophyllin with or without acyclovir cream has also been shown to be effective in treating the lesions.[60,62] Surgical excisions of the symptomatic lesions have resulted in temporary relief with recurrences.[59] Detecting and resolving the cause of immune suppression is the most important factor in the treatment of this condition.

NEOPLASTIC WHITE LESIONS
Leukoplakia

The term "leukoplakia" literally means a "white patch." Various attempts have been made at defining this lesion. The present definition accepted by most clinicians is "a predominantly white lesion of the oral mucosa that cannot be characterized as any

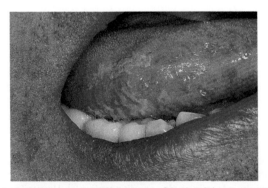

Fig. 5. Corrugated asymptomatic irregular areas of leukoplakia in a middle-aged human immunodeficiency virus–positive man. (*Courtesy of* Dr Steven Hess, Creighton University School of Dentistry.)

other definable lesion."[63] Leukoplakia is considered to be a premalignant lesion.[64–70] "Premalignant" means that this lesion is a step toward development of oral carcinoma. Various studies show that 4% to 6% of leukoplakic lesions give rise to oral carcinomas.[64–70] Leukoplakia is a strictly "clinical" term and is a diagnosis of exclusion. The lesions to be excluded are other white lesions such as lichen planus, lupus erythematosus, leukoedema, white sponge nevus, frictional keratosis, cheek/lip biting, and lesions associated with contact stomatitis.[71] This distinction typically can be accomplished by a biopsy and the association with causative factors.[71]

The condition is prevalent in males usually older than 40 years.[63,67,68] Common locations include tongue, floor of the mouth, and buccal mucosa.[63,67,68,72] The number of lesions per patient is higher amongst smokers.[72]

Etiology
The established causative factors for white lesions such as alcohol, tobacco, candidiasis. electrogalvanic, herpes simplex, and papilloma viruses should exclude the diagnosis of leukoplakia. It has been reported that a significant number of leukoplakic patients are smokers.[73,74] These smoking-related lesions have a lower malignant potential, and they tend to develop more on the floor of the mouth and regress partially or completely on cessation of habit.[68,72,75]

Alcohol consumption serves as a promoter for the conversion of the leukoplakic lesions to oral carcinomas. There is a strong synergism effect with tobacco.[72,75]

Several studies have tried to establish whether candidiasis causes leukoplakia or if it is a superimposed infection of a preexisting lesion.[65,76] Treatment of candidiasis leads to conversion of a nonhomogeneous leukoplakic lesion to a homogeneous one, and regression has also been seen in some cases.[76,77]

Extensive studies to establish the implications of human papilloma virus (HPV) in the etiology and malignant transformation of premalignant lesions have been done and are ongoing.[70,78] Microanalysis has confirmed that high-risk HPVs (16 and 18) were more frequently associated with oral squamous cell carcinomas than low-risk HPVs. The likelihood of detecting HPV in a premalignant lesion is 2 to 3 times greater than in a normal mucosa.[78] One study claimed that HPV in oral leukoplakia is not a prognostic indicator for malignant transformation.[79]

Technically, as per the definition of leukoplakia, these tobacco-induced and candidiasis-induced leukoplakias should not be included in the clinical diagnosis of leukoplakia.[80] However, if after cessation of smoking and treatment of candidiasis the lesions persist, they may fulfill the terminology of leukoplakia.

Clinical features
Clinical appearance of leukoplakia ranges from "homogeneous" (**Fig. 6A–F**) to "nodular or speckled" (see **Fig. 6G** and H) to "verruciform"(see **Fig. 6I**) to "proliferative verrucous" leukoplakia. Homogeneous leukoplakia is characterized by a thick, well-defined slightly elevated, fissured, wrinkled, or corrugated surface. These lesions are predominantly white and usually asymptomatic. The lesions may remain unchanged or may regress (one-third) or progress to the nodular or speckled form.[6,67] Nodular or speckled leukoplakia (nonhomogeneous) is characterized by keratotic white nodules or patches distributed over an atrophic erythematous background. These nodules may be irregular, flat, nodular, or exophytic, and are associated with complaints of mild pain or discomfort.[68] Verruciform leukoplakia is characterized by a white lesion with a papillary or pebbly or "bumpy" surface. These lesions are usually seen in sixth to eighth decade of life, and are generally

asymptomatic.[69] Proliferative verruciform leukoplakia is characterized by a widespread and multifocal appearance, and almost invariably develops into oral carcinomas.[69,81]

Histologic features

To fulfill a diagnosis of leukoplakia, no other definable lesion should be observed microscopically. Benign lesions display hyperkeratosis with or without acanthosis (**Fig. 7**A–C). A variable number of chronic inflammatory cells is seen in the underlying connective tissue (see **Fig. 7**B). In one study, 80% of the lesions biopsied were benign.[82] Epithelial dysplasia is commonly found in nonhomogeneous lesions.[83,84] These lesions often give rise to oral carcinomas, but it should be kept in mind that a large number of oral carcinomas also develop in lesions without previous diagnosis

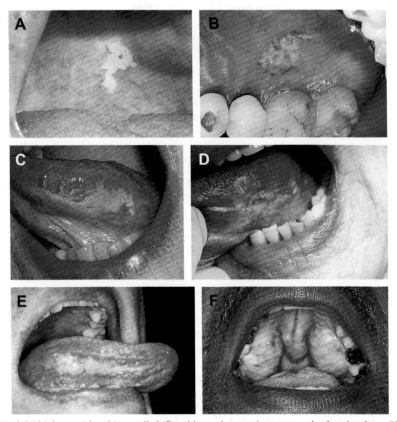

Fig. 6. (*A*) Thick grayish-white well-defined hyperkeratotic area on the hard palate. Biopsy revealed verrucoid hyperkeratosis. (*B*) Homogeneous or thick leukoplakia presented as a well-defined, elevated, corrugated white lesion on the junction of hard and soft palate. Moderate dysplasia was seen on microscopic evaluation. (*C*) Homogeneous or thick leukoplakia on the lateral border of the tongue. Mild dysplasia was seen on microscopic evaluation. (*D*) Early or thin leukoplakia on the ventral surface of the tongue. Squamous cell carcinoma later developed in this area. (*E*) Verruciform leukoplakia seen in the left maxillary vestibule. Verrucopapillary hyperkeratosis was seen on microscopic evaluation. (*F*) Granular leukoplakia seen on posterior hard palate. This irregular white patch exhibited early squamous cell carcinoma on microscopic evaluation.

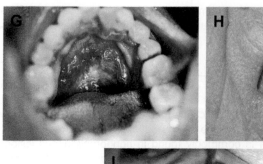
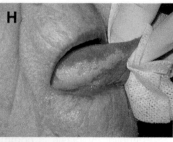
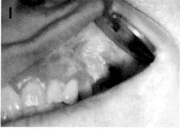

Fig. 6. (*G*) Thick leukoplakia on floor of the mouth in a heavy smoker. Microscopic evaluation revealed moderate dysplasia. (*H*) Thick homogeneous leukoplakia seen on the lateral and ventral surface of the tongue. (*I*) Thin or early leukoplakia on the palate. Lesion is smooth, white, and well demarcated.

of epithelial dysplasia (see **Fig. 7**D–F; **Box 1**).[85] The term carcinoma in situ (CIS) is used when the entire thickness of the epithelium is involved. CIS does not exhibit frank invasion of the lesion into the underlying connective tissue (see **Fig. 7**G).

Differential diagnosis
Lichen planus, cheek biting, frictional keratosis, smokeless tobacco-induced keratosis, nicotinic stomatitis, leukoedema, white sponge nevus, candidiasis, and lupus.

Treatment
Leukoplakias have a relatively low risk of malignant transformation. Hence, the recommended treatment should produce the fewest adverse effects. Initial treatments involve the elimination of all possible etiologic factors. If the lesion regresses, no further treatment is indicated.[86] Persistent lesions warrant a biopsy. "Benign" biopsy diagnosis may over time undergo dysplastic changes, therefore regular follow-up of these lesions is of utmost importance.

The presence of epithelial dysplasia increases the risk of malignant transformation. Surgery remains as the treatment of choice in most cases.[87] Other treatment modalities include laser surgery, cryosurgery, retinoids, β-carotene, bleomycin, calcipotriol, photodynamic therapy, and vitamin A.[88] No definite measures have been devised for the prevention of development of leukoplakia or oral carcinoma. Avoidance of smoking and alcohol, and consumption of fresh fruits and vegetables may have a protective effect. Oral cancer screening programs can help in early diagnosis of these lessons, and improve the prognosis and treatment success.[87,88]

Proliferative Verrucous Leukoplakia

The term proliferative verrucous leukoplakia (PVL) was coined in 1985 by Hansen and colleagues[66] because of the persistent and progressive nature of this white

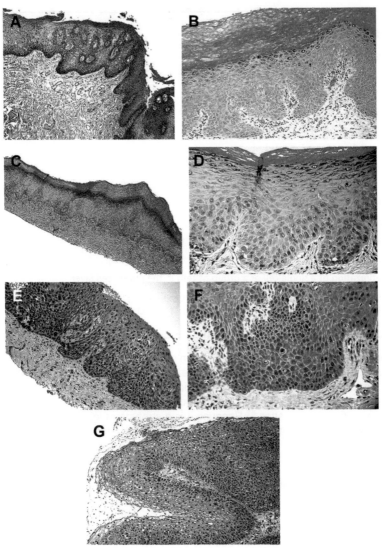

Fig. 7. (A) Hyperkeratosis with a frayed and shaggy surface suggestive of traumatic keratosis. No atypia is noted in the specimen (hematoxylin and eosin stain, original magnification ×10). (B) Severely thickened orthokeratin with a prominent granular cell layer. No appreciable atypia is seen (hematoxylin and eosin stain, original magnification ×20). (C) Verrucoid and papillary hyperkeratosis with mild atypical changes. This microscopic appearance is typically seen in biopsies from lesions such as in A (hematoxylin and eosin stain, original magnification ×5). (D) Mild dysplasia with hyperkeratosis. Dysplastic features are in general limited to the lower (basal) third of the epithelium. See also **Box 1** (hematoxylin and eosin stain, original magnification ×20). (E) Moderate to severe dysplasia with dysplastic alterations extending to the full thickness of the epithelium in some foci. (hematoxylin and eosin stain, original magnification ×20). (F) Abnormal mitoses, increased nuclear/cytoplasmic ratios, nuclear hyperchromatism seen extending to the middle third of dysplastic epithelium. Biopsy taken from lesion noted in **Fig. 6G** (hematoxylin and eosin stain, original magnification ×20). (G) Carcinoma in situ with dysplastic changes extending through full thickness of the epithelium with minimal keratinization noted on surface (hematoxylin and eosin stain, original magnification ×10).

Box 1
Criteria for epithelial dysplasia

- Loss of polarity of basal cells
- The presence of more than one layer of cells having a basaloid appearance
- Increased nuclear-cytoplasmic ratio
- Drop-shaped rete ridges
- Irregular epithelial stratification
- Increased number of mitoses
- Abnormal mitoses
- The presence of mitotic figures in the upper half of the epithelium
- Cellular and nuclear pleomorphism
- Nuclear hyperchromatism
- Enlarged nuclei
- Loss of intercellular adherence
- Keratinization of a single cell or a group of cells in the prickle cell layer

Data from Kramer IR, Lucas RB, Pindborg JJ, et al. Definition of leukoplakia and related lesions: an aid to studies on oral precancer. Oral Surg Oral Med Oral Pathol 1978;46: 518–39; with permission.

---

leukoplakic lesion. Several studies have been conducted to determine the cause and in a few of those, HPV types 16 and 18 have been associated, but to date the exact cause remains unclear.[89–91] Tobacco smoking does not seem to play a role.[81] PVL is more prevalent in women in their sixth decade of life, with the gingiva and tongue being the most common sites.[81] Because it is a subtype of idiopathic leukoplakia, it is also a premalignant lesion with a very high tendency for malignant transformation.[66,81]

Clinical features
PVL may be solitary or multiple, with wide clinical manifestations ranging from a flat verrucous appearance in its early stages to a more exophytic appearance with an erythematous component in the late stages (**Fig. 8**). The most remarkable feature is its relentless and progressive growth and recurrence despite treatment.[92] Regional lymph node involvement has been seen as a late feature in one study.[92]

Histologic features
PVL is a continuously developing lesion with the early lesions exhibiting only hyperkeratosis and late lesions representing epithelial dysplasia, verrucous carcinoma, or squamous cell carcinoma–like changes.[93]

Differential diagnosis
Idiopathic leukoplakia, erythroleukoplakia, verrucous hyperplasia, verrucous carcinoma, keratoacanthoma, oral florid papillomatosis, papilloma, and papillary squamous cell carcinoma.

Treatment
Treatment modalities ranging from surgery, irradiation, and chemotherapy have been implemented, but in most cases the lesion is persistent and recurrent. Close clinical follow-up every 6 months is strongly recommended.

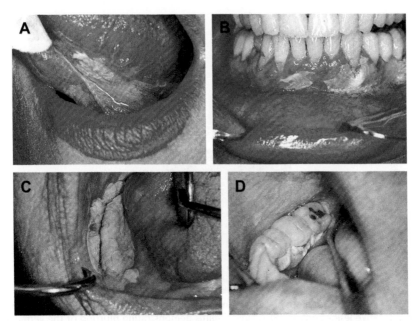

Fig. 8. (*A*) Characteristic diffuse, large, and corrugated leukoplakic areas involving the ventral surface of the tongue as well as the floor of the mouth. These lesions represent proliferative verruciform leukoplakia. (*B*) Thick white verruciform leukoplakic areas seen as multiple keratotic plaques with rough surface on the anterior mandibular gingiva, which is a frequent site of involvement. (*C*) Verruciform leukoplakia involving the mandibular alveolar ridge, mandibular vestibule, and right buccal mucosa. (*D*) Large areas of thick keratotic plaques seen on the lingual marginal gingiva of right posterior teeth, the retromolar pad, and the buccal mucosa.

Actinic Cheilitis

Actinic cheilitis is characterized by accelerated tissue degeneration as a result of excessive exposure to ultraviolet sunlight.[94] This irreversible and premalignant lesion is typically found on the vermillion border of lower lip of fair-skinned middle-aged individuals with an outdoor occupation.[95] Recent studies have shown fibroblast growth factor receptor 3 gene (FGFR3) mutations in actinic cheilitis as well as in squamous cell carcinoma.[96] A small percentage (6%–10%) of these lesions progresses to squamous cell carcinoma (**Fig. 9**A).[97]

Clinical features

Most cases exhibit blurring of the vermillion border of the lips, with the lesions ranging from solitary well-demarcated lesions to multiple poorly demarcated lesions.[95,97,98] Lesions may be keratotic, atrophic, infiltrative, erosive, erythematous, scaly, mildly puffy, and/or superficially fissured (see **Fig. 9**).[95] Symptoms such as burning and itching have also been reported.[95,98]

Histologic features

The epithelial changes range from simple hyperorthokeratosis without dysplasia to CIS.[94,95,97,98] Varying degrees of cytologic atypia such as increased nuclear/cytoplasmic ratios, loss of cellular polarity and orientation, and nuclear and cellular

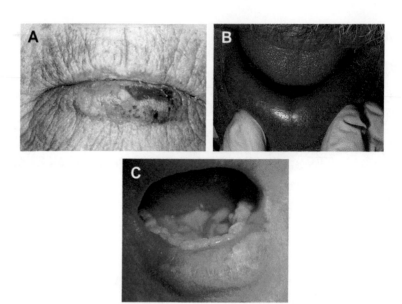

Fig. 9. (*A*) Areas of squamous cell carcinoma arising in actinic keratosis. Multiple areas of scaly, ulcerative lesions noted. (*B*) Actinic cheilitis demonstrating blurring of the vermillion border of the lower lip, with keratotic as well as atrophic areas. (*C*) Actinic cheilitis demonstrating blurring of the vermillion border of the lip, with a smooth surface and pale white keratotic lesions.

pleomorphism are found within the epithelium.[97] Solar elastosis, chronic inflammation, and vasodilatation are also characteristic of actinic cheilitis.

Differential diagnosis
Dry and chapped lips, traumatic lesions, and squamous cell carcinoma.

Treatment
Surgical intervention is the current treatment of choice.[99] Chemotherapy with 5-fluorouracil, CO_2 laser, and cryotherapy have also been recommended.[99] Patients should be advised to use lip balm with sunscreen, and periodic follow-up is recommended.[99]

Oral Submucosal Fibrosis

Oral submucosal fibrosis (OSMF) is a progressive, chronic, and premalignant condition characterized by fibroelastic changes and inflammation in the mucosa.[100,101] The etiology is still unclear, but a strong correlation exists with consumption of spicy food, chilies, and/or areca nuts, as well as vitamin B deficiency and protein malnutrition.[102,103] A genetic predisposition involving human lymphocytic antigen (HLA) A10, DR3, DR7, and probably B7 has been found.[104] OSMF is seen typically on the buccal mucosa, labial mucosa, soft palate, floor of the mouth, and tongue. High prevalence is seen in populations of the Indian subcontinent, affecting persons of all ages and both genders (**Fig. 10**A).[102–104]

Clinical features
OSMF is characterized by a burning sensation of the oral mucosa while eating hot or spicy foods.[103,104] Vesicles, excessive salivation, ulcers, dryness of the mouth, and pigmentation changes have also been reported.[100,103] More advanced lesions

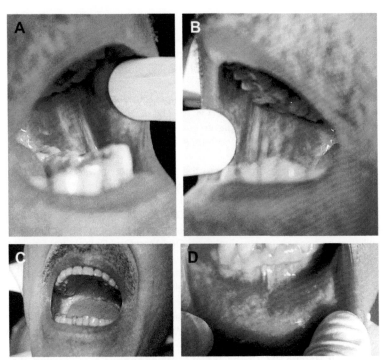

Fig. 10. (*A*) East Indian man with at least 8-year history of chewing betel nuts, demonstrating limited opening of the mouth and poorly demarcated white keratotic areas on the buccal mucosa. (*B*) Fibrous bands in buccal mucosa are evident in same patient as *A*. (*C*) Limited opening of the mouth. The patient reported pain and burning of the oral mucosa on consumption of spicy foods. Same patient as in *A*. (*D*) Submucosal fibrous bands demonstrated on the lower labial mucosa in a patient with oral submucosal fibrosis. Same patient as in *A*. (*Courtesy of* Dr Eric Fox, oral surgeon, Coral Springs FL, USA.)

demonstrate palpable fibrous bands leading to significant restriction in oral opening, speech, swallowing, and decrease in salivary flow (see **Fig. 10**B–D).[100,102–104]

Histologic features
Early findings include presence of chronic inflammatory cells, with several eosinophils in the lamina propria.[105] Epithelial atrophy, hyalinized subepithelial collagen, and loss of vascularity is seen in established cases. Fibrosis of minor salivary glands is also evident.[105]

Differential diagnosis
Amyloidosis, generalized fibromatosis, scleroderma, and oral lichen planus.

Treatment
Most patients present with moderate to severe disease, and treatment focuses on improving mouth movement and relieving symptoms.[102,104] Submucosal injections of steroids and collagenases, as well as topical steroid application, oral iron preparations, and topical vitamin A applications have been tried for palliative relief.[104,106] Severe cases need surgical intervention.[104,106] Patients require close follow-up because of the high potential of malignant transformation, as shown by different studies of biologic markers.[106]

REFERENCES

1. Hernandez-Martin A, Fernandez-Lopez E, de Unamuno P, et al. Diffuse whitening of the oral mucosa in a child. Pediatr Dermatol 1997;14(4):316–20.
2. Martin JL. Leukoedema: a review of the literature. J Natl Med Assoc 1992; 84(11):938–40.
3. Martin JL. Leukoedema: an epidemiological study in white and African Americans. J Tenn Dent Assoc 1997;77(1):18–21.
4. Axell T, Henricsson V. Leukoedema—an epidemiologic study with special reference to the influence of tobacco habits. Community Dent Oral Epidemiol 1981; 9(3):142–6.
5. van Wyk CW. An investigation into the association between leukoedema and smoking. J Oral Pathol 1985;14(6):491–9.
6. Neville BW, Damm DD, Allen CM, et al. Oral and maxillofacial pathology. 3rd edition. Philadelphia: WB Saunders; 2009. p. 9,743, 46–47.
7. Shibuya Y, Zhang J, Yokoo S, et al. Constitutional mutation of keratin 13 gene in familial white sponge nevus. Oral Surg Oral Med Oral Pathol Oral Radiol Endod 2003;96(5):561–5.
8. Terrinoni A, Candi E, Oddi S, et al. A glutamine insertion in the 1A alpha helical domain of the keratin 4 gene in a familial case of white sponge nevus. J Invest Dermatol 2000;114(2):388–91.
9. Jorgenson RJ, Levin S. White sponge nevus. Arch Dermatol 1981;117(2):73–6.
10. Morris R, Gansler TS, Rudisill MT, et al. White sponge nevus. Diagnosis by light microscopic and ultrastructural cytology. Acta Cytol 1988;32(3):357–61.
11. Martelli H Jr, Pereira SM, Rocha TM, et al. White sponge nevus: report of a three-generation family. Oral Surg Oral Med Oral Pathol Oral Radiol Endod 2007; 103(1):43–7.
12. Otobe IF, de Sousa SO, Migliari DA, et al. Successful treatment with topical tetracycline of oral white sponge nevus occurring in a patient with systemic lupus erythematosus. Int J Dermatol 2006;45(9):1130–1.
13. McLean IW, Riddle PJ, Schruggs JH, et al. Hereditary benign intraepithelial dyskeratosis. A report of two cases from Texas. Ophthalmology 1981;88(2):164–8.
14. Shields CL, Shields JA, Eagle RC Jr. Hereditary benign intraepithelial dyskeratosis. Arch Ophthalmol 1987;105(3):422–3.
15. Jham BC, Mesquita RA, Aguiar MC, et al. Hereditary benign intraepithelial dyskeratosis: a new case? J Oral Pathol Med 2007;36(1):55–7.
16. Sadeghi EM, Witkop CJ. Ultrastructural study of hereditary benign intraepithelial dyskeratosis. Oral Surg Oral Med Oral Pathol 1977;44(4):567–77.
17. Allingham RR, Seo B, Rampersaud E, et al. A duplication in chromosome 4q35 is associated with hereditary benign intraepithelial dyskeratosis. Am J Hum Genet 2001;68(2):491–4.
18. Baykal C, Kavak A, Gulcan P, et al. Dyskeratosis congenita associated with three malignancies. J Eur Acad Dermatol Venereol 2003;17(2):216–8.
19. Bhattacharyya I, Cohen DM, Silverman S Jr. Red and white lesions of the oral mucosa. In: Greenberg MS, Glick M, editors. Burkett's oral medicine: diagnosis and treatment. 10th edition. Hamilton (ON): Lippincott-Raven; 2003. p. 87.
20. Fernandes Gomes M, Pinheiro de Abreu P, de Freitas Banzi C, et al. Interdisciplinary approach to treat dyskeratosis congenita associated with severe aplastic anemia: a case report. Spec Care Dentist 2006;26(2):81–4.
21. Handley TP, Ogden GR. Dyskeratosis congenita: oral hyperkeratosis in association with lichenoid reaction. J Oral Pathol Med 2006;35(8):508–12.

22. Kanegane H, Kasahara Y, Okamura J, et al. Identification of DKC1 gene mutations in Japanese patients with X-linked dyskeratosis congenita. Br J Haematol 2005;129(3):432–4.
23. Leachman SA, Kaspar RL, Fleckman P, et al. Clinical and pathological features of pachyonychia congenita. J Investig Dermatol Symp Proc 2005;10(1):3–17.
24. Pradeep AR, Nagaraja C. Pachyonychia congenita with unusual dental findings: a case report. Oral Surg Oral Med Oral Pathol Oral Radiol Endod 2007;104(1):89–93.
25. McKusick VA. Mendelian inheritance in man; a catalog of human genes and genetic disorders. 12th edition. Baltimore (MD): John Hopkins University Press; 1998.
26. Thormann J, Kobayasi T. Pachyonychia congenita Jadassohn-Lewandowsky: a disorder of keratinization. Acta Derm Venereol 1977;57(1):63–7.
27. Fujimoto W, Nakanishi G, Hirakawa S, et al. Pachyonychia congenita type 2: keratin 17 mutation in a Japanese case. J Am Acad Dermatol 1998;38(6 Pt 1):1007–9.
28. McLean WH, Rugg EL, Lunny DP, et al. Keratin 16 and keratin 17 mutations cause pachyonychia congenita. Nat Genet 1995;9(3):273–8.
29. Hannaford RS, Stapleton K. Pachyonychia congenita tarda. Australas J Dermatol 2000;41(3):175–7.
30. Milstone LM, Fleckman P, Leachman SA, et al. Treatment of pachyonychia congenita. J Investig Dermatol Symp Proc 2005;10(1):18–20.
31. Parlak AH, Koybasi S, Yavuz T, et al. Prevalence of oral lesions in 13- to 16-year-old students in Duzce, Turkey. Oral Dis 2006;12(6):553–8.
32. Seoane Leston JM, Aguado Santos A, Varela-Centelles PI, et al. Oral mucosa: variations from normalcy, part I. Cutis 2002;69(2):131–4.
33. Wood NK, Goaz PW. White lesions of the oral mucosa. In: Wood NK, Goaz PW, editors. Differential diagnosis of oral lesions. St. Louis (MO): Mosby; 1997. p. 96–8.
34. Bouquot JE, Gorlin RJ. Leukoplakia, lichen planus, and other oral keratoses in 23,616 white Americans over the age of 35 years. Oral Surg Oral Med Oral Pathol 1986;61(4):373–81.
35. Kafas P, Stavrianos C. Thermal burn of palate caused by microwave heated cheese-pie: a case report. Cases J 2008;1(1):191.
36. Rossie KM, Guggenheimer J. Thermally induced 'nicotine' stomatitis. A case report. Oral Surg Oral Med Oral Pathol 1990;70(5):597–9.
37. Walsh PM, Epstein JB. The oral effects of smokeless tobacco. J Can Dent Assoc 2000;66(1):22–5.
38. Baruchin AM, Lustig JP, Nahlieli O, et al. Burns of the oral mucosa. Report of 6 cases. J Craniomaxillofac Surg 1991;19(2):94–6.
39. Fanibunda KB. Adverse response to endodontic material containing paraformaldehyde. Br Dent J 1984;157(7):231–5.
40. Gernhardt CR, Eppendorf K, Kozlowski A, et al. Toxicity of concentrated sodium hypochlorite used as an endodontic irrigant. Int Endod J 2004;37(4):272–80.
41. Maron FS. Mucosal burn resulting from chewable aspirin: report of case. J Am Dent Assoc 1989;119(2):279–80.
42. Moghadam BK, Gier R, Thurlow T. Extensive oral mucosal ulcerations caused by misuse of a commercial mouthwash. Cutis 1999;64(2):131–4.
43. Murrin JR, Abrams H, Barkmeier WW. Chemical burn of oral tissue caused by dental cavity varnish. Report of a case. Ill Dent J 1978;47(10):580–1.

44. Rees TD, Orth CF. Oral ulcerations with use of hydrogen peroxide. J Periodontol 1986;57(11):689–92.
45. Leao JC, Gueiros LA, Segundo AV, et al. Uremic stomatitis in chronic renal failure. Clinics (Sao Paulo) 2005;60(3):259–62.
46. McCreary CE, Flint SR, McCartan BE, et al. Uremic stomatitis mimicking oral hairy leukoplakia: report of a case. Oral Surg Oral Med Oral Pathol Oral Radiol Endod 1997;83(3):350–3.
47. Halazonetis J, Harley A. Uremic stomatitis. Report of a case. Oral Surg Oral Med Oral Pathol 1967;23(5):573–7.
48. Ross WF 3rd, Salisbury PL 3rd. Uremic stomatitis associated with undiagnosed renal failure. Gen Dent 1994;42(5):410–2.
49. Kellett M. Oral white plaques in uraemic patients. Br Dent J 1983;154(11):366–8.
50. Antoniades DZ, Markopoulos AK, Andreadis D, et al. Ulcerative uremic stomatitis associated with untreated chronic renal failure: report of a case and review of the literature. Oral Surg Oral Med Oral Pathol Oral Radiol Endod 2006;101(5):608–13.
51. Hovinga J, Roodvoets AP, Gaillard J. Some findings in patients with uraemic stomatitis. J Maxillofac Surg 1975;3(2):125–7.
52. Larato DC. Uremic stomatitis: report of a case. J Periodontol 1975;46(12):731–3.
53. Kabani S, Greenspan D, deSouza Y, et al. Oral hairy leukoplakia with extensive oral mucosal involvement. Report of two cases. Oral Surg Oral Med Oral Pathol 1989;67(4):411–5.
54. Schiodt M, Greenspan D, Daniels TE, et al. Clinical and histologic spectrum of oral hairy leukoplakia. Oral Surg Oral Med Oral Pathol 1987;64(6):716–20.
55. Triantos D, Porter SR, Scully C, et al. Oral hairy leukoplakia: clinicopathologic features, pathogenesis, diagnosis, and clinical significance. Clin Infect Dis 1997;25(6):1392–6.
56. Brandwein M, Nuovo G, Ramer M, et al. Epstein-Barr virus reactivation in hairy leukoplakia. Mod Pathol 1996;9(3):298–303.
57. Greenspan JS, Greenspan D, Lennette ET, et al. Replication of Epstein-Barr virus within the epithelial cells of oral "hairy" leukoplakia, an AIDS-associated lesion. N Engl J Med 1985;313(25):1564–71.
58. Reichart PA, Langford A, Gelderblom HR, et al. Oral hairy leukoplakia: observations in 95 cases and review of the literature. J Oral Pathol Med 1989;18(7):410–5.
59. Herbst JS, Morgan J, Raab-Traub N, et al. Comparison of the efficacy of surgery and acyclovir therapy in oral hairy leukoplakia. J Am Acad Dermatol 1989;21(4 Pt 1):753–6.
60. Lozada-Nur F, Costa C. Retrospective findings of the clinical benefits of podophyllum resin 25% sol on hairy leukoplakia. Clinical results in nine patients. Oral Surg Oral Med Oral Pathol 1992;73(5):555–8.
61. Schofer H, Ochsendorf FR, Helm EB, et al. Treatment of oral 'hairy' leukoplakia in AIDS patients with vitamin A acid (topically) or acyclovir (systemically). Dermatologica 1987;174(3):150–1.
62. Moura MD, Guimaraes TR, Fonseca LM, et al. A random clinical trial study to assess the efficiency of topical applications of podophyllin resin (25%) versus podophyllin resin (25%) together with acyclovir cream (5%) in the treatment of oral hairy leukoplakia. Oral Surg Oral Med Oral Pathol Oral Radiol Endod 2007;103(1):64–71.

63. Kramer IR, Lucas RB, Pindborg JJ, et al. Definition of leukoplakia and related lesions: an aid to studies on oral precancer. Oral Surg Oral Med Oral Pathol 1978;46(4):518–39.

64. Bouquot JE, Weiland LH, Kurland LT. Leukoplakia and carcinoma in situ synchronously associated with invasive oral/oropharyngeal carcinoma in Rochester, Minn., 1935–1984. Oral Surg Oral Med Oral Pathol 1988;65(2):199–207.

65. Field EA, Field JK, Martin MV. Does Candida have a role in oral epithelial neoplasia? J Med Vet Mycol 1989;27(5):277–94.

66. Hansen LS, Olson JA, Silverman S Jr. Proliferative verrucous leukoplakia. A long-term study of thirty patients. Oral Surg Oral Med Oral Pathol 1985; 60(3):285–98.

67. Lumerman H, Freedman P, Kerpel S. Oral epithelial dysplasia and the development of invasive squamous cell carcinoma. Oral Surg Oral Med Oral Pathol Oral Radiol Endod 1995;79(3):321–9.

68. Schepman KP, van der Meij EH, Smeele LE, et al. Malignant transformation of oral leukoplakia: a follow-up study of a hospital-based population of 166 patients with oral leukoplakia from The Netherlands. Oral Oncol 1998;34(4): 270–5.

69. Silverman S Jr, Gorsky M. Proliferative verrucous leukoplakia: a follow-up study of 54 cases. Oral Surg Oral Med Oral Pathol Oral Radiol Endod 1997;84(2): 154–7.

70. Sugerman PB, Shillitoe EJ. The high risk human papillomaviruses and oral cancer: evidence for and against a causal relationship. Oral Dis 1997;3(3):130–47.

71. van der Waal I, Schepman KP, van der Meij EH, et al. Oral leukoplakia: a clinico-pathological review. Oral Oncol 1997;33(5):291–301.

72. Freitas MD, Blanco-Carrion A, Gandara-Vila P, et al. Clinicopathologic aspects of oral leukoplakia in smokers and nonsmokers. Oral Surg Oral Med Oral Pathol Oral Radiol Endod 2006;102(2):199–203.

73. Banoczy J, Gintner Z, Dombi C. Tobacco use and oral leukoplakia. J Dent Educ 2001;65(4):322–7.

74. Downer MC, Evans AW, Hughes Hallet CM, et al. Evaluation of screening for oral cancer and precancer in a company headquarters. Community Dent Oral Epidemiol 1995;23(2):84–8.

75. Lewin F, Norell SE, Johansson H, et al. Smoking tobacco, oral snuff, and alcohol in the etiology of squamous cell carcinoma of the head and neck: a population-based case-referent study in Sweden. Cancer 1998;82(7):1367–75.

76. Cawson RA, Binnie WH. Candida, leukoplakia and carcinoma: a possible relationship. In: Mackenzie I, Dabelsteen E, Squier CA, editors. Oral premalignancy. Proceedings of the first Dows symposium. Iowa: University of Iowa Press; 1980. p. 59–66.

77. Holmstrup P, Bessermann M. Clinical, therapeutic, and pathogenic aspects of chronic oral multifocal candidiasis. Oral Surg Oral Med Oral Pathol 1983; 56(4):388–95.

78. Miller CS, Johnstone BM. Human papillomavirus as a risk factor for oral squamous cell carcinoma: a meta-analysis, 1982–1997. Oral Surg Oral Med Oral Pathol Oral Radiol Endod 2001;91(6):622–35.

79. Yang SW, Lee YS, Chen TA, et al. Human papillomavirus in oral leukoplakia is no prognostic indicator of malignant transformation. Cancer Epidemiol 2009;33(2): 118–22.

80. Axell T, Pindborg JJ, Smith CJ, et al. Oral white lesions with special reference to precancerous and tobacco-related lesions: conclusions of an international

symposium held in Uppsala, Sweden, May 18–21 1994. International Collaborative Group on Oral White Lesions. J Oral Pathol Med 1996;25(2):49–54.

81. Cabay RJ, Morton TH Jr, Epstein JB. Proliferative verrucous leukoplakia and its progression to oral carcinoma: a review of the literature. J Oral Pathol Med 2007; 36(5):255–61.

82. Waldron CA, Shafer WG. Leukoplakia revisited. A clinicopathologic study 3256 oral leukoplakias. Cancer 1975;36(4):1386–92.

83. Kaugars GE, Burns JC, Gunsolley JC. Epithelial dysplasia of the oral cavity and lips. Cancer 1988;62(10):2166–70.

84. Pindborg JJ, Jolst O, Renstrup G, et al. Studies in oral leukoplakia: a preliminary report on the period prevalence of malignant transformation in leukoplakia based on a follow-up study of 248 patients. J Am Dent Assoc 1968;76(4): 767–71.

85. Pindborg JJ, Daftary DK, Mehta FS. A follow-up study of sixty-one oral dysplastic precancerous lesions in Indian villagers. Oral Surg Oral Med Oral Pathol 1977;43(3):383–90.

86. Al-Drouby HA. Oral leukoplakia and cryotherapy. Br Dent J 1983;155(4):124–5.

87. Marley JJ, Linden GJ, Cowan CG, et al. A comparison of the management of potentially malignant oral mucosal lesions by oral medicine practitioners and oral & maxillofacial surgeons in the UK. J Oral Pathol Med 1998;27(10): 489–95.

88. Lodi G, Sardella A, Bez C, et al. Interventions for treating oral leukoplakia. Cochrane Database Syst Rev 2006;4:CD001829.

89. Bagan JV, Jimenez Y, Murillo J, et al. Lack of association between proliferative verrucous leukoplakia and human papillomavirus infection. J Oral Maxillofac Surg 2007;65(1):46–9.

90. Bagan JV, Jimenez Y, Murillo J, et al. Epstein-Barr virus in oral proliferative verrucous leukoplakia and squamous cell carcinoma: a preliminary study. Med Oral Patol Oral Cir Bucal 2008;13(2):E110–113.

91. Klanrit P, Sperandio M, Brown AL, et al. DNA ploidy in proliferative verrucous leukoplakia. Oral Oncol 2007;43(3):310–6.

92. Zakrzewska JM, Lopes V, Speight P, et al. Proliferative verrucous leukoplakia: a report of ten cases. Oral Surg Oral Med Oral Pathol Oral Radiol Endod 1996;82(4):396–401.

93. Batsakis JG, Suarez P, el-Naggar AK. Proliferative verrucous leukoplakia and its related lesions. Oral Oncol 1999;35(4):354–9.

94. Gupta PC, Mehta FS, Daftary DK, et al. Incidence rates of oral cancer and natural history of oral precancerous lesions in a 10-year follow-up study of Indian villagers. Community Dent Oral Epidemiol 1980;8(6):283–333.

95. Cavalcante AS, Anbinder AL, Carvalho YR. Actinic cheilitis: clinical and histological features. J Oral Maxillofac Surg 2008;66(3):498–503.

96. Chou A, Dekker N, Jordan RC. Identification of novel fibroblast growth factor receptor 3 gene mutations in actinic cheilitis and squamous cell carcinoma of the lip. Oral Surg Oral Med Oral Pathol Oral Radiol Endod 2009;107(4):535–41.

97. Menta Simonsen Nico M, Rivitti EA, Lourenco SV. Actinic cheilitis: histologic study of the entire vermilion and comparison with previous biopsy. J Cutan Pathol 2007;34(4):309–14.

98. Kaugars GE, Pillion T, Svirsky JA, et al. Actinic cheilitis: a review of 152 cases. Oral Surg Oral Med Oral Pathol Oral Radiol Endod 1999;88(2):181–6.

99. Robinson JK. Actinic cheilitis. A prospective study comparing four treatment methods. Arch Otolaryngol Head Neck Surg 1989;115(7):848–52.

100. Murti PR, Bhonsle RB, Pindborg JJ, et al. Malignant transformation rate in oral submucous fibrosis over a 17-year period. Community Dent Oral Epidemiol 1985;13(6):340–1.
101. Pindborg JJ, Sirsat SM. Oral submucous fibrosis. Oral Surg Oral Med Oral Pathol 1966;22(6):764–79.
102. Canniff JP, Harvey W, Harris M. Oral submucous fibrosis: its pathogenesis and management. Br Dent J 1986;160(12):429–34.
103. Javed F, Chotai M, Mehmood A, et al. Oral mucosal disorders associated with habitual gutka usage: a review. Oral Surg Oral Med Oral Pathol Oral Radiol Endod 2010;109:857–64.
104. Mehrotra D, Pradhan R, Gupta S. Retrospective comparison of surgical treatment modalities in 100 patients with oral submucous fibrosis. Oral Surg Oral Med Oral Pathol Oral Radiol Endod 2009;107(3):e1–10.
105. Isaac U, Issac JS, Ahmed Khoso N. Histopathologic features of oral submucous fibrosis: a study of 35 biopsy specimens. Oral Surg Oral Med Oral Pathol Oral Radiol Endod 2008;106(4):556–60.
106. Zhou S, Qu X, Yu Z, et al. Survivin as a potential early marker in the carcinogenesis of oral submucous fibrosis. Oral Surg Oral Med Oral Pathol Oral Radiol Endod 2010;109(4):575–81.

Vesiculobullous Eruptions of the Oral Cavity

Sherif Said, MD, PhD*, Loren Golitz, MD

KEYWORDS

• Oral • Vesiculobullous • Ulcerative • Pemphigus • Pemphigoid

---

Causes of vesiculobullous eruptions in the oral cavity encompass many entities that are usually of autoimmune- or immune-mediated etiology. Correlation of the clinical and immunologic findings is essential for the accurate classification and diagnosis and management of these cases. In this ensuing article, these entities are discussed in a classification that mainly reflects the prevailing histologic appearance of the different disease processes.

ORAL INTRAMUCOSAL BULLOUS DISEASES (PEMPHIGUS)
Definition

Pemphigus is a group of rare chronic autoimmune disorder characterized by blistering of the stratified squamous epithelium of the skin and mucosal surfaces and encompasses a number of subtypes, which include pemphigus vulgaris (PV) and pemphigus vegetans (PVeg), both commonly involve the oral mucosa; immunoglobulin (Ig) A pemphigus that also manifests oral lesions; and pemphigus foliaceous and its variant pemphigus erythematosus (Senear-Usher syndrome), which are rarely manifested orally and are primarily cutaneous.

Paraneoplastic pemphigus (PP), usually seen in association with lymphoproliferative diseases, is another important variant that can affect the oral cavity as well as drug-induced pemphigus.

Typically, a person develops a single variant of pemphigus, but cases of transition to other variants have been described.

Pemphigus Vulgaris

Incidence
PV is rare with an incidence of only 0.1 to 0.5 cases per 100,000 persons per year worldwide; however, it is the most common pemphigus variety affecting the oral

---

Financial Disclosure and conflict of intrest obligations: None for both authors.
Department of Pathology, University of Colorado Denver, Mail Stop F768, 12605 East 16th Avenue, Room 3014, Aurora, CO 80045, USA
* Corresponding author.
E-mail address: Sherif.said@ucdenver.edu

mucosa.[1] This disorder manifests in the fifth to sixth decades of life, with a slight female predilection.[2,3] Rare juvenile cases have also been reported.[1,4] PV has strong genetic associations with certain ethnic groups (Ashkenazi Jews and people of Mediterranean and South Asian origin).[5,6]

Clinical presentation

Oral involvement is the hallmark of PV and is seen in 90% of patients (**Fig. 1**). Indeed, 50% to 70% of cases present primarily with oral disease long before cutaneous manifestations appear (>1 year). However, those presenting with cutaneous manifestations also eventually show oral manifestations.[1,3,4,7] All other body mucosal sites (including pharyngeal, esophageal, nasal, vaginal, rectal, and urinary) can also be involved with the disease.

Lesions present as flaccid fluid-filled blisters or bullous lesions that eventually break, forming red, painful, erosive, irregular, ragged-edge, and ulcerated lesions. The buccal, palatal, ventral aspects of tongue and lip mucosa are commonly affected,[3,6,8–12] and wide oral mucosa involvement can be seen in severe cases.

Gingival lesions are uncommon at the onset but may frequently appear on gingiva as isolated blisters and erosions mainly located in the free gingiva and are hardly recognizable as bullous lesions. However, in advanced cases, erosive or desquamative gingivitis is seen.[13–15] If left untreated, new bullae forms as the older ones rupture; however, at the onset of the disease, these lesions present in a recurrent pattern and become persistent with time. Ulcers heal slowly, and scarring is rare.

These lesions translate themselves into typical symptoms of odynophagia, dysphagia, and severe discomfort experienced by the patient. A positive Nikolsky sign (slight rubbing of the skin or mucous membrane can lead to bullae formation or sloughing of the squamous epithelium) can be elicited in the mucous membrane or skin of affected individuals.

PV is a serious disease that is potentially fatal if blistering forms large denuded areas on the skin and mucous membranes.[12,16] If left untreated, this condition has a mortality rate of 50% at 2 years, which reaches almost 100% at 5 years.[17]

PV may be seen in association with other autoimmune disorders, including rheumatoid arthritis, myasthenia gravis, lupus erythematosus, and pernicious anemia.

Etiology

The causative factors in PV are largely idiopathic; however, some precipitating factors have been identified, including

1. Genetic factors. As mentioned earlier, certain ethnic groups have a particular predilection for the disease. Associations with HLA antigen have also been recognized in

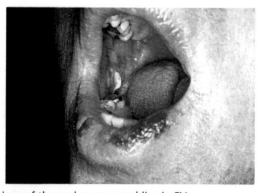

Fig. 1. Painful erosions of the oral mucosa and lips in PV.

these groups, particularly HLA-0DR4 (DRB1*0402) in the Ashkenazi Jewish population, Europeans, and Asians with DRw14 (DRB1*1041) and DQB1*0503.[18–22]

2. Diet. Garlic in particular has been identified as an important dietary factor.[23]

3. Drugs. Drugs are a rare cause of PV, which include angiotensin-converting enzyme inhibitors (eg, captopril, enalapril, fosinopril), thiols (eg, cephalosporins, penicillamine, penicillin), antiinflammatory drugs (eg, aspirin, nonsteroidal antiinflammatory drugs [NSAIDs]), and a variable array of drugs (eg, levodopa, nifedipine, propranolol, rifampicin).[24] Traditional cosmetic substances have been implicated in Tunisia as a cause of pemphigus.[25]

4. Viruses. The role of viruses in PV has been proposed mainly in relation to human herpesviruses (HHVs),[26,27] particularly HHV-8[28,29]; however, no confirmed role has been found yet.[26]

5. Several other factors have been implicated to cause PV, including smoking and exposure to pesticides. A role of increased estrogen hormone has also been suggested.[30]

Pathogenesis

Loss of squamous cell-cell adhesion through damaged or defective desmosomal proteins, leading to vesiculation, bullae formation with subsequent rupture, and formations of erosions/ulcers, broadly describes the sequence of the pathogenic events in PV.

The oral squamous epithelium is similar to its skin counter part, however, with different desmosomal components. The oral epithelium expresses mainly cadherin-type cell adhesion molecule desmoglein 3 (Dsg3) that binds squamous cell to each other, whereas the skin expresses both Dsg1 and Dsg3 consequently, resulting in different disease manifestations.[12] Patients with predominant oral manifestations express only Dsg3 antibodies.[31] In oral PV, there is deposition of IgG class autoantibodies intercellularly against Dsg3. In patients with oral and cutaneous manifestations, the fact that the skin integrity is more maintained by Dsg1 than by Dsg3 makes the oral manifestations predominant until the Dsg1 antibodies also appear, resulting in severe cutaneous manifestations.[32] In active disease, IgG4 autoantibodies are formed, and during remission, IgG1 predominates.[33]

HLA class II alleles seem to be particularly important in the recognition of Dsg3 by T lymphocytes. The autoantibodies bind to Dsg3 and Dsg1 and form intercellular immune complexes that activate the complement by inflammatory mediators and activated T cells, resulting in damage to the intercellular junction, leading to cell apoptosis by proteinases, Fas, and caspase, eventually causing cleavage/blistering.[34–36]

Histologic features

The hallmark of PV is the formation of bullae immediately above the basal cell layer (suprabasal bullae) (**Fig. 2**). The sequence of events starts with slight intercellular edema within the epithelial layer with subsequent acantholysis low in the stratum spinosum, with cleft formations and eventually suprabasilar bullae formation.

A single row of cuboidal basal cells remains below the bullae, giving the characteristic "tombstone" appearance (**Fig. 3**). Papillae lined by a single layer of cuboidal cells and with a core formed by projecting submucosa are seen. No significant inflammation is seen early in the disease; however, focal eosinophilic infiltrate may be seen in the epidermis before acantholysis (eosinophilic spongiosis).

The formed acantholytic cells become hyperchromatic and swollen with high nuclear cytoplasmic ratio and are identified in smears collected from the lesions aiding in the lesion diagnosis. These cells are known as Tzanck cells.

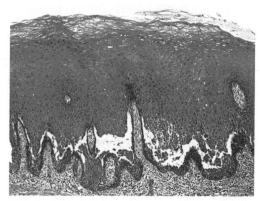

Fig. 2. Oral mucosal biopsy result showing an intraepithelial acantholytic bulla in PV.

Diagnosis

In addition to the clinical features, the following steps are used in the diagnosis of PV

1. Perilesional tissue biopsy and histopathologic examination
2. Direct immunofluorescence (DIF) microscopy or immunohistochemistry showing intercellular deposits of IgG and complement C3, which are more sensitive than conventional histopathology (**Fig. 4**)
3. Assays by indirect immunofluorescence (IIF) microscopy of serum antibody titers or by the use of specific enzyme-linked immunosorbent assays (ELISA).

Treatment and prognosis

Systemic immunosuppression is the mainstay of treatment to bring the disease process under control and to achieve complete and long-standing remission. With the proper immunosuppressive therapy, about half the patients achieve complete and long-standing remission after about 5 years.[34,37]

Systemic corticosteroids seem to be the mainstay of treatments.[11] Other treatments include plasmapheresis[38] alone or in association with cyclosporin or cyclophosphamide (Kiel synchronization protocol). Others drugs include dapsone, chlorambucil, cyclophosphamide, azathioprine, gold, minocycline, and methotrexate. However,

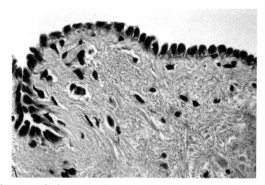

Fig. 3. Suprabasilar acantholysis, producing a "tombstone" appearance, composed of epidermal basal cells in PV.

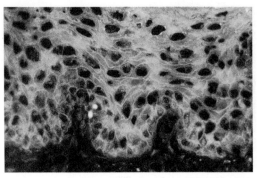

Fig. 4. A tissue biopsy result showing intercellular immunofluorescence with IgG in PV.

many of these drugs have adverse effects, and most clinicians focus on corticosteroid therapy.[34]

Other emerging recent agents include intravenous immunoglobulins in steroid-resistant PV,[39] mofetil,[40] tacrolimus,[41] and cholinergic agonists.[42] Immunoadsorption[43] and immunomodulation[44] are other new treatment modalities.

Pemphigus Vegetans

Incidence
PVeg, a variant of PV, is a rare cause of pemphigus that constitutes 1% to 2% of all pemphigus cases. However, if this condition occurs, it almost always involves the oral cavity.[1] The age of onset is usually between 40 and 50 years; however, any age group, including children, can be involved.[45]

Clinical presentation
Similar to PV, more than half the cases of PVeg show oral manifestations preceding cutaneous ones and those with cutaneous lesions eventually have oral involvement.[46]

PVeg has 2 types, Neumann and Hallopeau,[47] of which the Neumann subtype is more common. Some studies have questioned this classification.[46] In the Neumann type, the lesions are similar to those of PV. In the Hallopeau type, there are pustular lesions with a benign course and few relapses.[47,48] Both lesions develop hyperpigmented verrucous vegetative plaques (**Fig. 5**) with pustules and hypertrophic granulation tissue at the periphery. It is these verrucous vegetations that characterize PVeg and are painful, foul smelling in the cutaneous sites, and inflamed and vary in size from small lesions to larger-size areas. The propensity for bullae formation in PVeg is generally lower than that of PV.

In addition to the oral mucosal lesions, the tongue seems to acquire a cerebriform appearance with numerous sulci and gyri. The cutaneous lesions are also typically seen in the intertriginous locations (eg, axilla, groin).[49]

Pathogenesis and etiology
As in PV, autoantibodies are mainly formed against cell adhesion molecule Dsg 3. In cutaneous involvement, Dsg1 is also seen in a similar fashion to PV. Desmocollin 1 and 2 and periplakin have also been reported.[50–52] The autoantibodies seen are IgG type, mostly IgG4 and, to a lesser degree, IgG1. A combination of IgA and IgG has also been reported in a rare case.[52]

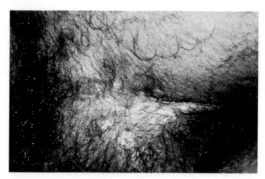

Fig. 5. An intertriginous verrucous plaque in PVeg.

The etiopathogenesis of Pveg is not clear, captopril and intranasal heroine use has been reported.[49]

Histologic features and diagnosis

The Neumann type shows histologic features similar to those seen in PV; however, eosinophilic spongiosis, in which the pustules seen in the early vegetations are filled with eosinophils, is a more prominent feature (**Fig. 6**). Older vegetations (**Fig. 7**) tend to demobstrate papillomatosis and hyperkeratosis and are less diagnostic.

The Hallopeau type show shows similar changes; however, the intraepidermal eosinophilic abscesses formed tend to be larger and more numerous.

Diagnostic laboratory findings are similar to those of PV.

Treatment and prognosis

Systemic glucocorticoids are the treatment of choice. Oral administration of corticosteroids alone may not induce remission, and addition of immunosuppressive agents (eg, cyclophosphamide, azathioprine, etretinate) may improve remission rates.[53]

Concerning prognosis, patients with Neumann type have a course similar to that of those with PV. Those patients with Hallopeau type have fewer, if any, relapses and usually respond to even lower doses of corticosteroids.

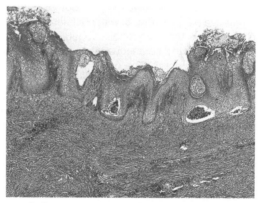

Fig. 6. A skin biopsy result showing verrucous plaque with microabscesses containing eosinophils in PVeg.

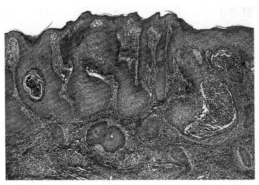

Fig. 7. An older verrucous plaque in PVeg, showing marked epithelial hyperplasia and eosinophilic vesicles.

Paraneoplastic Pemphigus

Background
Anhalt and colleagues,[54] in 1990, first described PP and put the original criteria for diagnosis, which includes

- Painful mucosa eruptions, with polymorphous skin eruptions in the setting of confirmed or occult malignancy
- Histopathologic changes ,such as acantholysis, keratinocyte necrosis, and interface dermatitis
- DIF observation of epidermal, intercellular, and basement membrane immunoreactants, mostly IgG and C3
- IIF observation of circulating antibodies directed against squamous, simple, columnar, and transitional epithelium
- Immunoprecipitation with a complex of 4 proteins (desmoplakin I, envoplakin, desmoplakin, and periplakin).

In 1993, Camisa and Helm[55] also suggested a set of major and minor criteria. In 2004, Anhalt[56] suggested minor criteria for diagnosis, including

- Painful progressive stomatitis
- Histopathologic changes of acantholysis or lichenoid dermatitis
- Demonstration of antiplakin antibodies
- Demonstration of an underlying neoplasm (mostly hematologic malignancies).

A recent literature review[57] lists benign and malignant neoplasms that can be associated with PP, including Hematologic (84% of reported cases)

- Non-Hodgkin lymphoma (most frequent)
- Chronic lymphocytic leukemia
- Thymoma
- Castleman disease
- Waldenström macroglobulinemia
- Hodgkin lymphoma
- Monoclonal gammopathy
- Systemic mastocytosis.

Nonhematologic (16%)

- Carcinomas (squamous cell carcinoma of tongue, vagina, and skin; broncho-genic carcinoma; endometrial carcinoma)
- Sarcomas (liposarcoma, poorly differentiated sarcomas, leiomyosarcoma, dendritic cell sarcoma, malignant nerve sheath tumor).

Incidence
The exact incidence of PP is not clear from the existing literature, but an article in 2004 puts the number of reported cases at least at 150 cases.[57] The mean age of occurrence is 60 years, with patients varying from ages 7 to 75 years. Men and women seem to be equally affected.

Clinical manifestations
Oral involvement is seen in 100% of reported cases.[57] Extensive erosions and shallow ulcerations of the oral mucosa are usually seen. Involvement of the nasopharynx, tonsils, and esophagus in the head and neck region as well as conjunctival lesions may be observed.[58] Initial presentation with oral lesions is present in 45% of cases.[59] Cutaneous lesions have been reported in most cases and present in 5 different morphologies, such as pemphiguslike (**Fig. 8**), pemphigoidlike, graft-versus-host disease (GVHD)-like, erythema multiforme–like, and lichen planus type.[60] Other organ systems affected include the respiratory and the gastrointestinal tracts.

Pathogenesis and etiology
PP is thought to be caused by evoking both cellular and humoral immune response against tumor antigens that lead to blistering in the mucosal and epithelial surfaces. The antibodies formed are directed against desmoplakin I, desmoplakin II, periplakin, and envoplakin. Patients with PP also have antibodies to Dsg 3.

Histologic features and diagnosis
The histologic changes are similar to those observed in PV (**Fig. 9**). However, changes similar to those seen in erythema multiforme have been reported.[61] As mentioned earlier, the diagnosis depends on major and minor criteria; 3 major or 2 major and 2 minor criteria are required for the diagnosis. As in PV, immunoglobulins and complements are deposited in the epidermis in an intercellular pattern (**Fig. 10**). The immunoprecipitation pattern is characteristic of PP.

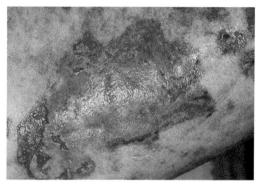

Fig. 8. A ruptured cutaneous bulla in PP.

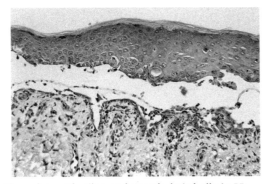

Fig. 9. An intraepidermal, suprabasilar, and acantholytic bulla in PP.

Treatment and prognosis
Treatment of PP is difficult, and the disease has poor prognosis with a survival rate of few months.[58] Treatment of the original tumor may improve symptoms. Corticosteroid use, alone or in combination with other medications (eg, cyclosporines, cyclophosphamides, plasmapheresis, immunophoresis), has been reported with limited success.

IgA Pemphigus
IgA pemphigus is a newly characterized, rare group of immune-mediated intraepidermal blistering skin (**Fig. 11**) and mucous membrane diseases and is characterized by tissue-bound and circulating IgA autoantibodies. These diseases commonly affect the oral cavity. Histologically, epidermal acantholysis and neutrophilic infiltration predominates (**Fig. 12**). The pathomechanisms of initiating the IgA autoantibodies to target desmosomal components (**Fig. 13**) (Dsg3, desmocollin 1, and desmocollin 2) are not characterized yet.[34] The clinical course of IgA-mediated pemphigus seems to be less aggressive than IgG-mediated pemphigus, with no significant morbidity.

Drug-Induced Pemphigus
Many of the drugs inducing pemphigus have been discussed under PV. Most of the patients generally improve and experience regression on cessation of the inducing drug.

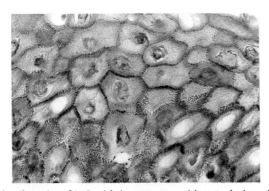

Fig. 10. Intercellular deposits of IgG with immunoperoxidase technique in PP.

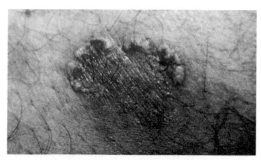

Fig. 11. Cutaneous vesicles and pustules in IgA pemphigus.

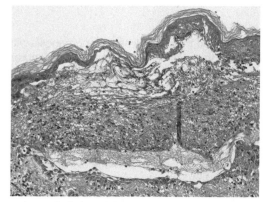

Fig. 12. Intraepidermal acantholytic vesicles containing neutrophils in IgA pemphigus.

ORAL SUBMUCOSAL BULLOUS DISEASES (PEMPHIGOIDES)
Definition

Pemphigoid is a group of chronic immune-mediated subepithelial blistering diseases that includes[62] cicatricial pemphigoid (CP), renamed mucous membrane pemphigoid (MMP), which is the most common form; bullous pemphigoid (BP); pemphigoid (herpes) gestationis; lichen planus pemphigoides; dermatitis herpetiformis (DH); linear IgA disease; epidermolysis bullosa acquisita (EBA); and bullous systemic lupus erythematosus (LE). Subepithelial bullous blistering has also been seen in PP-related cases.

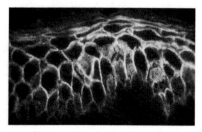

Fig. 13. Intercellular deposits of IgA antibodies in a skin biopsy of IgA pemphigus.

In pemphigoid, IgG autoantibodies can be directed against various antigens of the epithelial basement membrane.[63] In this article, the 2 most common types of pemphigoid that can affect the oral cavity, namely CP and BP, are addressed.

Cicatricial Pemphigoid (also known as Mucous Membrane Pemphigoid)

Incidence
CP is a rare condition that mainly affects the mucosal surfaces, particularly the oral mucosa (**Fig. 14**). This condition usually affects women more than men (1.5:1 ratio), with an age range of 50 to 62 years according to some studies.[64] However, the exact incidence and prevalence is unknown, but there does not seem to be a racial or geographic preference. Recent molecular characterizations of the disease have revealed the heterogeneity of CP.[62,63,65]

Clinical presentation
The heterogeneity of CP reflects itself in the variations of its clinical presentations. Patients can present with oral lesions, alone or with involvements of other mucous membranes or of skin, or systemic manifestations. Ocular involvement is a particularly serious complication (**Figs. 15** and **16**).

The oral mucosa is the initial site of lesions in most cases in which bullous[66] or vesicular lesions can occur at any of its sites. Blisters and bullae eventually rupture, leaving irregularly shaped painful erosions, which sometimes results in scarring of the mucous membrane; hence the name cicatricial with the formation of adhesions in severe cases. If the gingiva is affected, desquamative gingivitis is seen,[67] which varies from mild to severe forms.

Lesions can be limited to the oral cavity or can also affect the mucosa in other body sites (nose, esophagus, larynx, eyes, anus).[62] Up to 40% of patients who present with oral CP can develop ocular disease that can result in severe conequences, such as scarring of the conjunctiva with scleral fusion, inverted eye lid (entropion), and trichiasis. These developments can all eventually lead to opacification and blindness.[68,69] Skin involvement is usually seen in one-third of cases and can be limited to face, neck, scalp, axilla, trunk, and extremities.[70] A Nikolsky sign, as observed with PV, can be seen with CP.

Association with other autoimmune disorders and also sometimes with B-cell lymphoproliferative disorders has been observed.

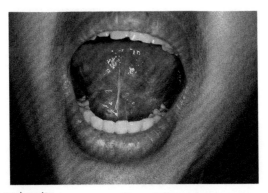

Fig. 14. CP of the oral cavity.

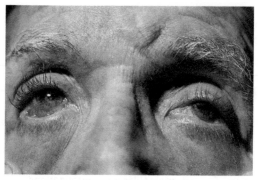

Fig. 15. Inflammation and ectropion of the eyes in CP.

Pathogenesis and etiology

The initiating events for CP are not usually known. However, in some instances, a factor, such as, a drug may be the initiating agent (eg, a medication such as furosemide).

CP is associated with autoantibodies to several components of the basement membrane autoantigens,[62] such as BP antigen (BPAg) 2[71,72] and less often to BPAg1,[72] laminin 5 (epiligrin), laminin 6, type VII collagen,[73] or β4 subunit of $\alpha_6\beta_4$ integrin.[74] HLA-DQB1*0301[75] may play a role in T-lymphocyte recognition of these antigens.

The autoantibodies formed are usually IgG and C3, but IgA or IgM may also be encountered, which may be a result of the heterogeneity of antigens.[62,76]

Complement activation with resultant increase in cytokines and other enzymes along with basal cell detachment may be one of the mechanisms involved.[62,77]

Histologic features and diagnosis

Subepithelial split with mild, chronic, inflammatory, cell infiltrate (lymphocytes, plasma cells, eosinophils, and neutrophils) may be observed (**Fig. 17**). The tissue, as in all these cases, should be taken from the tissue next to the ulcerated area.

DIF studies show deposits, usually IgG and C3, in a homogeneous linear fashion in the basement membrane zone along the epitheliomesenchymal junction.

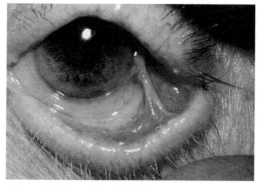

Fig. 16. Ectropion and synechia formation in CP.

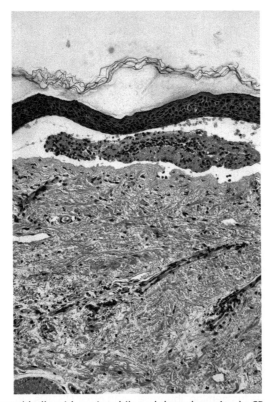

Fig. 17. Subepidermal bulla with eosinophils and dermal scarring in CP.

IIF and immunoblot assays are used to detect circulating antibodies. Using salt-split mucosa provides more sensitive assay results and shows IgG in the bullous floor. Other tests include direct and indirect immunoelectron microscopy, immunoblotting, immunoprecipitation, and ELISA.

Treatment and prognosis

Patients with only oral lesions have good prognosis and have been treated with topical drugs (corticosteroids, calcineurin anatagonists).[62] Patients with lesions that are not limited to the oral cavity have a more problematic disease process and have been treated with systemic drugs, including dapsone, corticosteroids, azathioprine, cyclophosphamide, methotrexate, mycophenolate mofetil, sulfasalazine, and other drugs.[62]

Patients who do not respond to the conventional treatments, such as high-dose systemic corticosteroids, immunosuppressant, or both, can be treated using intravenous immunoglobulins. Plasmapheresis has also been used in treating some patients. Surgical intervention is sometimes required to repair scars or other severe complications. However, surgical intervention should be advisably used because it may aggravate the disease.

Bullous Pemphigoid

Incidence

BP is uncommon in the United States, and its incidence is not clear. In Europe, this condition is recognized as the most common subepidermal bullous disease. It affects mostly patients older than 60 years, with equal sex predilection. Infant and childhood BP has also been reported.[78] No definitive racial or ethnic link has been identified. Primarily a skin disease, BP can affect the mucosal surfaces in 10% to 40% of cases.

Clinical presentation

BP has been reported in the oral cavity in up to 40% of the patients in some series, but presence of the condition in the oral cavity is not usually the presenting symptom, and the presenting symptom is usually limited to the oropharynx.[79] Most of the cases present with skin lesions; however, ocular involvement can also be seen rarely. The onset may be acute or subacute. Pruritus and widespread tense blisters are usually seen on an erythematous skin (**Fig. 18**). The blisters are usually tense and eventually they rupture, become flaccid and ulcerate, resulting in an ulcerated erythematous area.[80] The size of the blisters is variable from small vesicles to larger bullae.

Several distinct clinical forms of BP occur, including[79,81,82]

- Generalized bullous form, oral and ocular involvement usually occurs with this form
- Vesicular form
- Vegetative plaque form
- Generalized erythroderma form
- Urticarial form from which bullae eventually arise
- Nodular form
- Acral form
- Infant form.

Pathogenesis and etiology

BP has been reported to be induced by ultraviolet radiation, radiotherapy, and some drugs or medications furosemide, ibuprofen, and other NSAIDs, antibiotics, penicillamine, and captopril, among others.[83,84]

In BP autoantibodies, usually IgGs are formed against specific hemidesmosomal BP antigens BP230 (BPAg1) and a transmembrane protein with a collagenous extracellular domain BP 180 (BPAg2).[85] BPAg2 has been identified as the major antigen involved in the development of BP, and serum autoantibodies against BPAg2 has been correlated with the disease activity.[86] Other autoantibodies against α_6 integrin[87] and laminin 5[88] have also been observed.

Some cytokines and chemokines have been found to play a role in BP, including eotaxin, interleukin 16, MIG, CCL17, and CCL22.[89,90]

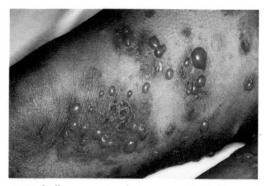

Fig. 18. BP showing tense bullae on an erythematous urticarial base of skin.

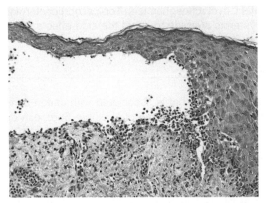

Fig. 19. A subepidermal bulla with a viable roof and numerous eosinophils in BP.

Histologic features and diagnosis

The samples for biopsies, like in other bullous diseases, are obtained from the perilesional tissue of a new blister. A classic biopsy specimen shows a subepidermal or submucosal bulla with a viable roof. The associated inflammatory infiltrate is mixed and is particularly rich in eosinophils, which is contained in the bullous cavity (**Fig. 19**). Mast cells and basophils can predominate early in the course of the disease. A cell-poor BP with minimal cellular infiltrate has also been observed.

DIF studies usually demonstrate IgG and C3 deposition in a linear fashion (**Fig. 20**) along the junction of the epithelium and subepithelium. DIF assay on a salt-split skin demonstrates IgG in the blister roof in patients with BP, which differentiates BP from CP and EBA.

IIF and immunoblot assays are used to detect circulating antibodies. Other tests include direct and indirect immunoelectron microscopy, immunoblotting, immunoprecipitation, and ELISA.

Treatment and prognosis

In most patients with BP who are treated for the condition, the disease remits within 1.5 to 5 years. However, BP can be life threatening in debilitated patients. Treatment modalities include antiinflammatory agents (eg, corticosteroids, dapsone, tetracyclines) and immunosuppressant agents (eg, azathioprine, methotrexate,

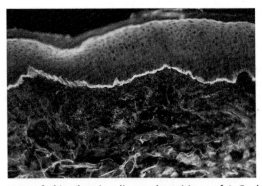

Fig. 20. DIF microscopy of skin showing linear depositions of IgG along the basement membrane zone in BP.

mycophenolate mofetil, cyclophosphamide). Topical corticosteroids have been advocated in place of systemic steroids to avoid the side effects of systemic treatment, particularly in the elderly.

Dermatitis Herpetiformis

Incidence

DH is an autoimmune disorder that is associated with gluten-sensitive enteropathy. DH occurs more frequently in the people of Northern European descent and is rare in Asians and Africans. The prevalence of DH is approximately 10 per 100,000 cases worldwide. HLA-DQA1*0501, HLA-DR3, HLA-B8, and HLA-B1*02, which encodes HLA-DQ2, heterodimers have been linked to prevalence.[91] A male to female ratio of 1.5:1 or 2:1 is seen,[92] usually affecting people mostly in the second to fourth decades of life.[93] However, any age, including children's age groups, may be affected.

Oral involvement in DH is extremely rare,[94] and patients with linear IgA bullous dermatosis (discussed later) are more likely to have oral involvement.

Clinical presentation

The history is typically of intensely pruritic papulovesicular eruptions on the extensor surfaces of the arms, knees, back, and buttocks. Gluten, as mentioned, exacerbates symptoms. Periods of exacerbation and remissions are typical of the disease. Oral involvement, as mentioned, is infrequent and men are more likely affected than women.[94] Observation of vesicles and bullae in the oral mucosa is rather difficult because these structures tend to rupture or excoriate quickly, leaving tender ulcers.

Pathogenesis and etiology

Etiologically, DH is considered as one of the manifestations of celiac disease.[95] The presence of granular IgA deposits in normal-appearing perilesional skin is detected by DIF assay in 92.4% of patients. Most of these deposits are located in the dermal papillae. Of the cases, 10% show continuous granular deposits at the basement membrane in both papillary and nonpapillary lesions.[96] C3 deposits can also be seen.

Histologic features and diagnosis

Accumulation of neutrophils in the dermal papillae are noted, which can eventually form papillary microabscesses that causes vacuolization, with separation and blister formation between the tips of the epidermis and the papillae. Coalesced blisters may give rise to larger tense blisters with an increased number of eosinophils in the blister. Biopsy samples should be taken from the perilesional mucosa rather than from the blister site for more accurate diagnosis.

Most patients with oral DH have a histologic evidence of enteropathy. In addition to the granular and linear IgA deposits observed in this disease, serum markers, such as IgA endomysial antibodies, can be seen.

Treatment and prognosis

DH is a lifelong disease with variable severity. Patients on a gluten-free diet and who can tolerate dapsone treatment[97] usually have a good prognosis. Patients who also have gluten-sensitive enteropathies accompanying DH are at risk of developing lymphoma.[98]

Linear IgA Disease

Incidence

Linear IgA disease is a rare autoimmune subepithelial disease that predominantly involves the skin with bimodal presentation (age group of 6 months to 10 years in children and 14–83 years in adults); however, oral involvement has been reported in this entity in up to 70% of patients with the disease.[99] The incidence of the disease has been only sporadically reported in different parts of the world; for example, the incidence in Utah (United States) is 0.6 per 100,000 cases and in France is 0.13 per 100,000 cases.[100] A slight female predominance has been reported (1.6:1).

According to a recent review article,[99] approximately 17 cases predominantly with oral involvement are reported in the literature, with the age range of these cases being between 29 and 79 years (10 women and 7 men). This finding suggests that IgA disease can manifest primarily as an oral presentation and not only second to a predominant skin presentation.

Clinical presentation
In most cases of linear IgA disease, the dermatologic manifestations are the main ones, with clear and/or hemorrhagic round or oval vesicles or bullae on normal, erythematous, or urticarial skin; erythematous papules; or blanching macules and papules. When this is the case, the oral manifestations tend to be minor. However, when the oral manifestations are the predominant, they include vesicles and bullae, painful ulcers and erosions, erosive cheilitis, desquamative gingivitis, and white patches with erythema,[99] and these manifestations may be severe enough to be histologically and clinically confused with other entities, especially CP and erosive lichen planus. In the 17 reported cases of predominant oral presentation, gingival erythema and desquamative gingivitis were observed. Ocular lesions also occur.

Pathogenesis and etiology
The cause of the disease is related to an environmental trigger, such as infectious agents (eg, herpesvirus, varicella, and agents causing typhoid and upper respiratory tract infections), or drug (eg, vancomycin, captopril, ampicillin sodium, phenytoin, amoxicillin, cyclosporines) or can be associated with lymphoproliferative disease (eg, Hodgkin and non-Hodgkin lymphomas, chronic lymphocytic leukemia) and different types of cancers (eg, thyroid, colon, uterine) that lead to the production of IgA autoantibodies against different antigenic sites in the basement membrane, including the lamina lucida, sublamina densa, or both locations, and formation of the characteristic linear IgA deposits. These antigenic sites include a 97-kDa protein antigen, which may be the extracellular portion of BPAg2.[101] Other antigens include a 120-kDa antigen, a 230-kDa antigen (BPAg1), and a 250-kDa antigen.[102]

Histologic features and diagnosis
The early changes show neutrophilic infiltrate aligned along the basement membrane (**Fig. 21**), with basal vacuolar degeneration. Neutrophilic microabscesses may be encountered in the dermal papillae. As the lesion progresses, subepidermal separation and blister formation without necrosis of the epithelial roof of the blister is seen, with predominantly polymorphic infiltrate that may show eosinophils.

DIF assay shows linear IgA in the basement membrane zone. Some patients show both linear IgA and IgG deposition, and IgM has been rarely reported. Of the patients, 50% have detectable IgA serum antibodies that bind to the basement membrane zone.

Treatment and prognosis
Most reported cases respond to dapsone (alone or with corticosteroids)[103] or sulfapyridine. Other drugs include sulfamethoxypyridazine, colchicine, dicloxacillin, mycophenolate mofetil, and intravenous immunoglobulins. Withdrawal of the precipitating

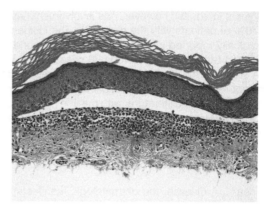

Fig. 21. Linear IgA dermatosis showing a band of neutrophils in a subepidermal bulla.

drug in drug-induced cases effectively reverses the course of the disease. In severe cases, oral corticosteroids may be used.

Remission has been reported in most cases of children within 2 years; however, adult diseases tend to run a more protracted course and the remission rate is less than that of the children. Oral lesions, such as desquamative gingivitis, lead to scarring and teeth damage. Extension to the larynx, pharynx, nose, and esophagus has also been reported.

Oral Lichen Planus

Definition
Oral lichen planus (OLP) is a chronic T-cell–mediated autoimmune disease in which autocytotoxic T lymphocytes trigger apoptosis of epithelial cells, causing white striations, papules, or plaques in the oral mucosa and gingiva, which may or may not be accompanied by erythema, blisters, and erosions.

Incidence
OLP is a common disorder seen worldwide, usually in adults older than 40 years, and is more common in women than in men (2:1) and affects all racial groups.[104,105] Younger age groups and children age groups can also be affected. OLP affects 1% to 2% of the general adult population, although the prevalence is not studied in many world locations.[106]

Clinical appearance
The presentation of OLP is variable. Some patients may be unaware of their condition and are discovered during routine clinical examination, whereas some complain of oral discomfort and soreness, particularly with atrophic erosive lesions. On occasions, lesions appear after variable types of dental procedures or after administration of systemic drugs (eg, NSAIDs, sulfonylureas, antimalarials, β-blockers). Concomitant skin lesions are seen in 44% of patients, and genital involvement is also encountered in 25% of women and in 2% of men with OLP. Other sites involved include the scalp (lichen planopilaris), nails, larynx, conjunctiva, and esophagus. Genital lesions, mostly seen in women, are also seen.[104]

Oral mucosal lesions usually occur on the buccal mucosa (**Fig. 22**), gingiva, tongue (mainly dorsum), labial mucosa, and vermilion of the lower lip.[104,107,108] Desquamative gingivitis may occur in some cases that appear similar to keratinous lesions (eg, leukoplakia).[109]

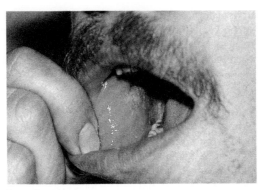

Fig. 22. OLP of the buccal mucosa.

The lesions may appear in different forms or a mixture of the following forms: white striations (Wickham striae) or reticular form, white papules, white plaques, erythema (mucosal atrophy), blisters and bullae formation/erosions (**Fig. 23**), and shallow ulcers.

OLP is characterized by remissions and exacerbation periods, which lasts for many years, and seem to be precipitated in periods of stress.

Pathogenesis and etiology

The precise cause of OLP in not well defined. Several associated factors have been observed, including mechanical trauma; systemic drugs[110] (β-blockers, sulfonylureas, ACE inhibitors, and some antimalarial drugs); human papillomavirus, herpesvirus 6, hepatitis C virus infections[111]; and contact sensitivity (dental amalgam resins, toothpaste flavorings).[112] OLP has also been observed as one of the manifestations that can be observed in GVHD.[113]

A T-cell–mediated autoimmune process in which cytotoxic CD8$^+$ T cells trigger the apoptosis of epithelial cells is theorized as one of the mechanisms of OLP.

Histologic features and diagnosis

Histologic examination of the affected squamous mucosa is the more-effective way for diagnosing OLP and usually reveals a bandlike subepithelial mononuclear cell infiltrate (T-lymphocytes and histocytes), intraepithelial T-cell infiltrate, and degenerating basal cells keratinocytes (Civatte bodies) that appear as homogenous eosinophilic globules. Sawtooth rete pegs, acanthosis, and parakeratosis are also observed.

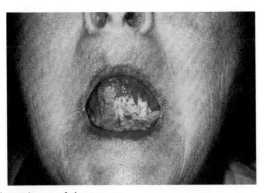

Fig. 23. Erosive lichen planus of the tongue.

The degenerating basal cells can cause notable disruption of the epithelial subepithelial adhesion resulting in cleft; blisters and bullae formation (bullous lichen planus) may be seen on clinical examination.

DIF testing is not useful in diagnosing the disease because it shows nonspecific findings, and paradoxically, specific findings may indicate a bullous etiology different from OLP.

Treatment and prognosis

Topical corticosteroids are the main line of treatment. Oral rinses containing dexamethasone, triamcinolone, and clobetasol can also be used. Several systemic immunosuppressive agents have been used, including dapsone, azathioprine, and cyclosporine, among others.

OLP is a chronic disease condition that can be long lasting (up to 20 years), particularly the erosive forms. Oral squamous cell carcinoma develops in fewer than 5% of patients with lichen planus.[104]

CONDITIONS THAT CAN CAUSE ORAL MUCOSAL BASAL CELL LAYER LIQUEFACTION OR VACUOLIZATION
Lupus Erythematosus

LE is a systemic autoimmune disease that affects the connective tissue and multiple vital organs and presents with classic signs and symptoms set by the American College of Rheumatology.

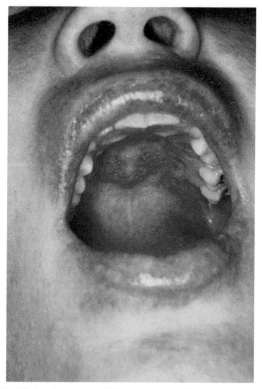

Fig. 24. Systemic LE with involvement of the palate and lips.

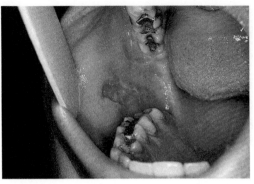

Fig.25. Discoid LE showing sharply marginated ulcer of the buccal mucosa.

Oral lesions, if they occur in LE, usually involve the palatal (**Fig. 24**) and gingival mucosa with occasional ulcerations (**Fig. 25**). The histologic findings show alternating areas of epithelial acanthosis and atrophy with focal basal cell liquefaction (**Fig. 26**) and occasional intraepithelial vesicles with subepithelial lymphocytic infiltrate, with upward migration of the lymphocytes and also deep lymphocytic infiltrate in the lamina propria.

DIF assays of the affected mucosa show granular deposits of one or more immunoreactants (IgG, IgM, or C3).

Erythema Multiforme (EM)

Erythema multiforme occurs in 3 forms:

- Erythema multiforme minor, usually herpes simplex associated (fever, malaise, and multiform lesions of skin and mucous membranes). Oral lesions occur in 25% of cases, with the lips being the most frequent involvement site, followed by the buccal mucosa, tongue, and soft palate. The oral lesions start as erythematous patches that gradually become painful ulcers.
- Stevens-Johnson syndrome (**Fig. 27**), a more sever form usually representing adverse drug reaction (stomatitis, purulent conjunctivitis, and multiform skin lesions). In 20% of cases severe, lesions occur in the oral cavity and eyes, with vesicular or bullous lesions that eventually become painful ulcers

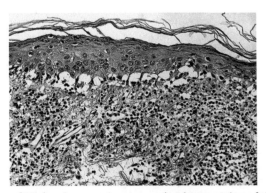

Fig. 26. Skin biopsy of LE showing prominent vacuolar degeneration of the basal cell layer.

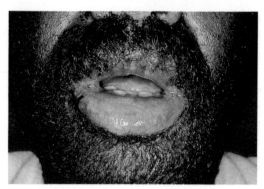

Fig. 27. Erythema multiforme (Stevens-Johnson syndrome) with extensive erosions of the lips and oral mucosa.

- Toxic epidermal necrolysis (TEN), the most severe form, also usually represents adverse drug reaction (detachment of full-thickness epidermis, partially or totally necrotic with eventual sloughing). The oral mucosa and the pharyngeal mucosa are very frequently affected in TEN.

The histologic appearance of lesional biopsy samples is similar in all entities and is not helpful in predicting the causative factor. Basal cell vacuolization with lymphocytic infiltrate and individual cell necrosis out of proportion to the number of lymphocytes occur. The dermal infiltrate is at the dermoepidermal junction as well as around the upper dermal vessels.

Graft Versus Host Disease (GVHD)

The median onset of GVHD is 6 months after transplantation. Oral manifestations of GVHD can be seen in up to 80% of patients with xerostomia (caused by minor salivary gland in a fashion similar to that seen in Sjögren syndrome) and oral ulcers and infections. The histologic appearance, as mentioned under OLP, is of interface lesions with basal cell degeneration, intracellular edema, and lymphocytic infiltrate in the submucosa.

REFERENCES

1. Becker BA, Gaspari AA. Pemphigus vulgaris and vegetans. Dermatol Clin 1993; 11:453–62.
2. Camacho-Alonso F, Lopez-Jornet P, Bermejo-Fenoll A. Pemphigus vulgaris. A presentation of 14 cases and review of the literature. Med Oral Pathol Oral Cir Bucal 2005;10:282–8.
3. Lamey PJ, Rees TD, Binnie WH, et al. Oral presentation of pemphigus vulgaris and its response to systemic steroid therapy. Oral Surg oral Med Oral Pathol 1992;74:54–7.
4. Rabinowitz LG, Esterly NB. Inflammatory bullous diseases in children. Dermatol Clin 1993;11:565–81.
5. Tron F, Gilbert D, Mouquet H, et al. Genetic factors in pemphigus. J Autoimmun 2005;24:319–28.
6. Pisanty S, Sharav Y, Kaufman E, et al. Pemphigus vulgaris: incidence in Jews of different ethnic groups according to age, sex and initial lesion. Oral Surg oral Med Oral Pathol 1974;38:382–7.

7. Koulou L, Stanley JR. Clinical, histologic, and immunopathologic comparison of pemphigus vulgaris, and pemphigus foliaceous. Semin Dermatol 1988;7:82–90.
8. Zagarelli D, Zagarelli E. Intraoral pemphigus vulgaris. Oral Surg oral Med Oral Pathol 1977;44:384–93.
9. Shah RM, Billmoria KF. Oral pemphigus vulgaris. Clinico-pathological followup of 34 cases. J Oral Med 1983;38:170–3.
10. Kanwar AJ, Dhar S. Oral pemphigus vulgaris. Pediat Dermatol 1995;12:195–7.
11. Scully C, Paes De Almeida O, Porter SR, et al. Pemphigus vulgaris: the manifestations and long term management of 55 patients with oral lesions. Br J Dermatol 1999;140:84–9.
12. Scully C, Callacombe SJ. Pemphigus Vulgaris: update on etiopathogenesis, oral manifestations and managements. Crit Rev Oral Biol Med 2002;13:397–408.
13. Shklar G, Frim S, Flynn E. Gingival lesions of pemphigus. J periodontal 1978;49:428–35.
14. Markitziu A, Pisanty S. Gingival pemphigus vulgaris. Oral Surg oral Med Oral Pathol 1983;55:250–2.
15. Mignogna MD, Lo Muzio L, Bucci E. Clinical features of gingival pemphigus vulgaris. J Clin Periodontol 2001;28:489–93.
16. Weinberg MA, Insler MS, Campen RB. Mucocutaneous features of autoimmune blistering diseases. Oral Surg oral Med Oral Pathol Oral Radiol Endod 1997;84:517–34.
17. Mimouni D, Anhalt GJ. Pemphigus. Dermatol Ther 2002;15:362–8.
18. Lombardi ML, Mercuro O, Tecame G, et al. Molecular analysis of HLA DRB1 and DQB1 in Italian patients with pemphigus vulgaris. Tissue Antigens 1996;47:228–30.
19. Mobini N, Padilla Jr T, Ahmed AR. Long-term remission in selected patients with pemphigus vulgaris treated with cyclosporine. J Am Acad Dermatol 1997;36:264–6.
20. Delgado JC, Hameed A, Yunis JJ, et al. Pemphigus vulagris autoantibody response is linked to HLA-DQB1*0503 in Pakistani patients. Hum Immunol 1997;57:110–9.
21. Loiseau P, Lecleach L, Prost C, et al. HLA class II polymorphism contributes to specify desmoglein derived peptides in pemphigus vulgaris and pemphigus foliaceous. J Autoimmun 2000;15:67–73.
22. Glorio R, Rodriguez CG, Haas R, et al. HLA haplotypes and class II molecular alleles in Argentinian patients with pemphigus vulgaris. J Cut Med Surg 2002;6(No.5):422–6.
23. Tur E, Brenner S. Diet and pemphigus. In pursuit of exogenous factors in pemphigus and fogo selvagem. Arch Dermatol 1998;134:1406–10.
24. Ruocco E, Aurilia A, Ruocco V. Precautions and suggestions for pemphigus patients. Arch Dermatol 2001;203:201–7.
25. Bastuji-Garin S, Turki H, Mokhtar I, et al. Possible relation of Tunisian pemphigus with traditional cosmetics. Am J epidemiol 2002;155:249–56.
26. Ruocco V, Wolf R, Ruocco E, et al. Viruses in pemphigus: a casual or causal relationship? Int J Dermatol 1996b;35:782–4.
27. Takashi I, Kobyashi TK, Nakamura S, et al. Coexistence of pemphigus vulgaris and herpes simplex virus infection in oral mucosa diagnosed by cytology, immunohistochemistry and polymerase chain reaction. Diag Cytopathol 1998;19:446–50.
28. Memer OM, Rady PL, Goldblum RM, et al. Human herpes virus 8 DNA sequences in blistering skin from patients with pemphigus. Arch Dermatol 1997;133:1247–51.

29. Jang HS, Oh CK, Lim JY, et al. Detection of HHV 8 DNA in pemphigus and chronic blistering skin diseases. J Korean Med Sci 2000;15:442–8.
30. Brenner S, Tur E, Shapiro J, et al. Pemphigus Vulgaris: environmental factors, occupational, behavioral, medical, and qualitative food frequency questionnaire. Int J Dermatol 2001;40:562–9.
31. Harman KE, Seed PT, Gratian MJ, et al. The severity of cutaneous and oral pemphigus is related to desmoglein 1 and 3 antibody levels. Br. J Dermatol 2001;775–80.
32. Harman KE, Gratian MJ, Bhogal BS, et al. A study of desmoglobin 1 autoantibodies in pemphigus vulgaris: racial differences in frequency and the association with a more severe phenotype. Br J Dermatol 2000;143:343–8.
33. Tremeau-Martinage C, Oksman F, Bazex J. Immunoglobulin G subclass distribution of anti-intercellular substance antibodies in pemphigus. Ann Dermatol Venereol 1995;122:409–11.
34. Scully C, Mignogna M. Oral mucosal disease. Pemphigus. Br. J oral Maxillofac Surg 2008;46:272–7.
35. Anhalt GJ, Diaz LA. Prospects for autoimmune disease: research advances in pemphigus. JAMA 2001;285:652–4.
36. Frusic-Zoltkin M, Pergmentz R, Michel B, et al. The interaction of pemphigus autoimmunoglobulins with epidermal cells: activation of the fas apoptotic pathway and the use of caspase activity for pathogenicity tests of pemphigus patients. Ann N Y Acad Sci 2005;1050:371–9.
37. Herbst A, Bystryn JC. Patterns of remission in pemphigus vulgaris. J Am Acad Dermatol 2000;42:422–7.
38. Turner MS, Sutton D, Sauder DN. The use of plasmapheresis and immunosuppression in the treatment of pemphigus vulgaris. J Am Acad Dermatol 2000;43: 1058–64.
39. Akerman L, Minouni D, David M. Intravenous immunoglobulin for treatment of pemphigus. Clin Rev Allergy Immunol 2005;29:289–94.
40. Powell AM, Albert S, Alfares S, et al. An evaluation for the usefulness of mycophenolate mofetil in pemphigus. Br J Dermatol 2003;149:138–45.
41. Wu SJ, Tanphaichitr A. Recent advances in dermatology. Clin Paediatr Med Surg 2002;19:65–78.
42. Nguyen VT, Arrendondo J, Chernyavsky AI, et al. Pemphigus vulgaris acantholysis ameliorated by cholinergic agonists. Arch Dermatol 2004;140:327–34.
43. Frost N, Messer G, Fierbeck G, et al. Treatment of pemphigus vulgaris with protein immunoadsorption: case report of long term history showing favorable outcome. Ann NY Acad Sci 2005;1051:591–6.
44. Schmidt E, Herzog S, Brocker EB, et al. Longstanding remission of recalcitrant juvenile pemphigus vulgaris after adjuvant therapy and rituximab. Br J Dermatol 2005;153:449–51.
45. Sillevis Smitt JH, Mulder TJ, Albeda FW, et al. Pemphigus vegetans in a child. Br J dermatol 1992;127:280–91.
46. Jansen T, Messer G, Meurer M, et al. Pemphigus vegetans. Eine Historische Betrachtung. Hautarzt 2001;52:504–9.
47. Virgili A, Thrombelli L, Calura G, et al. Sudden vegetations of the mouth (Hallopeau type). Arch Dermatol 1992;128:398–402.
48. Ahmed AR, Blose DA. Pemphigus vegetans. Int J Dermatol 1984;23:135–41.
49. Markopoulos AK, Antoniades DZ, Zaraboukas T. Pemphigus vegetans of the oral cavity. Int J Dermatol 2006;45:425–8.

50. Hashimoto K, Hashimoto T, Higashiyama M, et al. Detection of antidesmocollins I and II autoantibodies in two cases of Hallopeau type pemphigus vegetans by immunoblot analysis. J Dermatol Sci 1994;7(2):100–6.
51. Cozzani E, Christana K, Mastrogiacomo A, et al. Pemphigus vegetans Neumann type with anti desmoglein and anti-periplakin autoantibodies. Eur J Dermatol 2007;17(6):530–3.
52. Morizane S, Yamamoto T, Hishamatsu Y, et al. Pemphigus vegetans with IgG and IgA antidesmoglein 3 antibodies. Br J Dermatol 2005;153(6):1236.
53. Ichimiya M, Yamamoto K, Muto M. Successful treatment of pemphigus vegetans by addition of etretinate to systemic steroids. Clin Exp Dermatol 1998;23: 178–80.
54. Anhalt GJ, Kim SC, Stanley JR, et al. Paraneoplastic pemphigus. An autoimmune mucocutaneous disease associated with neoplasia. N Eng J Med 1990; 323(25):1729–35.
55. Camisa C, Helm TN. Paraneoplastic pemphigus is a distinct neoplasia-induced autoimmune disease. Arch Dermatol 1993;129(7):883–6.
56. Anhalt GJ. Paraneoplastic pemphigus. J Investig Dermatol Symp Proc 2004; 9(1):29–33.
57. Kaplan I, Hodak E, Ackerman L, et al. Neoplasms associated with paraneoplastic pemphigus: a review with emphasis on non-hematologic malignancy and oral mucosal manifestations. Oral Oncol 2004;40:553–62.
58. Kimyai-Asadi A, Jih MH. Paraneoplastic pemphigus. Int J Dermatol 2001;40(6): 367–72.
59. Joly P, Richard C, Gilbert D, et al. Sensitivity and specificity of clinical, histologic, and immunologic features in the diagnosis of paraneoplastic pemphigus. J Am Acad Dermatol 2000;43(4):619–26.
60. Nguyen VT, Ndoye A, Bassler KD, et al. Classification, clinical manifestations, and immunopathological mechanisms of the epithelial variant of paraneoplastic autoimmune multiorgan syndrome: a reappraisal of paraneoplastic pemphigus. Arch Dermatol 2001;37(2):193–206.
61. Horn TD, Anhalt GJ. Histologic features of paraneoplastic pemphigus. Arch Dermatol 1992;128:1091–5.
62. Scully C, Muzio L. Oral mucosal disease: mucous membrane pemphigoid. Br J Oral Maxil Surg 2008;46:258–366.
63. Barnadas MA, Gonzalez MJ, Planaguma M, et al. Clinical, histopathologic, and therapeutic aspects of subepidermal autoimmune bullous diseases with IgG on the floor of salt-split skin. Int J Dermatol 2001;40:268–72.
64. Bagan J, Lo Muzio L, Scully C. Mucous membrane pemphigoid. Oral Dis 2005; 11:197–218.
65. Verdolini R, Cerio R. Autoimmune subepidermal bullous disease: the impact of recent findings for the dermatopathologist. Virchows Arch 2003;443:184–93.
66. Alkan A, Gunhan O, Otan F. A clinical study of oral mucous membrane pemphigoid. J Int Med Res 2003;31:340–4.
67. Scully C, Porter SR. The clinical spectrum of desquamative gingivitis. Semin Cut Med Surg 1997;16:308–13.
68. Higgins GT, Allan R, Hall R, et al. Development of ocular disease in patients with mucous membrane pemphigoid involving the oral mucosa. Br J Ophthalmol 2006;90:964–7.
69. Mutasim DF, Pelc NJ, Anhalt GJ. Cicatricial pemphigoid. Dermatol Clin 1993;11: 499–510.

70. Chan LS, Ahmed AR, Anhalt GJ. The first international consensus on mucous membrane pemphigoid: definition, diagnostic criteria, pathogenic factors, medical treatment, and prognostic indications. Arch Dermatol 2002;138: 370–9.

71. Bernard P, Prost C, Durepaire N, et al. The major cicatricial pemphigoid antigen is a 180-kD protein that shows immunologic cross-reactivities with the bullous pemphigoid antigen. J Invest Dermatol 1992;99:174–9.

72. Balding SD, Prost C, Diaz LA, et al. Cicatricial pemphigoid autoantibodies react at multiple sites on the BP180 extracellular domain. J Invest Dermatol 1996;106: 141–6.

73. Roh JY, Yee C, Lazarova Z, et al. The 120-kDa soluble ectodomain of type XVII collagen is recognized by autoantibodies in patients with pemphigoid and linear IgA dermatosis. Br J Dermatol 2000;143:104–11.

74. Bhol KC, Dans MJ, Simmons RK, et al. The autoantibodies to alpha 6 beta 4 integrin of patients affected by ocular cicatricial pemphigoid recognize predominantly epitopes within the large cytoplasmic domain of human beta 4. J Immunol 2000;165:2824–9.

75. Carrozzo M, Fasano ME, Broccoletti R, et al. HLA-DQB1 alleles in Italian patients with mucous membrane pemphigoid predominantly affecting the oral cavity. Br J Dermatol 2001;145:805–8.

76. Daniels TE, Quadra-white C. Direct immunofluorescence in oral mucosal disease: a diagnostic analysis of 130 cases. Oral Surg Oral Med Oral Pathol 1981;51:38–47.

77. Eversole LR. Immunopathology of oral mucosal ulcerative, desquamative, and bullous diseases. Selective review of the literature. Oral Surg Oral Med Oral Pathol 1994;77:555–71.

78. Gajic-Veljic M, Nikolic M, Medenica L. Juvenile bullous pemphigoid: the presentation and follow-up of six cases. J Eur Acad Dermatol Venereol 2010;24:69–72.

79. Laskaris G, Sklavounou A, Stratigos J. Bullous pemphigoid, cicatricial pemphigoid and pemphigus vulgaris. Oral Surg Oral Med Oral Pathol 1982;54:656–62.

80. Korman NJ. Bullous pemphigoid. Cutan Med Surg 1996;664–73.

81. Sun C, Chang B, Gu H. Non-bullous lesions as the first manifestation of bullous pemphigoid: a retrospective analysis of 24 cases. J Dermatolog Treat 2009; 20(4):233–7.

82. Waisbourd-Zinman O, Ben-Amitai D, Cohen AD, et al. Bullous pemphigoid in infancy: clinical and epidemiologic characteristics. J Am Acad Dermatol 2008; 58(1):41–8.

83. Ruocco V, Sacerdoti G. Pemphigus and bullous pemphigoid due to drugs. Int J Dermatol 1991;30:307–12.

84. Bastuji-Garin S, Joly P, Picard Dahan C, et al. Drugs associated with bullous pemphigoid. Arch Dermatol 1996;132:272–6.

85. Xu L, Robinson N, Miller SD, et al. Characterization of BALB/c mice B lymphocyte autoimmune responses to skin basement membrane component type XVII collagen, the target antigen of autoimmune skin disease bullous pemphigoid. Immunol Lett 2001;77(2):105–11.

86. Schmidt E, Obe K, Brocker EB, et al. Serum levels of autoantibodies to BP180 correlates with disease activity in patients with bullous pemphigoid. Arch Dermatol 2000;136(2):174–8.

87. Kiss M, Perenyi A, Marczinovits I, et al. Autoantibodies to human alpha6 integrin in patients with bullous pemphigoid. Ann N Y Acad Sci 2005;1051:104–10.

88. Bekou V, Thoma-Uszynski S, Wendler O, et al. Detection of laminin 5-specific auto-antibodies in mucous membrane and bullous pemphigoid sera by ELISA. J Invest Dermatol 2005;124(4):732–40.
89. Frezzolini A, Cianchini G, Ruffelli M, et al. Interleukin-16 expression and release in bullous pemphigoid. Clin Exp Immunol 2004;137(3):595–600.
90. Echigo T, Hasegawa M, Shimada Y, et al. Both Th1 and Th2 chemokines are elevated in sera of patients with autoimmune blistering diseases. Arch Dermatol Res 2006;298(1):38–45.
91. Hall RP. Dermatitis herpetiformis. J Invest Dermatol 1992;99:873–81.
92. Bardella MT, Fredella C, Saladino V, et al. Gluten intolerance: gender- and age-related differences in symptoms. Scand J Gastroenterl 2005;40(1):15–9.
93. Templet JT, Welsh JP, Cusack CA. Childhood dermatitis herpetiformis: a case report and review of the literature. Cutis 2007;80(6):473–6.
94. Lahteenoja H, Irjala K, Viander M, et al. Oral mucosa is frequently affected in patients with dermatitis herpetiformis. Arch Dermatol 1998;134(6):756–8.
95. Fry L, Kier P, McMinn R, et al. Small intestinal structure and function and hematological changes in dermatitis herpetiformis. Lancet 1967;2:729–34.
96. Van L, Browning JC, Krishnan RS, et al. Dermatitis herpetiformis: potential for confusion with linear IgA bullous dermatosis on direct immunofluorescence. Dermatol Online J 2008;14(1):21.
97. Coleman MD. Dapsone: modes of action, toxicity and possible strategies for increasing patient tolerance. Br J Dermatol 1993;129(5):507–13.
98. Sigurgeirsson B, Agnarsson BA, Lindelof B. Risk of lymphoma in patients with dermatitis herpetiformis. BMJ 1994;308(6920):13–5.
99. Betts A, Yeoman CM, Farthing PM. Oral mucosal involvement as the sole or main manifestation of linear IgA disease: case report and review of the literature. Oral Surgery 2009;2:198–204.
100. Bernard P, Vaillant L, Labeille B, et al. Incidence and distribution of subepidermal autoimmune bullous skin diseases in three French regions. Bullous Diseases French Study Group. Arch Dermatol 1995;131(1):48–52.
101. Zone JJ, Taylor TB, Meyer LJ, et al. The 97 kDa linear IgA bullous disease antigen is identical to a portion of the extracellular domain of the 180 kDa bullous pemphigoid antigen BPAg2. J Invest Dermatol 1998;110:207–10.
102. Hirako Y, Nishizawa Y, Sitaru C, et al. The 97-kD and 120-Kd (LAD-1) fragments of bullous pemphigoid antigen 180/type XVII collagen have different N-termini. J Invest Dermatol 2003;121:1554–6.
103. Sago J, Hall RP. Dapsone. Dermatol Ther 2002;15:340–51.
104. Eisen D. The clinical features, malignant potential and systemic associations of oral lichen planus: a study of 723 patients. J Am Acad Dermatol 2002;46:207–14.
105. Eisen D, Carrozzo M, Bagan Sebastian JV, et al. Oral lichen planus: clinical features and management. Oral Dis 2005;11:338–49.
106. Axéll T, Rundquist L. Oral lichen planus–a demographic study. Community Dent Oral Epidemiol 1987;15(1):52–6.
107. Scully C, Carrozzo M. Oral mucosal disease: Lichen planus. Br J oral Maxillo fac Surg 2008;46:15–21.
108. Silverman Jr S, Grosky M, Lozada-Nur F. A prospective follow-up study of 570 patients with oral lichen planus: persistence, remission, and malignant associations. Oral Surg Oral Med Oral Pathol 1985;60(1):30–4.
109. Scully C, Porter SR. The clinical spectrum of desquamative gingivitis. Semin Cutan Med Surg 1997;14:431–58.

110. Robertson WD, Wray D. Ingestion of medications among patients with oral keratosis including lichen planus. Oral Surg Oral Med Oral Pathol 1992;74:183–5.
111. Carrozzo M, Gandolfo S. Oral disease possibly associated with hepatitis C virus. Crit Rev Oral Biol Med 2003;14:115–27.
112. Thornhill MH, Pemberton MN, Simmons RK, et al. Amalgam contact hypersensitivity lesions and oral lichen planus. Oral Surg Oral Med Oral Pathol Oral Radiol Oral Endod 2003;95:291–9.
113. Nakamura S, Hiroki AS, et al. Oral involvement in chronic graft-versus-host disease after allogeneic bone marrow transplantation. Oral Surg Oral Med Oral Pathol Oral Radiol Oral Endod 1996;82:556–63.

Common Oral Manifestations of Systemic Disease

Nadim M. Islam, DDS, MS[a],*, Indraneel Bhattacharyya, DDS, MSD[b],
Donald M. Cohen, DMD, MS, MBA[b]

KEYWORDS

- Oral manifestations • Anemia • Rheumatoid arthritis
- Amyloidosis • Neoplasm • Crohn disease • Endocrine disease
- Pyostomatitis vegetans

HEMATOLOGIC DISEASES
Iron-Deficiency Anemia

Iron-deficiency anemia is one of the most common causes of anemia worldwide.[1] This type of anemia has a direct relationship between the lack of availability of iron in the body and the demand of red blood cells (RBCs). Oral manifestations may include angular cheilitis, atrophic glossitis, mucosal pallor, and generalized atrophy of the oral mucosa. The glossitis may include flattening of the papillae on the dorsum of the tongue (**Fig. 1**), and is often accompanied with a tenderness or a burning sensation.[2] This process may result in a smooth, erythematous tongue (**Fig. 2**) mimicking benign migratory glossitis, also known as "geographic tongue" or erythema migrans; the condition may affect 2% of the population.[2] Geographic tongue may lead to the presence of lesions on the tongue that are red and white, nonindurated, atrophic, but with a slightly elevated, white rim, and the site keeps changing over a period of time. Atrophic glossitis as noted with iron-deficiency anemia, however, does not shift position over time. Angular cheilitis involves the commissures of the lips and causes some degree of cracking. and is generally caused by *Candida albicans* infection.[3]

Plummer-Vinson syndrome or Paterson-Kelly syndrome is another type of iron-deficiency anemia that presents with glossitis, and is generally seen in women of Scandinavian and Northern European origin. Oral complications include dysphagia, pain on swallowing, presence of abnormal bands of tissue in the esophagus called "esophageal webs," and spoon-shaped configuration of nails called "koilonychias." The significance of the condition is that it is premalignant and is related to a high

a Department of Oral & Maxillofacial Pathology, Medicine & Radiology, Indiana University School of Dentistry, 1050 Wishard Boulevard, Room R4221, Indianapolis, IN 46202-2859, USA
b Department of Oral and Maxillofacial Diagnostic Sciences, Oral & Maxillofacial Pathology, University of Florida College of Dentistry, PO Box 100414, Gainesville, FL 32610, USA
* Corresponding author.
E-mail address: nmislam@iupui.edu

Otolaryngol Clin N Am 44 (2011) 161–182
doi:10.1016/j.otc.2010.09.006
0030-6665/11/$ – see front matter © 2011 Elsevier Inc. All rights reserved.

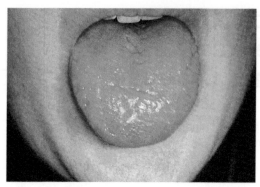

Fig. 1. Gross depapillation of the tongue dorsum in a patient with iron-deficiency anemia.

frequency of oral and esophageal squamous cell carcinomas that develop in these patients.[4] It is notable that if the anemia is recalcitrant, host resistance to infection may be significantly lowered.

Pernicious Anemia

Pernicious anemia is an uncommon condition, and recent evidence indicates a slight preponderance in the African American and Hispanic populations in the Unites States.[5] Pernicious anemia is a type of megaloblastic anemia, related to the lack of intrinsic factors in the stomach preventing the absorption of cobalamin (vitamin B12). Symptoms such as fatigue, weakness, shortness of breath, paresthesia, and tingling or numbness of extremities are not uncommon. Moreover, some patients present with memory loss, irritability, and depression.[5]

The oral manifestations include burning of the tongue, lips, and buccal mucosa as well as other mucosal sites. Focal or diffuse erythema of the tongue and mucosal atrophy is noted, depending on the duration and severity of the condition. An interesting term, "magenta tongue" (**Fig. 3**), is often used to describe the presentation. An easy differentiating feature from premalignant conditions that may present in a similar fashion is that the tongue lesions of pernicious anemia are mostly noted on the dorsum (**Fig. 4**), which is considered a low-risk area for development of squamous cell carcinoma.[5]

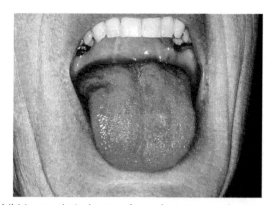

Fig. 2. Tongue exhibiting a relatively smooth, erythematous surface in a patient with iron-deficiency anemia.

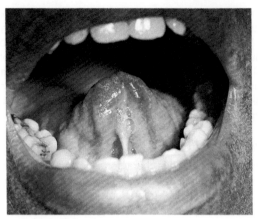

Fig. 3. The ventral surface of the tongue with intense red patches simulating areas of "magenta tongue" in a patient with pernicious anemia.

Leukemia

Leukemia has a variable presentation and may result in infiltration of the malignant cells in vital organs causing splenomegaly, hepatomegaly, and lymphadenopathy. Most clinical signs and symptoms are related to the reduced numbers of the white blood cells (WBCs) and RBCs. This crisis in turn reduces the oxygen-carrying capacity of the blood resulting in fatigue, easy tiring, and dyspnea.[6] Oral complications of leukemia include petechial hemorrhages of posterior hard palate and soft palate, and spontaneous gingival bleeding. The gingival bleeding is precipitated when the platelet count falls between 10,000 and 20,000/mm^3. Also noted are mucosal ulcers.[7] Rarely "numb chin syndrome" is appreciated, which is associated with the infiltration of the mental nerve by the malignant cells.[8] Areas of tissue destruction, necrosis, ulceration of the palate, and zygomycosis of the nasal cavity and the paranasal sinuses may be a significant finding.[9] Diffuse oral candidiasis is often a complication

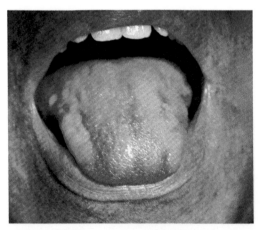

Fig. 4. Multifocal patchy erythematous zones on the tongue dorsum and lateral border in a patient with pernicious anemia.

of leukemia. Chemotherapeutics during the course of leukemia is one of the triggering factors in reactivation of herpes simplex virus (HSV), leading to the small vesicular type of oral mucositis. Viral herpetic gingivostomatitis may present on both the attached and mobile oral mucosa in contrast to only keratinized mucosa as observed in immunocompetent hosts.[10] The leukemic cells may also produce a diffuse, boggy, non-tender swelling with or without ulceration, which appears as a gingival enlargement or even a tumor-like growth containing a collection of leukemic cells called granulocytic sarcoma (**Fig. 5**) or extramedullary myeloid tumor.[10]

Langerhans Cell Histiocytosis (Histiocytosis X)

Langerhans cell histiocytosis (LCH) is characterized by abnormal monoclonal proliferation of antigen-presenting Langerhans cells. LCH may be focal or disseminated with extensive systemic involvement. LCH represents a spectrum of clinical disorders that are highly aggressive, destructive, and frequently fatal.[11] The common infantile form previously referred to as Letterer-Siwe disease is characterized by involvement of the viscera, and potentially causes death. Skin lesions are common and include papules, plaques, vesicles, and hemorrhagic nodules. The presence of alveolar bone loss in young children with premature primary teeth loss should raise the suspicion of the possibility of LCH.[12] Hand-Schüller-Christian disease is a more localized childhood disease with a triad of diabetes insipidus, lytic bone lesions, and proptosis. LCH can also occur in adolescents and adults. Of the bones of the jaw, the mandible, is the most frequently involved site.[13]

Oral manifestations of LCH include irregular ulcerations of the hard palate, which may be the primary manifestation of the disease. Gingival inflammation and ulcerated nodules, difficulty in chewing, and foul-smelling breath also occur. Large ulcerations with exposed bone, ecchymoses, gingivitis, and periodontitis followed by tooth loss are the hallmark of this condition. Radiographically, the teeth often appear to be "floating in air" and in some cases may present with a large radiolucent region (**Fig. 6**) exhibiting significant bone loss. These lesions may result in fractures and significant displacement of teeth.[13] Oral swellings or ulcerations resulting from mandibular or maxillary bone involvement may be common, and ulcerations may develop on the gingiva, palate, and floor of the mouth.[11–13] Sometimes a necrotizing gingivitis-like condition is noted with or without underlying bone destruction.

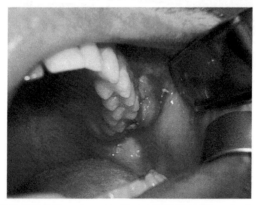

Fig. 5. An ulcerated gingival enlargement consistent with a leukemic "granulocytic sarcoma" noted on the left posterior buccal maxillary mucosa.

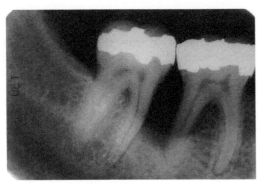

Fig. 6. Radiograph exhibiting significant bone loss in a patient with Langerhans cell disease.

Multiple Myeloma

Multiple myeloma usually involves the oral cavity in the later stages of the disease. The usual site of involvement is the jaws, mostly the mandible.[14–16] These lesions may cause significant facial asymmetry and swelling of the jaws (**Fig. 7**). This condition is associated with bone pain, numbness, mobility of teeth, and at times pathologic fractures.[17] If the disease is limited to only one site and exhibits a monoclonal, neoplastic proliferation of plasma cells in the bone it is termed plasmacytoma, being called extramedullary plasmacytoma when in the soft tissue. Radiographically multiple well-defined punched out lesions or even ragged radiolucencies of the skull and jaw are characteristic findings.[18] An interesting finding is amyloid deposits in the tongue leading to macroglossia, which in some cases prompts a biopsy ultimately leading to the final diagnosis.[19] The periorbital skin may in some cases also exhibit amyloid deposits appearing as waxy, firm, plaque-like lesions.[20]

AUTOIMMUNE CONDITIONS
Sjögren Syndrome

Sjögren syndrome (SS) is an autoimmune disease, affecting mostly women aged 50 years or older. There is a definite female sex predilection, with a 9:1 ratio as compared with males. SS is characterized by Sicca syndrome or the "primary Sjögren," comprising xerophthalmia and xerostomia. These SS patients frequently present with a parotid gland enlargement.[21] The secondary form of SS is often associated

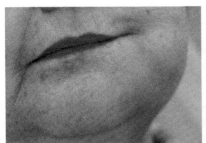
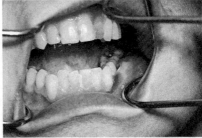

Fig. 7. Patient with multiple myeloma, with significant facial asymmetry of the left side and buccal mucosal swelling intraorally extending from the left canine to the posterior molar region.

with another concurrent autoimmune disease, mostly rheumatoid arthritis (RA) or systemic lupus erythematosus (SLE).

The oral manifestations in SS are generally related to the low salivary volume and comprise dysphagia, dysgeusia, difficulty in eating and speaking, as well as an increased rate of dental caries and susceptibility to infection.[22] The saliva is characteristically thick, ropey, and mucinous, or in some severe cases totally absent. The mucosal changes related to xerostomia include dry, red, and wrinkled mucosa. The tongue may appear "bald" or even "cobblestone-like" due to atrophy of the papilla. Cracks, fissures of the tongue, redness, and cheilitis are additional findings. Fungal infestation with *Candida albicans* is common in persons with SS. These patients also present with a relatively high incidence of dental caries because the amount of saliva is insufficient to dilute dietary sugar.[21,22] This increase in dental caries is especially noted around the cervical region of the teeth.[23] Inflammation of the parotid gland is a likely complication and is usually accompanied with fever and purulent discharge. Early recognition of SS is important, as this can lead to quick referral of the patient for early management of the dental caries that can progress fairly rapidly.[23,24] These SS patients are also at greater risk for the development of lymphoma, up to 40 times higher than the normal population.[25]

Kawasaki Disease

Kawasaki disease, also known as mucocutaneous lymph node syndrome, is a systemic vasculitis that affects medium- and large-sized arteries and lymph nodes, and is now considered to be the primary cause of childhood heart disease in the United States.[26] Though rare, if present it is usually noted in children younger than 5 years. An episode of acute edema, erythema of the hands and feet, pyrexia, oral erythema, and multiple rashes are almost always observed. A diagnostic criterion requires that the body temperature must exceed 38.5°C for minimum of 5 days. At least four of these five criteria have to be met to diagnose Kawasaki disease: (1) edema of extremity, erythema; (2) polymorphous exanthem; (3) bilateral conjunctival injection; (4) erythema and strawberry tongue; and (5) acute cervical lymphadenopathy.[26] The most striking oral finding includes swelling of papillae on the surface of the tongue (strawberry tongue) and intense erythema of the mucosal surfaces. The lips may be cracked, red, swollen, and often hemorrhagic and crusted.[26]

Scleroderma (Progressive Systemic Sclerosis; Hide-Bound Disease)

Scleroderma is a rare immunologically mediated condition characterized by deposition of extraordinary amounts of dense collagen in the tissues of the body. Skin is commonly involved, but almost all body organs eventually are affected. There is a 5:1 female predilection.[27]

When exposed to cold temperatures these patients show what is termed Raynaud phenomenon in their terminal phalanges. The blood supply to the fingers or toes, and in some cases the nose or earlobes, is reduced, the skin turns pale or white, and numb, and with further depletion of oxygen supply the skin turns blue and cyanotic (**Fig. 8**). The face appears smooth, taut, stretched, and mask-like, due to subcutaneous collagen deposition (**Fig. 9**). The "ala" of the nose becomes atrophic and exhibits a pinched appearance called "mouse facies." Serious sequelae of systemic sclerosis are fibrosis of lungs, heart, kidneys, and gastrointestinal tract, leading to organ failure mostly within 3 years of initial symptoms.[28,29] Gastrointestinal symptoms such as dysphagia and heartburn are not uncommon.

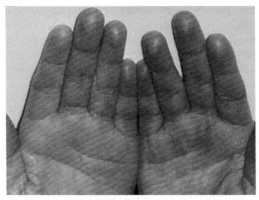

Fig. 8. Patient with scleroderma exposed to cold temperature exhibiting Raynaud phenomenon, with cyanotic fingers and palms.

The oral manifestations are variable. The lips appear pursed due to constriction of the mouth, thus making it difficult to open the mouth and resulting in what is termed microstomia, causing limited opening of mouth in about 70% of these patients. A "purse-string" appearance caused by creases and folds of skin radiating from the mouth may be noted. Xerostomia is a consistent finding, and some of these patients have concurrent secondary SS.[29] The tongue can lose mobility and generally has a smooth appearance. The collagen deposits invariably result in smoothening of the palatal rugae.[29] Diffuse widening of the periodontal ligament space is noted in the entire dentition. The mandible exhibits resorption of posterior part of the ramus, the coronoid process, the chin, and condyles on panoramic radiographs.[30]

Systemic Lupus Erythematosus

SLE is the most common of the so-called vascular collagen disorders in the United States, and more than 1.5 million people remain affected.[31] SLE is an immunologically mediated condition and has multiple clinical presentations. In SLE, apart from the renal and cardiac involvement, oral lesions are noted in 5% to 25% of the patients.

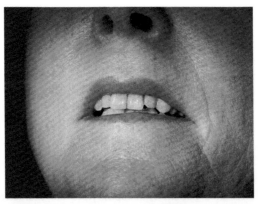

Fig. 9. "Mask-like" facial appearance caused by subcutaneous collagen deposition in a patient with scleroderma

The lesions affect the palate, buccal mucosa, and the gingivae; these may present as lichenoid areas that may be nonspecific in appearance, or even sometimes appear granulomatous. "Lupus cheilitis" involving the lower lip vermilion may be noted. Oral ulceration, pain, erythema, and hyperkeratosis as well as complaints of stomatodynia, dysgeusia, xerostomia, candidiasis, and periodontal disease are noted with some frequency in patients with SLE.[31]

Chronic cutaneous lupus erythematosus (CCLE) is limited to the skin and is also known as discoid lupus erythematosus (DLE). In this category the oral lesions are clinically identical to erosive lichen planus (**Fig. 10**), but these oral lesions are notably absent in the absence of skin lesions. Oral lesions are characteristically ulcerated, atrophic, and erythematous, exhibiting a central zone surrounded by white, fine, radiating striae that are often multiple (**Fig. 11**). Sometimes these may show a central stippled white dotted area. These oral lesions may be painful when exposed to acidic or salty foods in particular.[31] Oral lesions of the lichen planus are similar to those of DLE both clinically and histologically.[28]

Due to the similar clinical presentation, the lesions of SLE and CCLE must be diagnosed by applying strict histologic criteria, so as to distinguish one from the other.[28] The ulcerations are generally painless and may involve the palate.[32] Salivary gland hypofunction may be concurrently present in patients with SLE, leading to secondary SS and severe xerostomia.[33]

Rheumatoid Arthritis

RA is a chronic, autoimmune disorder causing nonsuppurative inflammatory destruction of the joints. About 3% of the United States population is afflicted by the condition. RA mostly affects women with a 3:1 sex predilection.[3] Some patients have a limited form of the disease with almost no debilitation, pain, or restricted movement. In others there is rapid progress to severely debilitating polyarthralgia.

In the head and neck region the temporomandibular joint (TMJ) is involved to some degree and has been noted in 40% of reported RA patients.[34] This involvement is usually bilateral and is a late finding in the course of the disease. It is usually evident as erosions in the condyle, with subsequent reduced range of motion of the mandible and pain with movement. The condition usually is not as severe as in the other joints that are involved but symptoms may include stiffness, crepitation, pain, or ache. The pain may be a result of pressure and clenching of teeth on one side, thereby inciting

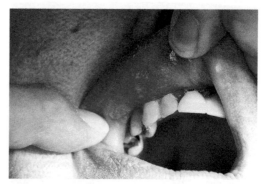

Fig. 10. Upper lip ulcer in a patient with lupus. Note the characteristic atrophic and erythematous area with a central zone, surrounded by white, fine, radiating striae, mimicking erosive lichen planus.

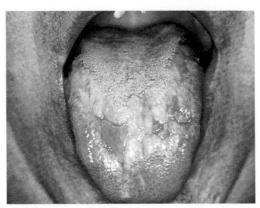

Fig. 11. Multiple granulomatous-appearing ulcerations on the tongue dorsum in a patient with systemic lupus erythematosus.

pain on the contralateral side. Gross destruction of the mandibular condyle may lead to mandibular micrognathia that presents with a receding chin and distinct malocclusion. Radiographically the condylar head may appear flattened with irregular surface features, and the temporal fossa surface may be eroded and exhibit some remodeling.[34] Many of these patients also have secondary SS.[35]

Amyloidosis

Amyloidosis represents a heterogeneous group of conditions characterized by the deposition of an extracellular proteinaceous material called amyloid.[36,37] This deposition may be associated with diseases such as multiple myeloma, RA, or chronic infections including tuberculosis. Amyloidosis may be of two types. Organ-limited amyloidosis has rarely been reported in the oral soft tissues. The second type is systemic amyloidosis, which may be in several forms such as primary, myeloma-associated, secondary, hemodialysis-associated, and hereditofamilial.[38]

The primary and myeloma-associated forms of amyloidosis usually affect older adults (average age 65 years). The initial signs and symptoms may be nonspecific. Eventually mucocutaneous lesions and macroglossia develop as a result of the deposition of the amyloid protein. Fatigue, weight loss paresthesia, hoarseness of voice, edema, and so forth may be the first indications of the disease. The skin lesions appear as smooth-surfaced, firm, waxy papules and plaques.[38] Macroglossia has been reported in 12% to 40% of these patients and presents as diffuse or nodular enlargement of the tongue. Sometimes oral amyloid nodules show ulceration and submucosal hemorrhage overlying the lesions.[36,37] Biopsy of rectal mucosa gingiva and labial salivary gland can be used to confirm the diagnosis.[39]

PULMONARY CONDITIONS
Wegener Granulomatosis

Wegener granulomatosis is a well-recognized disease process of unknown cause. The most acceptable hypothesis is that the disease is an abnormal immune reaction to a nonspecific infection, and/or it could be a type of hypersensitivity reaction to an inhaled antigen.[40] Wegener granulomatosis is a conglomerate of necrotizing granulomatous lesions of the respiratory tract, necrotizing glomerulonephritis, and systemic vasculitis of small-sized arteries and veins. The "limited form" of the disease generally spares the kidneys and shows only upper and lower respiratory tract involvement. If untreated at this stage, "generalized" Wegener granulomatosis rapidly develops, involves the kidneys causing irreparable glomerular damage, and proves fatal. The "superficial" form is classically limited to the skin and mucosa.[41]

Oral involvement in Wegener granulomatosis is not uncommon, and the characteristic "strawberry gingivitis" is a pathognomonic finding. This condition could be an early manifestation of the disease and almost always signals the onset of the renal involvement.[42] The gingiva presents with a florid and granular hyperplasia. It is swollen, reddened, with multiple short bulbous projections that are hemorrhagic (**Fig. 12**) and friable, and exhibit a red bumpy surface giving the strawberry-like appearance.[42] The buccal surface is frequently affected and lesions are characteristically confined to the attached gingiva (**Fig. 13**). This involvement starts at the interdental area and spreads laterally. The buccal mucosa or palate, when involved, has a nonspecific picture. Mobility of teeth resulting from underlying alveolar bone destruction is not uncommon.[42,43]

Other less common orofacial manifestations include facial paralysis, labial mucosal nodules, sinusitis-related toothaches, arthralgia of the TMJ, jaw claudication, oro-antral fistulae, and poorly healing extraction sites. The oral and skin manifestation may be a measure of patient outcome.[42,43]

Sarcoidosis

Sarcoidosis is a multisystem granulomatous disease of unknown etiology. There is strong evidence implicating degradation of antigenic material with the formation of noncaseating granulomatous inflammation. There is a definite racial bias, with blacks affected 13 to 17 times more often than whites.[3] The disease shows a female preponderance and a definite bimodal age distribution, one from 25 to 35 and the other between 45 and 65 years of age.[3] Sarcoidosis can affect any organ, but the lungs, lymph nodes, heart, spleen, eyes, kidneys, and the salivary glands remain the predominant sites. Bilateral hilar lymphadenopathy is evident in chest radiographs and 90% of

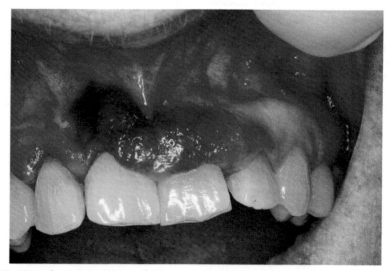

Fig. 12. "Strawberry gingivitis" of Wegener granulomatosis. Anterior maxillary gingiva exhibits a swollen, red area with short bulbous hemorrhagic projections.

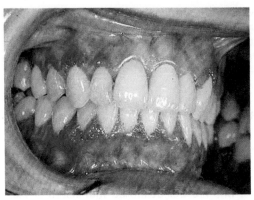

Fig. 13. Multifocal erythematous areas of Wegener granulomatosis affecting the buccal and facial attached gingiva.

the affected patients reveal abnormal chest radiographs during the course of the disease. Pulmonary manifestations include dyspnea, dry cough, chest pain, fever, malaise, fatigue, arthralgia, and weight loss.[44]

Cutaneous manifestations are noted in 25% of patients presenting as chronic violaceous indurated lesions called lupus pernio frequently on the nose, ears, lips, and face. Erythema nodosum are symmetric, elevated, indurated purplish plaques noted on the buttocks, limbs, and the back.[44] Ocular involvement is seen in 25% of the cases leading to keratoconjunctivitis sicca.[45]

Distinct and specific oral manifestations may include multiple nodules as well as painless ulcerations of the tongue (**Fig. 14**), gingiva, buccal mucosa, labial mucosa, and palate. In some cases the lesions have a granularity, may be hyperkeratotic, and present as brown-red or purple in color.[44] The lesions affecting the floor of mouth invariably involve the salivary glands in the area and lead to mucus extravasation. Lesions may be noted within the jaws in one-fourth of the reported intraoral cases. It is also well documented that intraoral lesions of sarcoidosis were the first clinical manifestation of the disease in the majority of the patient population.[44]

When bilateral hilar lymphadenopathy, erythema nodosum, and arthralgia are noted together it comprises a clinical condition known as Lofgren syndrome.[46] When the parotid gland is enlarged along with anterior uveitis, facial nerve palsy, and fever, the condition is termed Heerfordt syndrome.[46] Sarcoidosis may rarely involve the

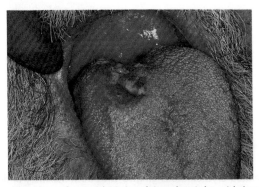

Fig. 14. Deep crater-like ulcer of sarcoidosis involving the right mid-dorsum of the tongue.

tongue causing swelling, enlargement, and subsequent ulcerations. Oral involvement in sarcoidosis usually manifests after systemic symptoms develop. Biopsy samples reveals noncaseating granulomas that are nonspecific, and hence granulomatous conditions like Wegener granulomatosis, Crohn disease, syphilis, or tuberculosis have to be excluded.[44–46]

ENDOCRINE DISORDERS
Diabetes Mellitus

Diabetes mellitus is a common disorder of carbohydrate metabolism. This condition is associated with many oral manifestations; however, most of these are evident in patients who have poorly controlled insulin-dependent diabetes (IDDM or type 1 diabetes) than in those who are well-controlled with insulin or those with noninsulin-dependent diabetes (NIDDM or type 2 diabetes). Postsurgical healing in these groups of patients is severely compromised and delayed.[47] Delay in healing with subsequent increased accumulation of plaque and food debris, higher susceptibility to infections, and pronounced hyperplasia of attached gingiva all play a significant role in the increased incidence of periodontal disease in diabetics.[48] A distinct type of erythematous gingiva with considerable degree of enlargement is noted as well (**Fig. 15**). Diabetes-related periodontal abscesses are not uncommon (**Fig. 16**). Periodontal involvement is frequent and progresses at a faster pace than in the uninvolved patient.[48] Diffuse, nontender, bilateral enlargement of the parotid glands, called diabetic sialadenosis, may be noted in both types of diabetics.[49] This condition is usually irreversible and even management of carbohydrate metabolism fails to restore the discrepancy. These patients are predisposed to a variety of oral candidal infections, usually presenting as a central papillary atrophy of the tongue dorsum in about 30% of these patients.[50] Xerostomia or the subjective feeling of dry mouth is appreciated in one-third of the patient population, which may result from an overall diminished flow of saliva and an increased salivary glucose level.[49–51] It has been well documented that there is a higher incidence of dental caries in patients with poorly controlled diabetes, which has been related to increased glucose levels in the saliva and the crevicular fluid.[52] Dysgeusia or altered taste and burning mouth syndrome are frequently reported with poorly controlled diabetes. The dry mouth is a potential breeding ground and remains predisposed to the development of oral infections. Fungal infection such as zygomycosis can be seen in uncontrolled diabetic

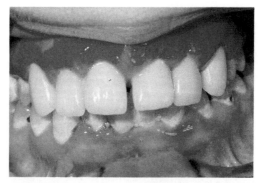

Fig. 15. Diabetes-related erythematous gingiva with both maxillary and mandibular anterior gingival involvement.

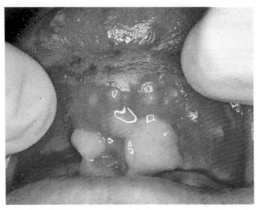

Fig. 16. Diabetes-related multiple periodontal abscesses noted on the maxillary anterior attached gingiva.

ketoacidotic patients. Erythema migrans or geographic tongue is a finding noted more frequently in patients with type 1 diabetes than in the general population.[53]

Hypothyroidism (Cretinism, Myxedema)

This condition is characterized by decreased levels of thyroid hormone. In infancy this affliction is termed cretinism. In adulthood the deficiency leads to marked deposition of glycosaminoglycans ground substance in the subcutaneous tissue, resulting in a nonpitting edema. This severe form of hypothyroidism is termed myxedema. The lips appear swollen and generally thickened because of the glycosaminoglycans deposition. Diffuse lingual enlargement is also appreciated. If the disease develops in early childhood, teeth fail to erupt but tooth formation proceeds at a normal pace.[54,55]

Hyperthyroidism (Thyrotoxicosis, Graves Disease)

Hyperthyroidism is a condition characterized by excess production of thyroid hormone. This excess production markedly increases the metabolism of the affected patient. Most of these changes are caused by Graves disease.[56] Other causes are hyperplasia of the thyroid gland tissue, and both benign and malignant thyroid tumors. The most common and obvious manifestation is the protrusion of the eyes, also caused by the deposition of glycosaminoglycans in the retro-orbital tissues; this is termed exophthalmos or proptosis. Other symptoms include nervousness, heart palpitations, heat intolerance, emotional lability, muscle weakness, and a warm smooth skin.[55]

Hypoparathyroidism

Reduced amount of production of parathyroid hormone (PTH) is known as hypoparathyroidism, which usually results from surgical removal of the parathyroid glands during thyroidectomy for other reasons or from autoimmune destruction of the parathyroid tissue. Rare syndromes such as DiGeorge syndrome and the endocrine-candidiasis syndrome may be associated with this condition.[57] One of the main findings of loss of the parathyroid gland is hypocalcemia. Chvostek's sign is a significant oral finding that is marked by twitching of the upper lip when the facial nerve is tapped just below the zygomatic process. A positive response suggests a latent degree of tetany. If the condition develops in early life or during tooth development, a pitting enamel hypoplasia and failure of tooth eruption may occur.[58]

Hyperparathyroidism

Excess production of PTH results in the condition called hyperparathyroidism. In the event of uncontrolled production of PTH it is called primary hyperparathyroidism, related to a parathyroid adenoma (80%–90% of cases) or hyperplastic parathyroid tissue (10%–15% of cases). When PTH is continuously produced in response to chronic low levels of serum calcium, usually in association with chronic renal disease, secondary hyperparathyroidism develops. The usual patients with primary hyperparathyroidism are women older than 60 years.[59] The patients present with the classic triad of "stones, bones, and abdominal groans." Stones are a tendency for development of renal calculi, as well as metastatic calcifications in the soft tissues. Bones relate to the osseous changes.[60] An early oral manifestation includes a radiographic presentation of generalized loss of the lamina dura of roots of teeth. The trabecular pattern of the bone is altered, resulting in a "ground-glass" appearance (**Fig. 17**).[60] In the more advanced stages of the disease there is development of the so-called brown tumors of hyperparathyroidism.[61] This name comes from the color of the tissue specimen, which is dark reddish-brown due to the abundant hemorrhage and hemosiderin deposition within the tumor. Radiographically these are well-demarcated unilocular or multilocular radiolucencies. The mandible, clavicle, ribs, and pelvic bones are the frequent locations. Significant cortical expansion is not a rarity with long-standing lesions.[61] Abdominal groans refer to pain emanating from the tendency of development of duodenal ulcers.[62]

Hypercortisolism (Cushing Syndrome)

Hypercortisolism, or Cushing syndrome, is a clinical condition that results from a sustained increase in blood glucocorticoid levels. This syndrome mostly results from corticosteroid therapy prescribed for other medical conditions, or may be related to an endogenous source such as an adrenal or pituitary gland tumor or even overproduction from the adrenal gland. Overproduction of adrenocorticotropic hormone (ACTH) from a pituitary tumor is called Cushing disease, a rare condition that affects young adult women.

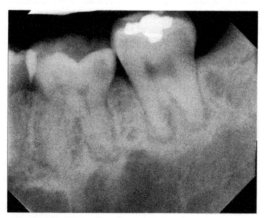

Fig. 17. Periapical radiograph exhibiting loss of the lamina dura of roots of molars with "ground-glass" appearance of the trabecular bone in a patient with hyperthyroidism secondary to chronic renal failure.

Oral manifestation includes prominent fatty tissue deposition in the facial area, resulting in a rounded facial appearance called "moon" facies.[63] A "buffalo hump" is noted, due to fat deposition in the dorsocervical spine region. There may be a variable degree of facial hirsutism noted on these patients. Osteoporosis leading to pathologic fractures of the mandible, maxilla, or alveolar bone as a result of trauma from impact may be a finding associated with this condition. Poor tendency of wound healing results in delayed healing of fracture, alveolar bone, and soft tissues after dental extractions.[64]

Hypoadrenocorticism (Addison Disease)

Reduced or insufficient production of adrenal corticosteroid hormone is usually related to the destruction of the adrenal cortex, and results in a condition termed primary hypoadrenocorticism or Addison disease.[65] This condition is related to auto-immune destruction, an infection such as tuberculosis, deep fungal involvement particularly in patients with acquired immunodeficiency syndrome, metastatic tumor, amyloidosis, sarcoidosis, or hemochromatosis. The secondary hypoadrenocorticism results from a malfunctioning pituitary gland. The striking orofacial manifestation is a "bronzing" hyperpigmentation of skin,[65] noted on sun-exposed areas and also over pressure points. This appearance is directly related to increased levels of β-lipotropin or ACTH, which stimulates melanocytes, in turn leading to the bronzing effect. Other oral presentations include a diffuse or patchy brown macular pigmentation most commonly on the buccal mucosa as well as on the floor of the mouth, ventral tongue, and other areas of the oral mucosa. The oral mucosal presentation often is the first manifestation of the disease and precedes the skin changes.[66]

METABOLIC DISORDERS
Mucopolysaccharidosis

This condition belongs to a heterogeneous group of metabolic disorders that are usually inherited in an autosomal recessive fashion. These disorders are all character-ized by the lack of any one of several normal enzymes needed to process the impor-tant intercellular substances known as glycosaminoglycans. These patients mostly display some degree of mental retardation. The facial features are relatively coarse, with heavy brow ridges. Cloudy degeneration of the corneas commonly leading to blindness is noted with some variability.[67]

The oral manifestations include some degree of macroglossia. Gingival hyperplasia is not uncommon and is noted particularly in the anterior region. The dental findings include numerous impacted teeth with prominent follicular spaces. Thin enamel with pointed cusps of posterior teeth is also noted in some cases.[67]

Hypophosphatasia

Hypophosphatasia is a rare metabolic bone disease and is thought to be of an auto-somal recessive trait pattern. The most important and one of the first presenting signs may be the premature loss of the primary teeth, particularly due to the lack of cementum on the root surfaces, and this occurs in the clinical setting of a lack of signif-icant inflammatory response. The deciduous incisor teeth are usually affected first and may be the only teeth involved. In some patients, this may be the only expression of the disease. In general, the severity of the condition is age dependent and the younger the age of onset, the more severe is the expression of the disease. Also noted are bony abnormalities that resemble rickets.[68]

Vitamin D–Resistant Rickets (Hereditary Hypophosphatemia)

Only after the use of vitamin D in the treatment of rickets became widespread was it found that this treatment strategy was not helping some patients even when vitamin D was used at the therapeutic dosage level. These patients turned out to have what has been termed vitamin D–resistant rickets. Such patients typically have an unusually short stature, with the lower body segment and the lower limbs shortened and bowed.[69] Dental findings include teeth with large pulp chambers, and pulp horns extending almost to the dentino-enamel junction. Of note, in these patients attrition causes the cuspal enamel to be worn down to the level of the pulp horn eventually causing pulpal exposure and pulp death. These exposures are small in size, and periapical abscesses and gingival sinus tracts may be formed that appear to affect normal teeth. Development of microclefts in the enamel may occur, allowing passage of oral microflora into the dentinal tubules and ultimately into the pulp.[69]

GASTROINTESTINAL DISEASES
Crohn Disease

Crohn disease is an inflammatory and/or immunologically mediated condition that generally affects the distal portion of the small bowel and the proximal colon. It is now well known that lesions may be noted anywhere from mouth to the anus.[70]

Oral manifestations are fairly nonspecific and include diffuse or nodular swelling of the oral and perioral tissues, a cobblestone appearance of the mucosa, and deep granulomatous-appearing ulcers. These ulcers are usually linear and are noted in the buccal vestibule. Diffuse swelling of one or both lips with associated angular cheilitis, painless localized swellings within the lips or face, and fissuring on the midline of the lower lip are some additional features.[70] Mucogingivitis is noted, best described as areas of patchy erythematous macules and plaques that involve the attached and unattached gingiva.[71] Soft fibrous hyperplastic tissue and mucosal tags are noted as well. An important aspect of this condition is the presence of ulcers that resemble aphthous stomatitis, and this is a consistent finding in most of the patients with this disease (**Fig. 18**). These patients present clinically with firm and palpable cervical lymph nodes. The oral lesions of Crohn disease precede the intestinal lesions by years, and in some cases are the only manifestation of the disease.[70]

Pyostomatitis Vegetans

Pyostomatitis vegetans is a relatively rare condition and is strongly believed to be an unusual oral expression of inflammatory bowel disease, particularly ulcerative colitis or

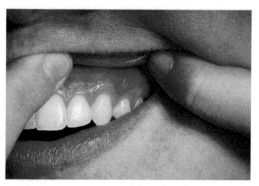

Fig. 18. An aphthous-like ulcer in a patient with Crohn disease.

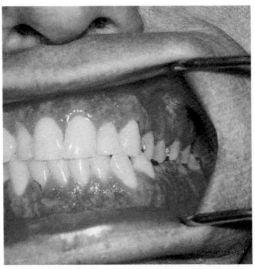

Fig. 19. A patient with pyostomatitis vegetans with characteristic yellowish, slightly elevated, linear, serpentine pustules set on an erythematous oral mucosa.

Crohn disease.[72] The classic oral manifestations include characteristic yellowish, slightly elevated, linear, serpentine pustules set on an erythematous oral mucosa (**Fig. 19**). The lesions primarily affect the buccal, labial, and vestibular mucosa (**Fig. 20**), the soft palate, and ventral tongue. These lesions are called "snail-track" ulcerations but in most instances these may not be true ulcers. The oral lesions may appear concomitantly with bowel symptoms or even precede the intestinal manifestations.[73]

NEOPLASTIC CONDITIONS
Metastatic Disease

Metastatic tumors to the oral region are rare but may involve both the soft and/or hard tissues,[74] and comprise about 1% of oral malignant neoplasms. These metastatic

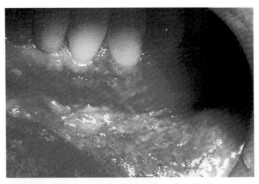

Fig. 20. Lesions of pyostomatitis vegetans affecting the labial as well as the vestibular mucosa and the attached gingiva.

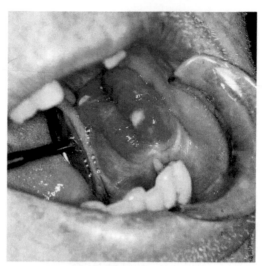

Fig. 21. Metastatic lung carcinoma presenting as an ulcerated, pyogenic granuloma-like growth associated with significant buccolingual cortical expansion.

lesions are noted more often to the jaws than to oral soft tissue. The most common site for oral soft tissue metastasis is the gingiva, and this site alone accounts for over 25% of all cases. The lesions appear more like common hyperplastic reactive lesions of the gingiva, mimicking a pyogenic granuloma that is often ulcerated.[75] Adjacent teeth may be loosened due to concomitant destruction of the underlying bone. These soft tissue metastases are more common in males than in females, and require a biopsy for definitive diagnosis. Metastatic tumors to the jaws are detected when the patient presents with swelling, pain, paresthesia, and even with what is termed as the "numb-chin syndrome," which is often noted when the lesion involves the mental nerve.[76] Radiographically these metastatic lesions are ill-defined radiolucencies with ragged, jagged, or irregular borders and sometimes may be mixed, both radiolucent and radiopaque in presentation. Breast carcinoma is the most commonly metastasizing tumor to the jaws, whereas lung carcinomas commonly go for the oral soft tissues (**Fig. 21**).[74] The most common bony site for metastasis is the molar region of the mandible and in almost one-third of reported cases; the oral metastatic lesion is the initial finding of the undiscovered malignancy.[75] Although rare, the possibility of an oral metastatic lesion should always be considered in cases of unexplained oral cavity growths or jaw radiolucencies. In summary, it is important to recognize that although rare, various tumors do metastasize to the oral cavity.[74,75]

SUMMARY

Systemic diseases may present with abnormalities in the head and neck region, particularly the oral cavity. Developing good differential diagnoses based on the presenting signs and symptoms is of prime importance. An early definitive diagnosis underscores initiation of correct treatment. The primary care physician, the dentist, and practicing otolaryngologist should be sentinel of these conditions for delivery of the highest possible standard of care. This article is not all-inclusive but clinical entities that present with significant oral manifestations are discussed.

ACKNOWLEDGEMENTS

Special thanks to Dr Donald M Cohen and Dr Indraneel Bhattacharyya of University of Florida, College of Dentistry for providing and sharing images used in the article.

REFERENCES

1. McFarlane DB, Pinderton PH, Dagg JH, et al. Incidence of iron deficiency, with and without anaemia, in women in general practice. Br J Haematol 1967;13:790–6.
2. Zegarelli DJ. Fungal infections of the oral cavity. Otolaryngol Clin North Am 1993; 26:1069–89.
3. Neville D, Allen B. Oral and maxillofacial pathology. 3rd edition. Saunders; 2009.
4. Zimmer V, Buecker A, Lammert F. Sideropenic dysphagia. Gastroenterology 2009;137:e1–2.
5. Toh BH, Alderuccio F. Pernicious anaemia. Autoimmunity 2004;37:357–61.
6. Lynch MA, Ship II. Initial oral manifestations of leukaemia. J Am Dent Assoc 1967;75:932–40.
7. Subramaniam P, Babu KL, Nagarathna J. Oral manifestations in acute lympho-blastic leukemic children under chemotherapy. J Clin Pediatr Dent 2008;32: 319–24.
8. Hiraki A, Nakamure S, Abe K, et al. Numb chin syndrome as an initial symptom of acute Lymphocytic leukemia: report of three cases. Oral Surg Oral Med Oral Pathol Oral Radiol Endod 1997;83:555–61.
9. Jones AC, Bentsen TY, Freedman PD. Mucormycosis of the oral cavity. Oral Surg Oral Med Oral Pathol 1993;75:455–60.
10. Da Silva-Santos PS, Silva BS, Coracin L, et al. Granulocytic sarcoma of the oral cavity in a chronic myeloid leukemia patient: an unusual presentation. Med Oral Patol Oral Cir Bucal 2010;15:e350–2.
11. Madrigal-Martínez-Pereda C, Guerrero-Rodríguez V, Guisado-Moya B, et al. Langerhans cell histiocytosis: literature review and descriptive analysis of oral manifestations. Med Oral Patol Oral Cir Bucal 2009;1(14):E222–8.
12. Moraes Pde C, Bönecker M, Furuse C, et al. Langerhans cell histiocytosis in a child: a 10-year follow-up. Int J Paediatr Dent 2007;17:211–6.
13. Mortellaro C, Pucci A, Palmeri A, et al. Oral manifestations of Langerhans cell histiocytosis in a pediatric population: a clinical and histological study of 8 patients. J Craniofac Surg 2006;17:552–6.
14. Mozaffari E, Mupparapu M, Otis L. Undiagnosed multiple myeloma causing extensive dental bleeding: report of a case and review. Oral Surg Oral Med Oral Pathol Oral Radiol Endod 2002;94:448–53.
15. Lee SH, Huang JJ, Pan WL, et al. Gingival mass as the primary manifestation of multiple myeloma: report of two cases. Oral Surg Oral Med Oral Pathol Oral Radiol Endod 1996;82:75–9.
16. Pinto LS, Campagnoli EB, Leon JE, et al. Maxillary lesion presenting as a first sign of multiple myeloma: case report. Med Oral Patol Oral Cir Bucal 2007;1(12):344–7.
17. Smith DB. Multiple myeloma involving the jaws. Oral Surg Oral Med Oral Pathol 1957;10:910–9.
18. Witt C, Borges AC, Klein K, et al. Radiographic manifestations of multiple myeloma in the mandible: a retrospective study of 77 patients. J Oral Maxillofac Surg 1997;55:450–3.
19. Reinish EI, Raviv M, Srolovitz H, et al. Tongue, primary amyloidosis, and multiple myeloma. Oral Surg Oral Med Oral Pathol 1994;77:121–5 17.

20. Epstein IB, Voss NJS, Stevenson-Moore P. Maxillofacial manifestations of multiple myeloma. Oral Surg Oral Med Oral Pathol 1984;51:267–71.
21. Hernández-Molina G, Avila-Casado C, Cárdenas-Velázquez F, et al. Similarities and differences between primary and secondary Sjögren's syndrome. J Rheumatol 2010;37:800–8.
22. Minozzi F, Galli M, Gallottini L, et al. Stomatological approach to Sjögren's syndrome: diagnosis, management and therapeutical timing. Eur Rev Med Pharmacol Sci 2009;13:201–16.
23. Newbrun E. Current treatment modalities of oral problems of patients with Sjögren's syndrome: caries prevention. Adv Dent Res 1996;10:29–34.
24. Atkinson JC, Fox PC. Sjögren's syndrome: oral and dental considerations. J Am Dent Assoc 1993;124:74–86.
25. Biasi D, Caramaschi P, Ambrosetti A, et al. Mucosa-associated lymphoid tissue lymphoma of the salivary glands occurring in patients affected by Sjögren's syndrome: report of 6 cases. Acta Haematol 2001;105:83–8.
26. Rowley AH, Shulman ST. Pathogenesis and management of Kawasaki disease. Expert Rev Anti Infect Ther 2010;8:197–203.
27. Chung L, Lin J, Furst DE, et al. Systemic and localized scleroderma. Clin Dermatol 2006;24(5):374–92.
28. Rose LF, Kaye D. Internal medicine for dentistry. 3rd edition. St. Louis (MO): Mosby Yearbook; 1990. p. 878–9, 93–94.
29. Nagy G, Kovacs J, Zeger M, et al. Analysis of the oral manifestations for systemic sclerosis. Oral Surg Oral Med Oral Pathol 1994;77:141–6.
30. Rout PG, Hamburger J, Potts AJ. Orofacial radiological manifestations of systemic sclerosis. Dentomaxillofac Radiol 1996;25:193–6.
31. Brennan MT, Valerin MA, Napeñas JJ, et al. Oral manifestations of patients with lupus erythematosus. Dent Clin North Am 2005;49:127–41.
32. Nico MM, Vilela MA, Rivitti EA, et al. Oral lesions in lupus erythematosus: correlation with cutaneous lesions. Eur J Dermatol 2008;18:376–81.
33. Grennan DM, Ferguson M, Williamson J, et al. Sjögren's syndrome in SLE. N Z Med J 1977;86:374–9.
34. Voog U, Alstergren P, Eliasson S, et al. Progression of radiographic changes in the temporomandibular joints of patients with rheumatoid arthritis in relation to inflammatory markers and mediators in the blood. Acta Odontol Scand 2004; 62:7–13.
35. Theander E, Jacobsson LT. Relationship of Sjögren's syndrome to other connective tissue and autoimmune disorders. Rheum Dis Clin North Am 2008;34:935–47.
36. Serdar A, Basak D, Sercan G, et al. Solitary amyloid tumor of the tongue base. Int J Otolaryngol 2009;2009:515068.
37. Elad S, Czerninski R, Fischman S, et al. Exceptional oral manifestations of amyloid light chain protein (AL) systemic amyloidosis. Amyloid 2010;17:27–31.
38. Sadek I, Mauermann ML, Hayman SR, et al. Primary systemic amyloidosis presenting with asymmetric multiple mononeuropathies. J Clin Oncol 2010;28(25): e429–32.
39. Do Amaral B, Coelho T, Sousa A, et al. Usefulness of labial salivary gland biopsy in familial amyloid polyneuropathy Portuguese type. Amyloid 2009;16:232–8.
40. Marzano AV, Fanoni D, Berti E. Oral and cutaneous findings are valuable diagnostic aids in Wegener's granulomatosis. Eur J Intern Med 2010;21:49.
41. Reboll R, Zapater E, Calabuig C, et al. Wegener's granulomatosis: description of a case with oral manifestation. Med Oral Patol Oral Cir Bucal 2010;15(4):e601–4.

42. Ruokonen H, Helve T, Arola J, et al. Strawberry like" gingivitis being the first sign of Wegener's granulomatosis. Eur J Intern Med 2009;20:651–3.
43. Stewart C, Cohen D, Bhattacharyya I, et al. Oral manifestations of Wegener's granulomatosis: a report of three cases and a literature review. J Am Dent Assoc 2007;138:338–48.
44. Marcoval J, Mañá J. Specific (granulomatous) oral lesions of sarcoidosis: report of two cases. Med Oral Patol Oral Cir Bucal 2010;15:e456–8.
45. Shenoy R, Al Burwani B. Necrotizing retinopathy simulating acute retinal necrosis causing rhegmatogenous retinal detachment in sarcoidosis: a case report. Eur J Ophthalmol 2010;20:218–20.
46. Poate TW, Sharma R, Moutasim KA, et al. Orofacial presentations of sarcoidosis— a case series and review of the literature. Braz Dent J 2008;25(205):437–42.
47. Miley DD, Terezhalmy GT. The patient with diabetes mellitus: etiology, epidemiology, principles of medical management, oral disease burden, and principles of dental management. Quintessence Int 2005;36:779–95.
48. Mealey BL, Oates TW. Diabetes mellitus and periodontal diseases; American Academy of Periodontology. J Periodontol 2006;77:1289–303.
49. Mandel L, Patel S. Sialadenosis associated with diabetes mellitus: a case report. J Oral Maxillofac Surg 2002;60:696–8.
50. Belazi M, Velegraki A, Fleva A, et al. Candidal overgrowth in diabetic patients: potential predisposing factors. Mycoses 2005;48:192–6.
51. Zachariasen RD. Xerostomia and the diabetic patient. J Gt Houst Dent Soc 1996; 67:10–3.
52. Falk H, Hugoson A, Thorstensson H. Number of teeth, prevalence of caries and periapical lesions in insulin-dependent diabetics. Scand J Dent Res 1989;97: 198–206.
53. Wysocki GP, Daley TD. Benign migratory glossitis in patients with juvenile diabetes. Oral Surg Oral Med Oral Pathol 1987;63:68–70.
54. Roberts CG, Ladenson PW. Hypothyroidism. Lancet 2004;363:793–803.
55. Topliss DJ, Eastman CJ. Diagnosis and management of hyperthyroidism and hypothyroidism. Med J Aust 2004;180:186–93.
56. Pearce EN. Diagnosis and management of thyrotoxicosis. BMJ 2006;332: 1369–73.
57. Spiegel AM. Hypoparathyroidism. In: Wyngaarden JB, Smith LH Jr, Bennett JC, editors. Cecil's textbook of medicine. Philadelphia: W.B. Saunders; 1992. p. 1419–20.
58. Walls AWG, Soames JV. Dental manifestations of autoimmune hypoparathyroidism. Oral Surg Oral Med Oral Pathol 1993;75:452–4.
59. Aggunlu L, Akpek S, Coskun B. Leontiasis ossea in a patient with hyperparathyroidism secondary to chronic renal failure. Pediatr Radiol 2004;34:630–2.
60. Solt DB. The pathogenesis, oral manifestations, and implications for dentistry of metabolic bone disease. Curr Opin Dent 1991;1(6):783–91.
61. Triantafillidou K, Zouloumis L, Karakinaris G, et al. Brown tumors of the jaws associated with primary or secondary hyperparathyroidism. A clinical study and review of the literature. Am J Otol 2006;27:281–6.
62. Hayes CW, Conway WF. Hyperparathyroidism. Radiol Clin North Am 1991;29: 85–96.
63. Newell-Price J, Bertagna X, Grossman AB, et al. Cushing's syndrome. Lancet 2006;367:1605–17.
64. Findling JW, Raff H. Cushing's syndrome: important issues in diagnosis and management. J Clin Endocrinol Metab 2006;91:3746–53.

65. Chakera AJ, Vaidya B. Addison disease in adults: diagnosis and management. Am J Med 2010;123:409–13.
66. Shah SS, Oh CH, Coffin SE, et al. Addisonian pigmentation of the oral mucosa. Cutis 2005;76:97–9.
67. Alpöz AR, Coker M, Celen E, et al. The oral manifestations of Maroteaux-Lamy syndrome (mucopolysaccharidosis VI): a case report. Oral Surg Oral Med Oral Pathol Oral Radiol Endod 2006;101:632–7.
68. Van den Bos T, Handoko G, Niehof A, et al. Cementum and dentin in hypophosphatasia. J Dent Res 2005;84:1021–5.
69. Batra P, Tejani Z, Mars M. X-linked hypophosphatemia: dental and histologic findings. J Can Dent Assoc 2006;72:69–72.
70. Fatahzadeh M, Schwartz RA, Kapila R, et al. Orofacial Crohn's disease: an oral enigma. Acta Dermatovenerol Croat 2009;17:289–300.
71. Ojha J, Cohen DM, Islam MN, et al. Gingival involvement in Crohn disease. J Am Dent Assoc 2007;138:1574–81.
72. Pazheri F, Alkhouri N, Radhakrishnan K. Pyostomatitis vegetans as an oral manifestation of Crohn's disease in a pediatric patient. Inflamm Bowel Dis 2010. [Epub ahead of print]. DOI: 10.1002/ibd.21245.
73. Femiano F, Lanza A, Buonaiuto C, et al. Pyostomatitis vegetans: a review of the literature. Med Oral Patol Oral Cir Bucal 2009;14:E114–7.
74. Lim SY, Kim SA, Ahn SG, et al. Metastatic tumours to the jaws and oral soft tissues: a retrospective analysis of 41 Korean patients. Int J Oral Maxillofac Surg 2006;35:412–5.
75. Van der Waal RI, Buter J, van der Waal I. Oral metastases: report of 24 cases. Br J Oral Maxillofac Surg 2003;41:3–6.
76. Yoshioka I, Shiiba S, Tanaka T, et al. The importance of clinical features and computed tomographic findings in numb chin syndrome: a report of two cases. J Am Dent Assoc 2009;140:550–4.

Oral Manifestations of Hematologic and Nutritional Diseases

Bethanee J. Schlosser, MD, PhD[a], Megan Pirigyi, BA[a],
Ginat W. Mirowski, DMD, MD[b],*

KEYWORDS

- Amyloidosis • Anemia • Leukemia • Lymphoma
- Vitamin deficiency • Glossitis • Anorexia • Bulimia

Oral manifestations of hematologic and nutritional deficiencies can affect the mucous membranes, teeth, periodontal tissues, salivary glands, and perioral skin. In this article the authors review common oral manifestations of hematologic conditions starting with disorders of the white blood cells including cyclic hematopoiesis (cyclic neutropenia), leukemias, lymphomas, plasma cell dyscrasias, and mast cell disorders. This review is followed by a discussion of the impact of red blood cell disorders including anemias, and less common red blood cell dyscrasias (sickle cell disease, hemochromatosis, and congenital erythropoietic porphyria) as well as thrombocytopenia. Several nutritional deficiencies exhibit oral manifestations. The authors specifically discuss the impact of water-soluble vitamins (B2, B3, B6, B9, B12, and C), fat-soluble vitamins (A, D, and K), and the eating disorders anorexia nervosa and bulimia nervosa on the oral tissues.

ORAL MANIFESTATIONS OF HEMATOLOGIC DISEASES

Common and rare hematologic disorders may exhibit nonspecific as well as pathognomonic oral manifestations. Mechanisms of oral pathology may include direct infiltration by abnormal hematologic cells, deposition of abnormal proteins, oral ulceration, and abnormal hematopoiesis. All hematopoietic lineages may present with oral findings depending on the specific disorder.

Funding support: None.
Financial disclosures and/or conflicts: The authors have nothing to disclose.
[a] Department of Dermatology, Northwestern University Feinberg School of Medicine, 676 North Street Clair, Suite 1600, Chicago, IL 60611, USA
[b] Department of Oral Pathology, Medicine, Radiology, Indiana University School of Dentistry, Indianapolis, IN, USA
* Corresponding author. Indiana University School of Dentistry, Indianapolis, IN 46032.
E-mail address: gmirowsk@iupui.edu

Otolaryngol Clin N Am 44 (2011) 183–203
doi:10.1016/j.otc.2010.09.007
0030-6665/11/$ – see front matter © 2011 Elsevier Inc. All rights reserved.

White Blood Cell Disorders

Cyclic hematopoiesis

Neutrophils, or polymorphonuclear leukocytes (PMNs), are an integral part of the innate immune system against bacterial pathogens, and typically account for 50% to 70% of the circulating white blood cell population. Neutrophil activation releases myeloperoxidase, a heme protein that produces cytotoxic oxidants and affects nitric oxide–dependent signaling within the vascular endothelium. Cyclic hematopoiesis (previously termed cyclic neutropenia, Online Mendelian Inheritance in Man [OMIM] #162800) is a rare disorder characterized by periodic failure of hematopoietic progenitor cells resulting in dramatic oscillations in neutrophil, monocyte, eosinophil, platelet, and reticulocyte counts.[1] Patients typically experience transient fever, oral ulcerations, and recurrent skin infections in conjunction with the neutropenia that occurs at intervals of 15 to 35 days (most commonly 21 days).[2–5] Both the autosomal dominant form of the disease and sporadic cases are caused by a mutation in the gene for neutrophil elastase (*ELA2*, chromosome 19p13.3).[3,6] These mutations disrupt granulopoiesis and induce apoptosis.[7]

Cyclic hematopoiesis most commonly presents in infants and children, although adult onset may occur.[8] In general, disease manifestations recede with age. Clinical presentation can vary in severity and tends to occur when the neutrophil count drops below 500 cells/μL. Systemic and extraoral manifestations include fever, lymphadenopathy, and skin and respiratory infections. The oral manifestations of cyclic hematopoiesis include recurrent aphthous stomatitis (RAS), recurrent gingivitis, and periodontitis.[9,10] RAS is one of the most common presenting symptoms in cyclic hematopoiesis; RAS arises during the nadir and resolves spontaneously as the neutrophil count improves.[2] The finding of RAS with or without periodontal disease, particularly in a child, should raise the suspicion of cyclic neutropenia.

Diagnostic evaluation entails serial measurement of circulating neutrophils. The diagnosis may be established by demonstrating at least 2 cycles of neutropenia.[11] Treatment involves regular administration of recombinant granulocyte colony-stimulating factor (G-CSF), which can diminish the frequency and severity of symptoms.

Leukemias

The leukemias are malignancies of hematopoietic cells characterized by the proliferation of malignant leukocytes and destruction of the bone marrow. The neoplastic immature leukocytes (blast cells) appear in the peripheral blood, often resulting in an impressive leukocytosis. The leukemias are classified according to the progenitor cell involved (lymphoid or myeloid lineage) and whether the disease follows an acute or chronic course. Clinical manifestations of leukemia may result from loss of normal leukocyte function, suppression of hematopoietic cell lines, or direct infiltration of leukemic cells into tissues. Consequently, the signs and symptoms are varied and may include fatigue, anemia, lymphadenopathy, recurrent infection, bone and abdominal pain, bleeding, and purpura.

Leukemia cutis, infiltration of the skin by leukemic cells, presents as firm and rubbery papules, plaques, and nodules, and may precede development of systemic leukemia. Ulcers and blisters occur less commonly. Myelogenous leukemias may present as dermal nodules termed chloromas or granulocytic sarcomas. On sectioning and exposure to air, these nodules develop a blue-green color due to the presence of myeloperoxidase within the leukemic cells.

Oral manifestations may occur in any of the leukemias, but they are more prevalent in acute (vs chronic) and myeloid (vs lymphoid) leukemias.[12] Oral examination of patients may reveal mucosal pallor due to anemia, or bleeding and petechiae of the palate, tongue, or lips as the result of underlying thrombocytopenia. Painful and deep oral ulcerations are common and may result from either neutropenia or direct infiltration by malignant cells.[11,13] Patients may also develop severe viral, fungal, and bacterial oral infections as a consequence of immunosuppression.[11]

Gingival hyperplasia results from leukemic infiltration of the gingivae. This infiltration is most common in the acute leukemias, particularly acute monocytic leukemia and acute promyelocytic leukemia.[2,14,15] Patients typically present with moderately edematous, erythematous, and friable gingivae that may encroach on the teeth. Gingival hyperplasia often improves markedly following appropriate chemotherapy.[14]

Lymphomas

Lymphomas are malignancies of lymphocytes and their precursor cells. These tumors develop in secondary lymphatic tissues, most commonly in the lymph nodes and less frequently in extranodal lymph tissues. One classification scheme differentiates Hodgkin lymphoma (HL) from non-Hodgkin lymphoma (NHL). HL predominantly affects adolescents and young adults with an additional prevalence peak in middle age. NHL typically presents in middle-aged to older individuals. Both HL and NHL occur more commonly in men.

Clinical manifestations are diverse but frequently include painless lymphadenopathy, hepatosplenomegaly, and secondary infections. The symptoms of fever, night sweats, and weight loss (B symptoms) as well as pruritus suggest advanced disease and a poor prognosis. The diagnosis is based on histologic and immunohistochemical findings in diseased tissue.

Oral manifestations of lymphoma are far more likely to occur in NHL, particularly Burkitt lymphoma and AIDS-associated B-cell lymphoma (**Fig. 1**).[16] In NHL, oral involvement preferentially affects the lymphoid tissues of Waldeyer's ring as well as the vestibule and gingivae.[17] Painless, soft masses, with or without traumatic ulceration, may also involve the palate, buccal mucosa, and gingivae.[18] The clinical differential diagnosis includes minor salivary gland neoplasms, Kaposi sarcoma, and infections.[19]

Burkitt lymphoma is an aggressive pediatric lymphoma that is commonly associated with oral manifestations. Epstein-Barr virus infection has been implicated in its pathogenesis. Burkitt lymphoma presents as a rapidly expanding mass causing bone and adjacent soft tissue destruction, resulting in painful loosening of the teeth; it more commonly affects the maxilla than the mandible.[18]

AIDS-associated B-cell lymphoma is typically a non-Hodgkin B-cell lymphoma that presents as a papule, nodule, or tumor with or without ulceration; this entity typically

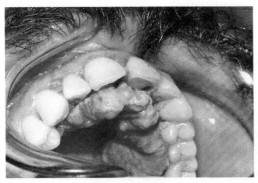

Fig. 1. Prominent gingival infiltration is evident in this human immunodeficiency virus–positive patient as a result of gingival infiltration by non-Hodgkin B-cell lymphoma.

affects Waldeyer's ring or the gingivae (see **Fig. 1**). AIDS-associated lymphoma manifests when the CD4 count is less than 50/μL and portends a poor prognosis.[20–22]

Amyloidosis

The amyloidoses are a group of disorders characterized by pathologic deposition of fibrillar proteins in various tissues.[23] Amyloidosis is classified according to the type of protein produced[23] and whether protein deposition is localized or systemic.[24] Amyloidosis may be a primary disorder (AL amyloidosis), or it can be a secondary manifestation of neoplastic (ie, multiple myeloma) or chronic inflammatory (ie, rheumatoid arthritis, tuberculosis) disorders. AL amyloidosis is the most common systemic amyloidosis and the amyloidosis that most frequently affects the oral cavity. Localized amyloidosis may also produce oral lesions.

AL amyloidosis is characterized by systemic deposition of immunoglobulin light or heavy chains, which may occur as a primary disease process or as the sequela of multiple myeloma. Due to its extensive range of organ and tissue involvement, the clinical manifestations of the disease are numerous. Some signs and symptoms include fatigue, weight loss, edema, renal failure, autonomic and peripheral neuropathy, and rapidly evolving congestive heart failure due to a restrictive cardiomyopathy.[25]

The oral manifestations of amyloidosis include macroglossia, edema, submucosal hemorrhage, glossodynia, taste disturbance, and xerostomia (due to destruction of salivary glands). Macroglossia is found in 20% of patients, making it the most widely documented oral finding; it is a distinctive feature of AL amyloidosis that is not typically found in the other systemic amyloidoses.[23] Patients with macroglossia present with enlargement (localized nodular or diffuse) and/or woody induration of the tongue. Scalloping of the lateral tongue borders may result from counterpressure exerted by the teeth as the tongue enlarges (**Fig. 2**). On occasion, macroglossia can be severe enough to compromise the airway and require surgical intervention.[26] In some patients with AL amyloidosis, firm, yellowish nodules composed of amyloid may also occur on the gingivae, buccal mucosa, or palate.[27]

Localized amyloidosis of the oral cavity is relatively rare, but patients typically present with one or more soft, red, yellow, purple, or blue nodules on the buccal mucosa, tongue, gingivae, or less commonly, the palate.[24]

Dogma suggests that diagnostic biopsy should be obtained from the rectum. However, oral biopsies are easier to obtain, less traumatic, and of equal yield

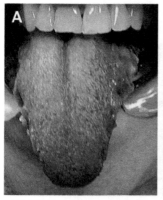 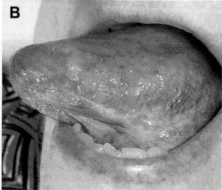

Fig. 2. (A) Mild scalloping of the lateral tongue borders and prominent palpable woody induration on examination were the presenting signs of systemic amyloidosis in this patient. (B) Lateral view of the tongue shows subtle nodules at sites of amyloid deposition.

compared with rectal biopsies.[28] Diagnosis of amyloidosis requires histologic exami-nation and demonstration of extracellular amyloid deposits. Histologic specimens are stained with Congo red and examined with polarized microscopy for the characteristic apple-green birefringence. Depending on the type of amyloidosis suspected, addi-tional immunohistochemical stains may include κ and λ light chain, β-amyloid A4 protein, transthyretin, and β2-microglobulin. Immunofixation electrophoresis of serum or urine may also be used to detect and characterize circulating proteins.[23]

Multiple myeloma

Multiple myeloma (MM) is a malignant plasma cell dyscrasia that results in the over-production of immunoglobulin light chains. MM typically presents in middle-aged and older adults, and is more prevalent in men and African Americans. Amyloidosis confers a poorer prognosis in patients with MM.[11,29,30] The most common presenting symptom is bone pain caused by osteolytic lesions or pathologic fractures. However, patients may also present with hypercalcemia, proteinuria, renal failure, anemia, or thrombocytopenia. The radiographic finding of multiple "punched-out" bone lesions is highly suggestive of advanced MM. Up to 30% of patients have involvement of the mandible with associated swelling, pain, paresthesias, and tooth loss.[18] Gingival bleeding or oral petechiae may be seen when marrow infiltration by malignant plasma cells causes thrombocytopenia.[11] In rare instances, MM can produce extramedullary plasmacytomas. When located in the oral cavity, plasmacytomas are most commonly found on the gingivae or hard palate, and appear as dome-shaped nodules that have a tendency to ulcerate.[11]

The diagnosis of MM requires evidence of end-organ damage (ie, lytic bone lesions, anemia, hypercalcemia, or renal insufficiency), bone marrow aspiration or biopsy to demonstrate plasma cell proliferation in the marrow, and the detection of monoclonal protein in the serum or urine. Treatment with cyclophosphamide and other chemother-apeutic agents may be associated with both cutaneous and oral mucosal manifesta-tions that are beyond the scope of this article.

Langerhans cell histiocytosis

Formerly known as histiocytosis X, Langerhans cell histiocytosis (LCH) is a rare disorder of unknown etiology that encompasses several different clinical entities involving the proliferation of Langerhans cells. The disease is characterized by destructive tissue infiltration by abnormal histiocytes mixed with lymphocytes and eosinophils. LCH has a broad spectrum of clinical manifestations depending on the site and extent of organ involvement.[11] Some patients have mild, localized pain caused by isolated bone lesions, whereas others develop rapidly progressive systemic disease involving nearly every organ system. Definitive diagnosis of LCH requires histologic confirmation.[31]

Ten percent to 20% of patients have lytic lesions of the maxilla or mandible, result-ing in edema and ulceration of the overlying mucosa, gingival inflammation, necrosis, and recession as well as increased tooth mobility and premature tooth loss.[11,31,32] Radiographic findings include localized osteolytic lesions, pathologic fractures, "floating teeth" in which the teeth appear to "float" within the radiographic lucency, and premature tooth loss. Ulceration of the oral mucosa in the absence of underlying bone lesions rarely occurs. These painful ulcers are most commonly located on the buccal mucosa or the posterior vestibule.[32] Evaluation of the patient with LCH should include whole-body radiographic skeletal survey or bone scintigraphy, and serum studies to assess for diabetes insipidus and hypercalcemia.

Systemic mastocytosis

Mastocytosis encompasses several distinct clinical entities characterized by abnormal proliferation of mast cells. Most cases of mastocytosis exclusively involve the skin, but systemic disease is characterized by involvement of bone marrow and other organs. Typical symptoms of mastocytosis are related to release of mast cell mediators, including histamine and various vasoactive factors. Consequently, clinical manifestations include urticaria, flushing, pruritus, diarrhea, palpitations, and syncope. In systemic mastocytosis, patients may present with bone pain, osteoporosis, lymphadenopathy, hepatosplenomegaly, and neuropsychiatric disturbances.

Oral manifestations of systemic mastocytosis are rare. However, painful osteolytic lesions of the mandible or maxilla have been reported, and they may be associated with ulceration and sinus tract formation.[33,34] Mast cell infiltration of the salivary and lacrimal glands may lead to the sicca syndrome, characterized by excessive dryness of the mouth and eyes.[35,36]

Systemic mastocytosis is defined by major and minor criteria: the major criterion is the presence of dense mast cell infiltrates in the bone marrow or extracutaneous organs, and the minor criteria include (1) presence of 25% abnormal or spindle-shaped mast cells on bone marrow aspirate or tissue biopsy, (2) c-Kit mutation at codon 816V, (3) expression of CD2 and/or CD25 on CD117+ mast cells, and (4) total serum tryptase levels persistently greater than 20 ng/mL.[37] The diagnosis requires evidence of either the major criterion and one minor criterion, or 3 minor criteria.[37]

Red Blood Cell Disorders

Anemia, regardless of cause, is associated with pallor, fatigue, dyspnea, tachycardia, glossitis, glossodynia, and stomatitis. In anemia due to deficiency of iron, folate, or vitamin B12, the oral findings may be the initial presentation, and may precede a decrease in hemoglobin or change in mean corpuscular volume.[16,38]

Iron-deficiency anemia

Iron-deficiency anemia, the most common cause of anemia worldwide, may result from insufficient dietary intake or malabsorption of iron, chronic blood loss, hemolysis, and pregnancy. As in other anemias, iron deficiency presents with pallor, fatigue, dyspnea, tachycardia, and telogen effluvium. Iron-deficiency anemia tends to produce nail findings such as splitting or spooning (koilonychia).

The most common oral manifestation of iron-deficiency anemia is mucosal pallor, most notable on the gingivae and vermilion lips. Angular cheilitis and atrophic glossitis (loss of filiform and fungiform papillae of the tongue, causing the tongue to appear smooth and red) are also important diagnostic clues. This atrophic glossitis may be preceded by glossodynia, burning sensation, or dysphagia.[11,38] Epidemiologic studies show variable association between iron deficiency and RAS, and repletion of iron stores may not affect the clinical course of RAS.[39,40] Iron deficiency is a predisposing factor for oral candidiasis.[16,38]

The combination of iron deficiency anemia, dysphagia, and esophageal strictures or webs comprises the Plummer-Vinson syndrome. This disorder is now rare but was previously found in middle-aged women with glossitis, glossodynia, angular cheilitis, and koilonychia. Plummer-Vinson syndrome is associated with an increased risk of oral and pharyngeal carcinoma.[18]

A diagnosis of iron-deficiency anemia is suggested by the finding of microcytic, hypochromic anemia in conjunction with decreased serum iron (<60 µg/dL), decreased serum ferritin (<15 µg/dL), and elevated total iron-binding capacity (>400 µg/dL).

In men and postmenopausal women, the diagnosis of iron deficiency anemia should prompt further investigation for possible gastrointestinal bleeding.

Megaloblastic anemia

Megaloblastic anemia is a consequence of defective DNA synthesis during erythropoiesis and most commonly results from vitamin B12 (cobalamin, cyanocobalamin) or folate deficiency. Potential causes of folate deficiency include inadequate dietary intake, malabsorption, or increased folate consumption that may occur during pregnancy, periods of rapid growth, or chronic inflammation. Vitamin B12 deficiency is less common but may be seen in the elderly, vegetarians, and patients with pernicious anemia, human immunodeficiency virus, or gastrointestinal disease. In addition to the usual clinical manifestations of anemia, vitamin B12 deficiency may cause neuropsychiatric findings such as ataxia, loss of vibratory sensation, dementia, or psychosis.

Megaloblastic anemia frequently causes atrophy of oral mucosa exhibited by glossitis and angular cheilitis. The tongue may be painful, and patients may note alterations in taste sensation. The tongue may be beefy red, and occasionally erythematous patches can be found on the buccal mucosa as well.[11] Folate and vitamin B12 deficiencies have also been implicated as contributing factors to RAS, and in some patients aphthae will improve following folate and vitamin B12 repletion.[38–41] The diagnosis of vitamin B12 deficiency can be distinguished from folate deficiency by direct measurement of serum vitamin B12 levels or the detection of elevated serum methylmalonic acid.

Sickle cell disease

Sickle cell disease (SCD) is an autosomal recessive disorder in which a hemoglobin mutation predisposes erythrocytes to deformation in the setting of low oxygen tension. The clinical manifestations of SCD are diverse, and may result from vaso-occlusion and infarction of tissues, hemolysis, or increased susceptibility to bacterial infection. In general, patients with SCD are at increased risk of osteomyelitis, which is thought to result from repetitive bone infarction providing a favorable environment for bacterial growth. Acute pain in the long bones, chest, or abdomen, fever, malaise, numbness, weakness and altered cognition may signify an acute sickle crisis.

The most common oral manifestations of SCD are pallor or jaundice of the oral mucosa due to hemolysis. The soft palate or floor of the mouth may be the most sensitive areas for detecting jaundice. Osteomyelitis of the mandible is a rare complication.[42,43] Infarction of branches of the mandibular nerve, due to vaso-occlusion, rarely causes persistent anesthesia of the teeth, gingivae, or oral mucosa.[44,45] In addition, SCD patients may develop sudden onset of pain or necrosis in previously healthy teeth.[46] The definitive diagnosis of SCD requires demonstration of hemoglobin S by hemoglobin electrophoresis.

Hemochromatosis

Hereditary hemochromatosis is an autosomal recessive disease caused by increased gastrointestinal absorption of iron in the gut resulting in systemic iron overload. This genetic disorder is most often caused by mutation in the *HFE* gene (6p21.3, OMIM #235200), but mutation in the hemojuvelin gen (*HJV*, 1q21) has also been described.[47] Hereditary hemochromatosis is characterized by the deposition of hemosiderin pigment in various tissues, which if left untreated may lead to diabetes mellitus, cirrhosis, heart failure, joint disease (preferentially affecting the second and third metacarpophalangeal joints), gonadal dysfunction, amenorrhea, and generalized bronze cutaneous hyperpigmentation.

The primary oral manifestation of hereditary hemochromatosis, or any state of iron overload, is blue-gray to brown hyperpigmentation that most commonly affects the palate, buccal mucosa, and gingivae.[17] This oral pigmentation, however, is seen in a minority of patients with hereditary hemochromatosis. When stained with Prussian blue, biopsy specimens may demonstrate iron deposits.

The diagnosis of hereditary hemochromatosis requires measurement of serum ferritin and transferrin saturation. Serum ferritin levels greater than 200 μg/L in premenopausal women and 300 μg/L in men and postmenopausal women indicate iron overload due to hemochromatosis. Transferrin saturation refers to the ratio of serum iron and total iron-binding capacity, and is more sensitive than serum ferritin as a screening tool for hemochromatosis. A fasting transferrin saturation greater than 45% to 50% is diagnostic for hemochromatosis. Genetic testing for *HFE* mutations should be considered in patients with laboratory or histologic evidence of iron overload, especially in the context of liver disease. Treatment consists of serial phlebotomy, and chelation therapy may also be indicated.

Congenital erythropoietic porphyria

Porphyrias are a heterogeneous group of genetic metabolic disorders involving disruption of the heme biosynthetic pathway. Porphyrias are categorized based on the enzymatic defect and organ systems affected. Congenital erythropoietic porphyria (CEP, OMIM #263700, also known as Gunther disease) is a very rare autosomal recessive disorder caused by a deficiency of uroporphyrinogen III synthase (*UROS* gene, 10q25.2-q26.3).[48] High amounts of uroporphyrin accumulate in all tissues and when concentrated in erythrocytes, osmotic fragility results in hemolysis. Hemolytic anemia may present as early as in utero, potentially resulting in hydrops fetalis or intrauterine fetal demise. Porphyrins deposited in bone impart orange-red fluorescence and result in severe bone loss, osteopenia, and acro-osteolysis. Pink to red discoloration of the urine is pathognomonic; pink staining of the diapers in infancy may be the initial presenting sign. Mucocutaneous manifestations are common, and the disease can have devastating sequelae.

CEP typically presents in infancy or early childhood with severe photosensitivity leading to burning, blistering, erosions, hyperpigmentation, milia, and scarring of sun-exposed skin. Mutilation deformity of the face and hands with syndactyly (mitten deformity) is notable. Hypertrichosis of the face and extremities is common; the pathogenesis of this clinical manifestation is not known. Porphyrin deposition also affects the conjunctiva and manifests as conjunctivitis, blepharitis, and scarring with ectropion. Corneal scarring with eventual blindness may occur.[49]

A pathognomonic oral manifestation of CEP is erythrodontia, a condition in which the teeth develop a red-brown discoloration and bright red fluorescence on Wood's lamp examination (**Fig. 3**).[16,50,51] This unusual finding is thought to result from

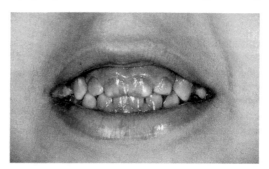

Fig. 3. Pathognomonic brown-red pigmentation of the teeth (erythrodontia) in a child with congenital erythropoietic porphyria. (*Courtesy* of Anthony J. Mancini, MD.)

increased binding of porphyrin to calcium phosphate in dentin and enamel.[51] Erythrodontia is not observed in other porphyrias.

Treatment includes strict avoidance of sun exposure and use of ocular lubricants. Red blood cell transfusion and bone marrow transplantation have been reported to be successful.

Platelet Disorders

Thrombocytopenia

A reduction in platelet number or function can occur through a variety of mechanisms, including autoimmune destruction (including connective tissue disease), splenic sequestration, bone marrow infiltration by tumor cells, infection (eg, infectious mononucleosis), and adverse drug reaction. Regardless of the cause, platelet disorders typically manifest with petechiae, purpura, and bleeding of the mucous membranes. Other presentations include epistaxis, hematuria, gastrointestinal bleeding, and on rare occasion, intracranial hemorrhage.

Gingival bleeding, either spontaneous or in response to minor trauma (ie, toothbrushing, flossing), is often the first sign of thrombocytopenia. The oral mucosa, most notably soft palate and buccal mucosa, may demonstrate petechiae and ecchymoses. Deep red to black hemorrhagic bullae may occur with very low platelet counts.[11]

ORAL MANIFESTATIONS OF NUTRITIONAL DISEASES

Vitamins and minerals are organic and inorganic substances, respectively, that are required for the health and function of epithelia including skin and mucous membranes. Nutritional deficiencies of vitamins and minerals can result from reduced intake, impaired absorption, or increased use (relative to the amount consumed). In economically disadvantaged communities, inadequate dietary consumption accounts for the majority of nutrient deficiencies. Eating disorders, fad diets, debilitated states, and alcoholism can also result in inadequate consumption of vitamins and minerals. Nutrient intake correlates with the number of posterior occluding pairs of natural teeth that an individual possesses.[52] Edentulous adults have been shown to have lower levels of retinol, β-carotene, ascorbate, tocopherol, and folic acid than dentate adults.[53]

The rate of epithelial cell turnover of the oral mucous membranes is much more rapid than that of skin (3–7 days[54] vs up to 28 days[55]). As a result, the oral cavity often demonstrates early signs and symptoms of metabolic alteration resulting from systemic diseases, medications, or nutritional deficiencies. Repetitive exposures and trauma that occur with normal daily activities (ie, eating, breathing, talking) may augment the impact of nutritional deficiencies on mucous membrane integrity. Oral commensal microflora and pathologic microorganisms can further challenge weakened mucous membranes.[54]

Water-soluble vitamins that have a role in the health and normal function of the oral mucosa, and therefore exhibit oral manifestations when deficient, include vitamins B2 (riboflavin), B3 (niacin), B6 (pyridoxine), B9 (folic acid), B12 (cobalamin), and C. Water-soluble vitamins are not stored in the body in large amounts and therefore must be obtained through dietary or supplement sources on a regular and frequent basis.[54] The lack of large body stores effectively prevents hypervitaminoses of water-soluble vitamins. By contrast, significant physiologic reservoirs of fat-soluble vitamins preclude the need for daily consumption but also predispose to potential toxicity. Fat-soluble vitamins that affect the oral mucosa include vitamins A, D, and K.

Water-Soluble Vitamins

Vitamin B1 (thiamine, thiamin, aneurin)

Vitamin B1 was the first B vitamin discovered. Vitamin B1 facilitates the conversion of carbohydrates to glucose and the intracellular metabolism of fats and proteins.[56] Dietary sources of vitamin B1 include yeast, wheat germ, whole-grain or enriched cereals, legumes, liver and other organ meats, lean meats (especially pork), blackstrap molasses, and soybeans. Vitamin B1 is easily destroyed on exposure to heat. Vitamin B1 is absorbed by the small intestine (predominantly the jejunum and ileum) through both passive and active transport mechanisms.[57] The half-life of thiamine is 9 to 18 days, and thiamine stores become depleted within 1 month.[58] Risk factors for vitamin B1 deficiency include alcoholism (which interferes with thiamine absorption), gastrointestinal disease (including prolonged diarrhea), renal dialysis, hyperemesis gravidarum, hyperthyroidism, lactation, diabetes mellitus, parenteral nutrition, anorexia nervosa, and a diet consisting predominantly of polished rice.[54] Thiamine deficiency results in beriberi and Wernicke-Korsakoff syndrome, neither of which have oral manifestations.

Vitamin B2 (riboflavin, lactoflavin)

Vitamin B2 is part of the coenzymes flavin mononucleotide (FMN) and flavin adenine dinucleotide (FAD), which aid enzymes in several intracellular metabolic oxidation/reduction reactions involved in cellular metabolism, the processing of carbohydrates, amino acids, and fats, and the regeneration of the free radical scavenger glutathione.[59] Riboflavin is found in milk, other dairy products, and dietary sources that contain significant amounts of vitamin B1. Unlike vitamin B1, however, vitamin B2 is heat-stable. Vitamin B2 is absorbed primarily in the proximal small bowel. Risk factors for vitamin B2 deficiency include alcoholism, gastrointestinal disease (ie, achlorhydria, malabsorption, diarrhea, and so forth), chlorpromazine use (due to increased excretion of riboflavin), and other nutrient deficiencies (ie, zinc, vitamin B3). Vitamin B2 deficiency is usually seen as a component of mixed B vitamin deficiency and classically manifests as the oculo-oro-genital syndrome.[60,61] Patients with this triad present with conjunctivitis, photophobia, and pruritic or burning, erythematous, scaling patches involving the genitalia (scrotum, penis, vulva) and perianal skin that may progress to superficial ulceration. Oral manifestations include erythema of the pharyngeal and oral mucous membranes, atrophic glossitis with a magenta color, glossodynia, cheilosis, and angular cheilitis.

The diagnosis of riboflavin deficiency is made clinically but may be assisted by the detection of an increased activation coefficient for red blood cell glutathione reductase activity. Rapid amelioration of signs and symptoms on administration of vitamin B2 (1–3 mg/d for children, 10–20 mg/d for adults) confirms the diagnosis.

Vitamin B3 (niacin, nicotinic acid)

Vitamin B3 and its amide form, niacinamide (nicotinamide), are required for normal cell function and metabolism. The amide derivatives, nicotinamide adenine dinucleotide (NAD) and nicotinamide adenine dinucleotide phosphate (NADP), play vital roles in pyridoxine nucleotide (cytosine, thymidine) synthesis, oxidation/reduction reactions involved in carbohydrate, amino acid, glycerol, and fatty acid metabolism, and adenine triphosphate (ATP) production. Sources of niacin include yeast, meats (eg, liver, lean pork, salmon, and poultry), cereals, legumes, and seeds. Niacin and niacinamide are absorbed through the intestinal epithelium via simple diffusion. Niacin is also produced de novo from tryptophan with the assistance of vitamin and mineral cofactors (vitamin B2, vitamin B6, copper, and iron). Predisposing factors for the development of vitamin B3 deficiency include alcoholism, gastrointestinal disease, consumption of a corn-dominant diet, drug therapy (ie, isoniazid, 5-fluorouracil, 6-mercaptopurine, and sulfapyridine), congenital defects of tryptophan transport in the intestine and/or kidneys (eg, Hartnup disorder, OMIM #234500),[62,63] and carcinoid syndrome in which tryptophan is converted preferentially to serotonin instead of niacin.[64,65]

Niacin deficiency, termed pellagra, exhibits diarrhea, photodistributed dermatitis, and dementia; death may occur. Early symptoms include malaise, apathy, and weakness. Gastrointestinal involvement may precede other organ systems and presents with nausea, abdominal pain, and diarrhea (typically watery, but bloody and mucoid may also be seen) with malabsorption. Initial cutaneous findings include erythema and edema accompanied by a burning sensation, with or without blisters (much like acute sunburn) symmetrically distributed at areas of sun exposure and/or trauma. Over time, progressive brittle scaling, lichenification, and hyperpigmentation of skin lesions occur. Neurologic symptoms may include paresthesias and muscle weakness with ataxia. Mental status changes, including apathy, depression, irritability, and poor concentration occur early in the course of disease and can progress to disorientation, delirium, and coma. Within the oral cavity, niacin deficiency exhibits mucosal edema, cheilosis, angular cheilitis, bright red glossitis, burning mouth, gingival erythema, and dental caries.[54]

Low serum levels of niacin, tryptophan, NAD, and NADP confirm the diagnosis of pellagra. Measurement of urinary niacin metabolites (eg, N-methylnicotinamide) may be more sensitive than measurement of serum NAD and NADP levels.[66] Oral administration of niacinamide (for adults, 100 mg every 6 hours until resolution of major acute symptoms followed by 50 mg every 8–12 hours until the skin normalizes; for children, 10–50 mg every 6 hours until disease resolution) effectively reverses the clinical signs and symptoms of pellagra. Patients with pellagra often suffer from other nutritional deficiencies mandating provision of a high-protein diet and B-complex vitamin supplementation.

Vitamin B5 (pantothenic acid)
Vitamin B5 is a component of coenzyme A and therefore plays an instrumental role in many cellular metabolic processes including fatty acid metabolism, cholesterol synthesis, and amino acid degradation. Key sources of pantothenic acid include meat (ie, beef, chicken, liver), eggs, tomatoes, broccoli, potatoes, and whole grains.[67] Pantothenic acid deficiency is rare due to its wide presence in foods and large body stores. Symptoms of vitamin B5 deficiency include numbness and burning paresthesias of the feet. Pantothenic acid deficiency does not exhibit oral manifestations.

Vitamin B6 (pyridoxine, pyridoxal, pyridoxamine)
Vitamin B6 has various forms and is involved in gluconeogenesis, amino acid decarboxylation, fatty acid metabolism, heme biosynthesis, and neurotransmitter synthesis.[54] As noted previously, vitamin B6 is an important cofactor in the conversion of tryptophan to niacin. Sources of vitamin B6 include meat, fish, eggs, milk, whole grains, vegetables, and nuts. Intestinal absorption of vitamin B6 occurs in the proximal jejunum. Advanced age, alcoholism, chronic renal failure and/or renal dialysis, liver disease, malnutrition, and intestinal malabsorption predispose to vitamin B6 deficiency. Increased pyridoxine requirements occur during pregnancy and lactation. Administration of isoniazid, D-penicillamine, hydralazine, L-dopa, or cycloserine may precipitate pyridoxine deficiency.[54]

Pyridoxine deficiency presents with weakness, dizziness, and fatigue resulting from the associated anemia. Bilateral distal extremity numbness followed by burning paresthesia with impaired proprioception and vibration, depression, confusion, and generalized seizures may also occur. Patients may experience anorexia, nausea, abdominal discomfort, and diarrhea. Examination may reveal a scaling, erythematous eruption, similar to seborrheic dermatitis, around the eyes, nose, and mouth. Oral manifestations include atrophic glossitis, cheilosis, angular stomatitis, and gingival erythema.[54]

Low plasma pyridoxal-5-phosphate levels confirm vitamin B6 deficiency. Pyridoxine replacement, the dose and administration route of which depend on the disease severity and underlying etiology, results in improvement over days to weeks. Secondary B vitamin deficiencies (eg, niacin) may result from pyridoxine deficiency, and the patient's comprehensive nutritional needs should be addressed.

Vitamin B7 (biotin, vitamin H)
Vitamin B7 is an essential cofactor for carboxylases involved in fatty acid synthesis, gluconeogenesis, and amino acid catabolism. Dietary sources of biotin include cooked egg yolks, sardines, nuts (almonds, peanuts, pecans, walnuts), and legumes. Inadequate dietary intake rarely causes biotin deficiency. Prolonged consumption of raw egg white, parenteral nutrition without biotin supplementation, and biotinidase deficiency (OMIM #253260) cause biotin deficiency.[68] In addition, long-term anticonvulsant therapy can deplete biotin stores.[69,70]

Neurologic symptoms include depression, hallucination, ataxia, and peripheral paresthesias. In infancy, hypotonia, lethargy, and developmental delay may occur. Biotin deficiency presents with alopecia, conjunctivitis, and periorificial dermatitis with erythema and fine scaling around the eyes, nose, mouth, genitalia, and anus. Biotin deficiency does not cause oral mucous membrane pathology.

Vitamin B9 (folic acid, folate)
Vitamin B9 is reduced by dihydrofolate reductase to the biologically active form, tetrahydrofolate (tetrahydrofolic acid). Tetrahydrofolate plays an integral role in the synthesis of purines, thymidine, and amino acids and therefore affects DNA, RNA, and protein production and cell division. As such, folate deficiency preferentially affects tissues with rapid rates of cell turnover and high DNA synthesis requirements (ie, bone marrow, gastrointestinal epithelium, and mucosa).

Folate is widely distributed among food groups but is found in significant amounts in green leafy vegetables (eg, spinach), yeast, legumes (eg, lima and kidney beans), peanuts, organ meats (eg, liver, kidney), and dairy products. Food preparation and cooking (eg, boiling) can significantly reduce folate content. Folate is absorbed in the proximal jejunum through both active and passive transport. Risk factors for vitamin B9 deficiency include low socioeconomic status, infancy and prematurity, advanced age, institutionalization, alcoholism, malnutrition, and gastrointestinal diseases (ie, celiac disease and inflammatory bowel disease) with resulting malabsorption, as well as pregnancy, lactation, and chronic hemolytic anemia (due to increased demand). Methotrexate, sulfasalazine, and valproic acid interfere with folate metabolism. Increased excretion of folate occurs in the context of vitamin B12 deficiency.

Folate deficiency results in megaloblastic anemia with or without thrombocytopenia and leukopenia as well as gastrointestinal and neurologic disturbances. Anorexia, abdominal pain, nausea, vomiting, and diarrhea are common. Neurologic sequelae include confusion, peripheral neuropathy, and seizures. Folate deficiency results in elevated serum homocysteine levels and predisposes to atherosclerosis.[71] During pregnancy, folate deficiency may result in spontaneous abortion, placental abruption, and congenital neural tube defects. Oral findings include atrophic glossitis with erythema and swelling of the tongue and angular cheilitis.[54] Patients may also report tongue soreness or burning and dysphagia.

Folate administration in the context of vitamin B12 deficiency can result in significant neurologic deterioration; therefore, patients with megaloblastic anemia should be evaluated with measurement of both serum folate and vitamin B12 levels. Folate supplementation corrects folate deficiency and prevents complications.

Vitamin B12 (cobalamin, cyanocobalamin)

Vitamin B12 is an important cofactor required for DNA synthesis. Dietary sources of vitamin B12 include milk, cobalamin-fortified cereals, eggs, and meat; plants have little cobalamin content. Ingested cobalamin in food is liberated by pepsin digestion in the gastric acidic milieu. Cobalamin is then bound by intrinsic factor (IF), a glycoprotein produced by gastric parietal cells. The IF-cobalamin complex eventually binds to and is internalized with the IF receptor on the epithelial cells of the duodenum and ileum. Intestinal cobalamin absorption also occurs less efficiently via passive diffusion. The elderly, strict vegetarians or vegans, and those who have undergone gastric or ileal resection are particularly susceptible to vitamin B12 deficiency. Pernicious anemia, the most common form of vitamin B12 deficiency, is caused by autoantibodies against IF and/or gastric parietal cells and appears to have a genetic predisposition.[38] Large body stores, half of which are located in the liver, delay clinical manifestations of cobalamin deficiency by 2 to 5 years.

Vitamin B12 deficiency results in megaloblastic anemia, which is indistinguishable from that of folate deficiency. Neurologic sequelae of cobalamin deficiency involve the brain, spinal cord (posterior and lateral columns), and peripheral and optic nerves. Symptoms include ascending numbness or paresthesias that begin in the distal extremities, ataxia and gait difficulties, limb weakness, and psychiatric and cognitive disturbances. Deficiency of cobalamin manifests orally as generalized stomatitis, taste disturbance, and a red, atrophic, beefy, burning tongue in which the loss of filiform papillae imparts a "bald" appearance.[54] Oral changes may occur in the absence of symptomatic anemia. Folate and vitamin B12 deficiencies have been implicated in RAS, with improvement of some patients' aphthae following repletion.[38–41]

The diagnosis of vitamin B12 deficiency is made when megaloblasts and hypersegmented neutrophils are noted on peripheral blood smear in the context of a low serum vitamin B12 level. Detection of either antiparietal cell antibodies or antibodies to IF confirms the diagnosis of pernicious anemia. In the absence of these autoantibodies, elevated serum gastrin levels demonstrate achlorhydria and suggest pernicious anemia. If the aforementioned laboratory evaluation is unrevealing, the Schilling test can be used to determine the etiology of cobalamin deficiency.[72] Depending on the pathogenesis of cobalamin deficiency, parenteral or oral cyanocobalamin administration can correct the hematologic, neurologic, and mucocutaneous abnormalities. Patients should be evaluated and treated for additional nutritional deficiencies, specifically folate. Patients with pernicious anemia exhibit increased risk of gastric carcinoma and carcinoid tumors, and should undergo close surveillance.[73,74]

Vitamin C (ascorbic acid, ʟ-ascorbic acid, ascorbate)

Vitamin C is a cofactor for norepinephrine synthesis, amidation of peptide hormones, carnitine biosynthesis, and tyrosine metabolism. Vitamin C is also an essential cofactor for prolyl hydroxylase and lysyl hydroxylase, and therefore plays an integral role in collagen formation. Vitamin C participates in redox reactions and acts as an antioxidant.[75] Vitamin C also enhances the absorption of iron in the small intestine. Humans are unable to synthesize ascorbic acid.[76] Excellent dietary sources of vitamin

C include citrus fruits, broccoli, tomatoes, green peppers, and cabbage. Vitamin C levels are depleted after 30 days if no exogenous vitamin C is consumed.[77] Risk factors for vitamin C deficiency include male gender, low dietary intake, and tobacco smoking (which reduces absorption and accelerates degradation of vitamin C).[78] Additional predisposing conditions include advanced age, alcoholism, low socioeconomic status, small bowel diseases, and chronic diarrhea. Pregnancy, lactation, type 1 diabetes mellitus, and hemodialysis exhibit increased demands for vitamin C.[79,80]

Early signs of vitamin C deficiency include lethargy and malaise. Shortness of breath, myalgias, and arthralgias also occur. Due to its essential role in collagen synthesis, vitamin C deficiency results in poor wound healing, dehiscence of established scars, and bony abnormalities. Capillary fragility manifests as perifollicular petechiae (most notable on the lower extremities and buttocks), generalized ecchymosis, and subperiosteal, retrobulbar, subarachnoid, and intracerebral hemorrhages. Capillary fragility may be demonstrated at the bedside using the Rumpel-Leede test (capillary fragility test, tourniquet test). Advanced scurvy presents with anemia, convulsions, neuropathy, jaundice (secondary to hemolysis), oliguria, and generalized edema, and may be fatal. Cutaneous findings include roughness and scaling with follicular accentuation, corkscrew hairs, and alopecia. Intraoral manifestations include mucosal petechiae, swollen and blue or red gingivae (hemorrhagic gingivitis), gingival bleeding, gingival hypertrophy, and interdental infarcts.[81,82] Loss of connective tissue and alveolar bone result in loosening and loss of the teeth.[83] Low dietary vitamin C intake confers an increased risk of 20% for developing periodontal disease.[83]

Symptoms of deficiency manifest at a vitamin C level of less than 2.5 mg/dL. Oral vitamin C (100 mg 3 times daily) results in rapid improvement; intestinal absorption is limited to 100 mg at a time. Parenteral administration should be used in patients with malabsorption. Prompt diagnosis and treatment can reverse signs and symptoms and prevent permanent sequelae.

Fat-Soluble Vitamins

Vitamin A (retinol)

Vitamin A encompasses a family of fat-soluble vitamins that include retinol (preformed vitamin A, obtained from animal sources), β-carotene (provitamin A, obtained from plant sources), and carotenoids. Retinol is the most biologically active form. Vitamin A plays an important role in epithelial integrity, vision, immune response, and reproduction as well as the growth and modeling of bones and teeth.[53] Rich sources of vitamin A include liver, cod liver oil, eggs, whole milk, and yellow-green leafy vegetables. Vitamin A is absorbed throughout the intestine and is stored in the liver (50%–80% of total body stores), lungs, kidneys, and adipose tissue. The bioavailability of vitamin A from animal sources is greater than that from plant sources. Predisposing conditions for vitamin A deficiency include malnutrition, alcoholism, fat malabsorption disorders, small bowel bypass surgery, impaired biliary or pancreatic secretions, and a vegan diet. Ethanol consumption inhibits the biochemical processing of retinol.

Vitamin A deficiency is associated with impaired cellular and humoral immunity as well as ocular, cutaneous, and mucosal changes. Xerophthalmia, abnormal keratinization of the cornea, nyctalopia (poor adaption to darkness), and blindness may result. Follicular hyperkeratosis (phrynoderma, toadskin), diffuse dryness and scaling, and wrinkling are typical cutaneous findings. Oral manifestations of vitamin A deficiency include xerostomia, periodontal disease, and increased rates of intraoral infection. In infants and children with vitamin A deficiency, impaired tooth development is noted. Laboratory evaluation of persons with suspected vitamin A deficiency should include serum retinol level, zinc level, iron studies (as low iron may worsen vitamin A deficiency), and complete blood count (to assess for anemia or infection). Treatment requires vitamin A supplementation, the dose of which varies with deficiency severity, and remediation of underlying contributing factors.

The large stores of vitamin A in conjunction with the body's inability to catabolize vitamin A predispose to potential toxicity. Hypervitaminosis A may be acute or chronic and occur in the setting of food fads (ie, excessive consumption of liver) and accidental overdose (carotenemia or other vitamin A ingestion). Clinical manifestations exhibit dose-dependent severity and include headache, anorexia, nausea, abdominal pain, myalgias, bone and joint pain, and irritability. Hepatic dysfunction and reduced bone mineral density may result. Women of reproductive age are at risk for retinoid embryopathy (hydrocephalus, central nervous system abnormalities, cerebellar malformation, microphthalmia, microtia/anotia, micrognathia, cleft palate, cardiac defects, hypoplastic or absent thymus) if toxicity occurs early in pregnancy. Generalized dryness of the skin and mucous membranes (conjunctivae, nasal mucosa) is characteristic. Oral manifestations of vitamin A toxicity include cheilitis, gingivitis, and impaired healing. Carotenemia (excessive consumption of β-carotene) manifests as yellow-orange discoloration of the skin; the sclera and oral mucous membranes, however, are not affected. Treatment of vitamin A intoxication includes discontinuation of vitamin A consumption and supportive care; signs and symptoms typically improve over several weeks.

Vitamin D (calciferol, cholecalciferol, ergocalciferol)

Vitamin D regulates calcium and phosphorus homeostasis via intestinal absorption and bone deposition and resorption. Ultraviolet B radiation (290–320 nm) transforms provitamin D_3 in the epidermis and dermis to previtamin D_3, which is then isomerized to vitamin D_3 (cholecalciferol). Alternatively, vitamin D_3 (cholecalciferol) and vitamin D_2 (ergocalciferol) may be absorbed from dietary sources. Vitamin D (which includes vitamin D_3 and vitamin D_2) must be sequentially hydroxylated in the liver and kidneys to be biologically active. Dietary sources of vitamin D are somewhat limited and include fish liver oils (ie, cod liver oil), fatty fish (ie, salmon, mackerel), egg yolks, and fortified milk. Vitamin D is absorbed in the small intestine. Risk factors for vitamin D deficiency include inadequate exposure to sunlight, advanced age, more darkly pigmented skin, institutionalization, malabsorption or resection of the small intestine, hepatic or renal disease, and exclusive breast feeding of infants. Medications that induce the activity of hepatic cytochrome P450 enzymes (ie, phenytoin, phenobarbital, and rifampin) increase the catabolism of vitamin D.

Rickets, vitamin D deficiency in children, presents with frontal bossing, pectus carinatum, kyphosis, and bowing of the legs with delayed gross motor milestones. Vitamin D deficiency in adults results in osteomalacia (poor mineralization of the skeletal matrix) with periosteal bone pain, myalgias, and proximal muscle weakness. Although lower levels of vitamin D may increase the likelihood of the loss of periodontal attachment, vitamin D deficiency lacks other oral mucosal findings.[84] Patients with hypervitaminosis D exhibit signs and symptoms of hypercalcemia.

Vitamin E (tocopherol)

Vitamin E is an antioxidant that prevents propagation of free radical damage to biologic membrane lipids. Vitamin E is found in a wide variety of dietary sources, notably oils and fats. Susceptible populations for vitamin E deficiency include premature infants and patients with fat malabsorption syndromes, impaired pancreatic or biliary secretion, lipid transport abnormalities, or genetic abnormalities of α-tocopherol transfer protein (α-TTP) (ie, ataxia with vitamin E deficiency, OMIM #277460).[85] Vitamin

E deficiency is rare and presents with peripheral neuropathy, muscle weakness, and cardiac arrhythmias. There are no oral manifestations of tocopherol deficiency.

Vitamin K (phylloquinone)

Vitamin K is an essential cofactor in the production of the procoagulant Factors II (prothrombin), VII, IX, and X, and the anticoagulant proteins, Protein C and Protein S. Vitamin K is found in significant amounts in green leafy vegetables (ie, collard greens, spinach, broccoli) and oils (ie, soybean, canola, olive). Vitamin K is absorbed predominantly in the terminal ileum. Risk factors for vitamin K deficiency include small bowel resection, chronic liver disease, cholestasis, lipid malabsorption, chronic illness, alcoholism, malnutrition, oral anticoagulant therapy (ie, warfarin, salicylates), or prolonged use of antibiotics. Newborns, especially those that are exclusively breast-fed, are also susceptible. The main clinical manifestation of vitamin K deficiency is bleeding, which can affect any site. Oral signs may include submucosal hemorrhage and gingival bleeding. Diagnostic testing reveals a low serum vitamin K level and prolonged prothrombin time. Asymptomatic vitamin K deficiency can be treated with oral phytonadione. Menadione, a synthetic, water-soluble form of vitamin K, is administered orally in patients with fat malabsorption. In more severe cases, intramuscular or subcutaneous vitamin K administration may be warranted.

ANOREXIA NERVOSA AND BULIMIA NERVOSA

Patients with eating disorders are particularly susceptible to nutritional deficiencies. Patients with anorexia nervosa (AN) and bulimia nervosa (BN) are prone to a variety of deficiencies that affect both the hard and soft tissues of the oral cavity including the teeth, bones, periodontal tissues, salivary glands, and mucous membranes.[86,87] Although AN and BN patients achieve weight management through different mechanisms, both disorders are rooted in altered perception of body image and a variety of stressors. Women account for 85% to 95% of patients with eating disorders, and AN is twice as common as BN.[88] According to the *Diagnostic and Statistical Manual of Mental Disorders IV*, AN is defined as a refusal to maintain body weight at or above a minimally normal weight for age and height (typically <85% ideal body weight), intense fear of gaining weight, disturbance in the way one's body weight or shape is experienced, and amenorrhea in postmenarchal females of at least 3 menstrual cycles.[89] Systemic signs of AN include hypothermia, peripheral edema, hypotension, and bradycardia. Diagnostic criteria for BN include recurrent episodes of binge eating with a perceived lack of control over eating during these episodes, recurrent inappropriate compensatory behavior to prevent weight gain, binging and compensatory activity at least twice a week for 3 months, and undue influence of body shape and weight on self-evaluation.[89] Patients with BN frequently have normal or above-normal weight. Cutaneous manifestations of eating disorders include xerosis, lanugo, alopecia, and poor skin turgor.[90] Mucosal findings include atrophy, glossitis, and gingivitis due to vitamin deficiencies.[87] Trauma secondary to purging may be associated with erythematous erosions on the soft palate, while repeated trauma of the purging finger against the maxillary teeth may result in hyperkeratosis and scarring of the dorsal aspects of the fingers and hands (Russell sign). Demineralization and loss of tooth enamel result from recurrent vomiting followed by toothbrushing in the presence of gastric acid. Other causes of enamel loss include regular consumption of carbonated beverages and mechanical erosion associated with toothbrushing. Patients with BN or the binge/purge subtype of AN may paradoxically present with "chubby cheeks," which are caused by parotid gland sialadenosis or necrotizing sialometaplasia.[87] The treatment of patients with eating disorders may be particularly challenging given the associated psychological conditions and multisystem involvement, and these patients may be best cared for in the context of a multidisciplinary clinic.

SUMMARY

This review of the oral manifestations of vitamin deficiencies and hematologic disorders reveals the importance of a careful and comprehensive history and physical examination in evaluating patients with these conditions. The overlapping, nonspecific signs and symptoms of vitamin deficiencies necessitate a complete evaluation of the patient's nutritional status before initiating any isolated replacement therapy. The signs and symptoms affecting the oral cavity in both hematologic and nutritional disorders are underappreciated but can have a profound impact on the quality of life and prognosis in these complex patients.

REFERENCES

1. Online Mendelian Inheritance in Man, OMIM (TM). Cyclic hematopoiesis. 2010. Available at: http://www.ncbi.nlm.nih.gov/omim/. Accessed June 29, 2010.
2. Patton LS. Hematologic diseases. In: Ship JA, Greenberg MS, Glick M, editors. Burket's oral medicine. 11th edition. Hamilton (ON): BC Decker Inc; 2008. p. 385–410.
3. Horwitz MS, Duan Z, Korkmaz B, et al. Neutrophil elastase in cyclic and severe congenital neutropenia. Blood 2007;109(5):1817–24.
4. Berliner N, Horwitz M, Loughran TP Jr. Congenital and acquired neutropenia. Hematology Am Soc Hematol Educ Program 2004;63–79.
5. Peng HW, Chou CF, Liang DC. Hereditary cyclic neutropenia in the male members of a Chinese family with inverted Y chromosome. Br J Haematol 2000;110(2):438–40.
6. Dale DC, Bolyard AA, Aprikyan A. Cyclic neutropenia. Semin Hematol 2002; 39(2):89–94.
7. Grenda DS, Murakami M, Ghatak J, et al. Mutations of the ELA2 gene found in patients with severe congenital neutropenia induce the unfolded protein response and cellular apoptosis. Blood 2007;110(13):4179–87.
8. Palmer SE, Stephens K, Dale DC. Genetics, phenotype, and natural history of autosomal dominant cyclic hematopoiesis. Am J Med Genet 1996;66(4):413–22.
9. Cohen DW, Morris AL. Periodontal manifestations of cyclic neutropenia. J Periodontol 1961;32:159–68.
10. Long LM Jr, Jacoway JR, Bawden JW. Cyclic neutropenia: case report of two siblings. Pediatr Dent 1983;5(2):142–4.
11. Eisen D, Lynch DP. Oral manifestations of systemic diseases. the mouth: diagnosis and treatment. St. Louis (MO): Mosby; 1998. 212–36.
12. Hou GL, Huang JS, Tsai CC. Analysis of oral manifestations of leukemia: a retrospective study. Oral Dis 1997;3(1):31–8.
13. McKenna SJ. Leukemia. Oral Surg Oral Med Oral Pathol Oral Radiol Endod 2000; 89(2):137–9.
14. Weckx LL, Hidal LB, Marcucci G. Oral manifestations of leukemia. Ear Nose Throat J 1990;69(5):341–2, 345–6.
15. Cooper CL, Loewen R, Shore T. Gingival hyperplasia complicating acute myelomonocytic leukemia. J Can Dent Assoc 2000;66(2):78–9.
16. Cawson RA, Odell EW. Cawson's essentials of oral pathology and oral medicine. 8th edition. Edinburgh (NY): Churchill Livingstone/Elsevier; 2008.

17. Bruch JM, Treister NS. Clinical oral medicine and pathology. New York: Humana Press; 2010.
18. Neville B, Damm DD, White DH. Lymphoreticular and hematopoietic diseases. color atlas of clinical oral pathology. 2nd edition. Ontario (Canada): BC Decker Inc; 2003. p. 313–32.
19. Kolokotronis A, Konstantinou N, Christakis I, et al. Localized B-cell non-Hodgkin's lymphoma of oral cavity and maxillofacial region: a clinical study. Oral Surg Oral Med Oral Pathol Oral Radiol Endod 2005;99(3):303–10.
20. Bower M. Acquired immunodeficiency syndrome-related systemic non-Hodgkin's lymphoma. Br J Haematol 2001;112(4):863–73.
21. Gabarre J, Raphael M, Lepage E, et al. Human immunodeficiency virus-related lymphoma: relation between clinical features and histologic subtypes. Am J Med 2001;111(9):704–11.
22. Pluda J, Yarchoan R. For HIV patients survival increases the risk of lymphoma. RN 1990;53(11):144.
23. Falk RH, Comenzo RL, Skinner M. The systemic amyloidoses. N Engl J Med 1997; 337(13):898–909.
24. Aono J, Yamagata K, Yoshida H. Local amyloidosis in the hard palate: a case report. Oral Maxillofac Surg 2009;13(2):119–22.
25. Stoopler ET, Sollecito TP, Chen SY. Amyloid deposition in the oral cavity: a retrospective study and review of the literature. Oral Surg Oral Med Oral Pathol Oral Radiol Endod 2003;95(6):674–80.
26. Mardinger O, Rotenberg L, Chaushu G, et al. Surgical management of macroglossia due to primary amyloidosis. Int J Oral Maxillofac Surg 1999;28(2):129–31.
27. Viggor SF, Frezzini C, Farthing PM, et al. Amyloidosis: an unusual case of persistent oral ulceration. Oral Surg Oral Med Oral Pathol Oral Radiol Endod 2009; 108(5):e46–50.
28. Hachulla E, Janin A, Flipo RM, et al. Labial salivary gland biopsy is a reliable test for the diagnosis of primary and secondary amyloidosis. A prospective clinical and immunohistologic study in 59 patients. Arthritis Rheum 1993;36(5):691–7.
29. Elad S, Czerninski R, Fischman S, et al. Exceptional oral manifestations of amyloid light chain protein (AL) systemic amyloidosis. Amyloid 2010;17(1):27–31.
30. Vela-Ojeda J, Garcia-Ruiz Esparza MA, Padilla-Gonzalez Y, et al. Multiple myeloma-associated amyloidosis is an independent high-risk prognostic factor. Ann Hematol 2009;88(1):59–66.
31. Milian MA, Bagan JV, Jimenez Y, et al. Langerhans' cell histiocytosis restricted to the oral mucosa. Oral Surg Oral Med Oral Pathol Oral Radiol Endod 2001;91(1):76–9.
32. Madrigal-Martinez-Pereda C, Guerrero-Rodriguez V, Guisado-Moya B, et al. Langerhans cell histiocytosis: literature review and descriptive analysis of oral manifestations. Med Oral Patol Oral Cir Bucal 2009;14(5):E222–8.
33. Castling B, Smith AT, Myers B. Involvement of the jaw bones in systemic mastocytosis. Br J Oral Maxillofac Surg 2006;44(2):87–8.
34. Medina R, Faecher RS, Stafford DS, et al. Systemic mastocytosis involving the mandible. Oral Surg Oral Med Oral Pathol 1994;78(1):28–35.
35. Bac DJ, van Marwijk Kooy M. Mastocytosis and Sjögren's syndrome. Ann Rheum Dis 1992;51(2):277–8.
36. Pal B. Systemic mastocytosis and Sjögren's syndrome. Ann Rheum Dis 1992; 51(10):1183.
37. Tharp MD. Mast cell disease. In: Callen J, Jorizzo JL, Bolognia JL, et al, editors. Dermatologic signs of internal disease. Philadelphia (PA): Elsevier; 2009. p. 349–54.

38. Lu SY, Wu HC. Initial diagnosis of anemia from sore mouth and improved classification of anemias by MCV and RDW in 30 patients. Oral Surg Oral Med Oral Pathol Oral Radiol Endod 2004;98(6):679–85.

39. Koybasi S, Parlak AH, Serin E, et al. Recurrent aphthous stomatitis: investigation of possible etiologic factors. Am J Otolaryngol 2006;27(4):229–32.

40. Piskin S, Sayan C, Durukan N, et al. Serum iron, ferritin, folic acid, and vitamin B12 levels in recurrent aphthous stomatitis. J Eur Acad Dermatol Venereol 2002;16(1):66–7.

41. Scully C, Gorsky M, Lozada-Nur F. The diagnosis and management of recurrent aphthous stomatitis: a consensus approach. J Am Dent Assoc 2003;134(2):200–7.

42. Patton LL, Brahim JS, Travis WD. Mandibular osteomyelitis in a patient with sickle cell anemia: report of case. J Am Dent Assoc 1990;121(5):602–4.

43. Shroyer JV 3rd, Lew D, Abreo F, et al. Osteomyelitis of the mandible as a result of sickle cell disease. Report and literature review. Oral Surg Oral Med Oral Pathol 1991;72(1):25–8.

44. Friedlander AH, Genser L, Swerdloff M. Mental nerve neuropathy: a complication of sickle-cell crisis. Oral Surg Oral Med Oral Pathol 1980;49(1):15–7.

45. Gregory G, Olujohungbe A. Mandibular nerve neuropathy in sickle cell disease. Local factors. Oral Surg Oral Med Oral Pathol 1994;77(1):66–9.

46. Kelleher M, Bishop K, Briggs P. Oral complications associated with sickle cell anemia: a review and case report. Oral Surg Oral Med Oral Pathol Oral Radiol Endod 1996;82(2):225–8.

47. Online Mendelian Inheritance in Man, OMIM (TM). Hemachromatosis. 2010. Available at: http://www.ncbi.nlm.nih.gov/omim/. Accessed July 1, 2010.

48. Online Mendelian Inheritance in Man, OMIM (TM). Congenital erythropoietic porphyria. 2009. Available at: http://www.ncbi.nlm.nih.gov/omim. Accessed July 3, 2010.

49. Altiparmak UE, Oflu Y, Kocaoglu FA, et al. Ocular complications in two cases with porphyria. Cornea 2008;27(9):1093–6.

50. Nunsley J, Grossman M, Piette W. Porphyrias. In: Callen J, Jorizzo J, Bolognia J, et al, editors. Dermatologic signs of internal disease. 4th edition. Philadelphia (PA): Saunders Elsevier; 2009. p. 223–4.

51. Fritsch C, Bolsen K, Ruzicka T, et al. Congenital erythropoietic porphyria. J Am Acad Dermatol 1997;36(4):594–610.

52. de Andrade FB, de Franca Caldas A Jr, Kitoko PM. Relationship between oral health, nutrient intake and nutritional status in a sample of Brazilian elderly people. Gerodontology 2009;26(1):40–5.

53. Krall EA, Henshaw M. The older dental patient. In: Palmer CA, Friedman GJ, Friedman DR, editors. Diet and nutrition in oral health. 2nd edition. Upper Saddle River (NJ): Pearson Prentice Hall; 2007. p. 379–96.

54. Boyd L, Palmer C. Nutrition and oral health. In: Brian JN, Cooper MD, editors. Complete review of dental hygiene. Upper Saddle River (NJ): Prentice-Hall; 2001. Chapter 5.

55. Weinberg MA. Anatomy of the periodontal structures: the healthy state. In: Weinberg MA, Westphal C, Froum SJ, et al, editors. Comprehensive periodontics for the dental hygienist. 2nd edition. Upper Saddle River (NJ): Pearson Prentice Hall; 2006. Chapter 1.

56. Lonsdale D. A review of the biochemistry, metabolism and clinical benefits of thiamin (e) and its derivatives. Evid Based Complement Alternat Med 2006;3(1):49–59.

57. Butterworth RF. Thiamin. In: Shils ME, Shike M, Ross AC, et al, editors. Modern nutrition in health and disease. 10th edition. Baltimore (MD): Lippincot Williams & Wilkins; 2006. p. 426–32.

58. Thiamine. Monograph. Altern Med Rev 2003;8(1):59–62.
59. Rivlin RS. Riboflavin (Vitamin B2). In: Zempleni J, Rucker RB, McCormick DB, et al, editors. Handbook of vitamins. 4th edition. Boca Raton (FL): CRC Press; 2007. p. 233–52.
60. Jacobs EC. Oculo-oro-genital syndrome: a deficiency disease. Ann Intern Med 1951;35(5):1049–54.
61. Friedli A, Saurat JH. Images in clinical medicine. Oculo-orogenital syndrome—a deficiency of vitamins B2 and B6. N Engl J Med 2004;350(11):1130.
62. Online Mendelian Inheritance in Man, OMIM (TM). Hartnup disorder. 2009. Available at: http://www.ncbi.nlm.nih.gov/omim. Accessed July 13, 2010.
63. Levy HL. Hartnup disorder. In: Scriver CR, Sly WS, Childs B, et al, editors. The metabolic and molecular bases of inherited disease. 8th edition. New York: McGraw-Hill Professional; 2003. p. 4957–69.
64. Castiello RJ, Lynch PJ. Pellagra and the carcinoid syndrome. Arch Dermatol 1972;105(4):574–7.
65. Shah GM, Shah RG, Veillette H, et al. Biochemical assessment of niacin deficiency among carcinoid cancer patients. Am J Gastroenterol 2005;100(10):2307–14.
66. Creeke PI, Dibari F, Cheung E, et al. Whole blood NAD and NADP concentrations are not depressed in subjects with clinical pellagra. J Nutr 2007;137(9):2013–7.
67. Trumbo PR. Pantothenic acid. In: Shils ME, Shike M, Ross AC, et al, editors. Modern nutrition in health and disease. 10th edition. Baltimore (MD): Lippincott Williams & Wilkins; 2006. p. 462–7.
68. Online Mendelian Inheritance in Man, OMIM (TM). Biotinidase deficiency. 2009. Available at: http://www.ncbi.nlm.nih.gov/omim/. Accessed July 6, 2010.
69. Mock DM, Dyken ME. Biotin catabolism is accelerated in adults receiving long-term therapy with anticonvulsants. Neurology 1997;49(5):1444–7.
70. Mock DM, Mock NI, Nelson RP, et al. Disturbances in biotin metabolism in children undergoing long-term anticonvulsant therapy. J Pediatr Gastroenterol Nutr 1998;26(3):245–50.
71. Varela-Moreiras G, Murphy MM, Scott JM. Cobalamin, folic acid, and homocysteine. Nutr Rev 2009;67(Suppl 1):S69–72.
72. Snow CF. Laboratory diagnosis of vitamin B12 and folate deficiency: a guide for the primary care physician. Arch Intern Med 1999;159(12):1289–98.
73. Hsing AW, Hansson LE, McLaughlin JK, et al. Pernicious anemia and subsequent cancer. A population-based cohort study. Cancer 1993;71(3):745–50.
74. Hagarty S, Huttner I, Shibata H, et al. Gastric carcinoid tumours and pernicious anemia: case report and review of the literature. Can J Gastroenterol 2000; 14(3):241–5.
75. Russell RM, Suter PM. Vitamin and trace mineral deficiency and excess. In: Fauci AS, Braunwald E, Kasper DL, et al, editors. Harrison's principles of internal medicine. 17th edition. New York: McGraw-Hill Companies, Inc; 2008. p. 445.
76. Leger D. Scurvy: reemergence of nutritional deficiencies. Can Fam Physician 2008;54(10):1403–6.
77. Levine M, Conry-Cantilena C, Wang Y, et al. Vitamin C pharmacokinetics in healthy volunteers: evidence for a recommended dietary allowance. Proc Natl Acad Sci U S A 1996;93(8):3704–9.
78. Mosdol A, Erens B, Brunner EJ. Estimated prevalence and predictors of vitamin C deficiency within UK's low-income population. J Public Health (Oxf) 2008;30(4): 456–60.
79. Biesalski HK. Parenteral ascorbic acid in haemodialysis patients. Curr Opin Clin Nutr Metab Care 2008;11(6):741–6.

80. Singer R, Rhodes HC, Chin G, et al. High prevalence of ascorbate deficiency in an Australian peritoneal dialysis population. Nephrology (Carlton) 2008;13(1): 17–22.
81. Moynihan PJ, Lingstrom P. Oral consequences of compromised nutritional well-being. In: Touger-Decker R, Sirois DA, Mobley CC, editors. Nutrition and oral medicine. Totowa (NJ): Humana Press; 2005. p. 107–28.
82. Li R, Byers K, Walvekar RR. Gingival hypertrophy: a solitary manifestation of scurvy. Am J Otolaryngol 2008;29(6):426–8.
83. Nishida M, Grossi SG, Dunford RG, et al. Dietary vitamin C and the risk for periodontal disease. J Periodontol 2000;71(8):1215–23.
84. Dietrich T, Joshipura KJ, Dawson-Hughes B, et al. Association between serum concentrations of 25-hydroxyvitamin D3 and periodontal disease in the US population. Am J Clin Nutr 2004;80(1):108–13.
85. Online Mendelian Inheritance in Man, OMIM (TM). Familial isolated deficiency of Vitamin E. 2003. Available at: http://www.ncbi.nlm.nih.gov/omim. Accessed July 15, 2010.
86. Yager J, Andersen AE. Clinical practice. Anorexia nervosa. N Engl J Med 2005; 353(14):1481–8.
87. Lo Russo L, Campisi G, Di Fede O, et al. Oral manifestations of eating disorders: a critical review. Oral Dis 2008;14(6):479–84.
88. Hoek HW, van Hoeken D. Review of the prevalence and incidence of eating disorders. Int J Eat Disord 2003;34(4):383–96.
89. American Psychiatric Association. American Psychiatric Association. Task force on DSM-IV. Diagnostic and statistical manual of mental disorders: DSM-IV. 4th edition. Washington, DC: American Psychiatric Association; 1994.
90. Coxson HO, Chan IH, Mayo JR, et al. Early emphysema in patients with anorexia nervosa. Am J Respir Crit Care Med 2004;170(7):748–52.

Burning Mouth Syndrome and Secondary Oral Burning

Jacob S. Minor, MD[a],*,
Joel B. Epstein, DMD, MSD, FRCD(C), FDS RCS(Ed)[b,c]

KEYWORDS

- Burning mouth syndrome • Glossodynia • Stomatopyrosis
- Neuropathy • Taste change • Xerostomia

Burning mouth syndrome (BMS) is an idiopathic condition causing a deep burning pain of the oral mucosa, despite an absence of identifiable dental or medical pathology, lasting at least 4 to 6 months.[1–7] BMS should be distinguished from secondary oral burning reported by patients with a variety of documented oral mucosal and medical conditions. BMS was first described by Fox[8] in 1935 and has gone by many aliases, including glossodynia, glossopyrosis, oral dysesthesia, sore tongue, stomatodynia, and stomatopyrosis.[9] The International Classification of Diseases (ICD-9) uses the term glossodynia with the descriptors glossopyrosis or painful tongue for code 529.6.[10] In this article BMS is used to refer to idiopathic oral burning not associated with oral mucosal or systemic conditions.

BMS is found in a 7:1 female to male ratio and approximately 90% of sufferers are perimenopausal women.[5] In one study of 130 patients, a burning sensation was noted in the tongue in 72%, in the hard palate in 25%, in the lips in 24%, and other sites such as buccal and labial mucosa, soft palate, and floor of mouth in 36%. Whereas some patients had burning confined to the tongue only, others had other or multiple sites of involvement.[11] Another study showed similar prevalence of tongue involvement, though with palate and lip involvement in only 5.7% of respondents.[12] In many cases symptomatic complaints are bilaterally distributed. Many patients also report

---

The authors have nothing to disclose.
[a] Department of Otolaryngology, University of Colorado at Denver, 12631 East 17th Avenue, B-205, Denver, CO 80045, USA
[b] Department of Oral Medicine and Diagnostic Sciences, College of Dentistry, University of Illinois at Chicago, MC 838, 801 South Paulina Street, Chicago, IL 60612, USA
[c] Department of Otolaryngology and Head and Neck Surgery, University of Illinois at Chicago, MC 838, 801 South Paulina Street, Chicago, IL 60612, USA
* Corresponding author.
E-mail address: jacob.minor@ucdenver.edu

Otolaryngol Clin N Am 44 (2011) 205–219
doi:10.1016/j.otc.2010.09.008
0030-6665/11/$ – see front matter © 2011 Elsevier Inc. All rights reserved.

associated symptoms of oral dryness and alteration in taste, such as a metallic bitter sensation, as well as worsening with stress, excessive speaking, or hot foods, and improvement with cold food, work, and relaxation.[5,7,13–15] Taste change and oral dryness may be associated with etiology in some cases. In general, BMS does not interfere with sleep, but may be present on waking or increase later in the day.[16] In the patients who report xerostomia, measurement of saliva may or may not confirm hyposalivation, suggesting that in some cases the sensation reported of dryness may be related to altered sensation and not a change in saliva.[14] Because of the lack of findings on physical examination, BMS may be a source of frustration for the caregiver, the patient, and significant others related to the patient.[1] This article surveys the current state of knowledge regarding BMS with the aim of assisting the practitioner in forming a strategy for diagnosis and management of this condition.

EPIDEMIOLOGY

Several studies have attempted to assess the prevalence of BMS in various populations. The largest United States study surveyed more than 42,000 households for various types of orofacial pain, and estimated a BMS prevalence of 0.7%.[17] This method, of course, precluded examination to rule out other pathology and oral burning. A Swedish study in 1999 surveying 669 men and 758 women found a prevalence of 1.6% among men and 5.5% among women, with increasing prevalence with age up to more than 12% among the oldest women.[12] Patients in this study were brought in for examination if they reported burning mouth symptoms. In that study no BMS was found in men younger than 40 or in women younger than 30 years. Other studies have also confirmed that BMS is predominant in women,[6,18,19] especially in those who are perimenopausal.[20]

ETIOLOGY

Although there is no confirmed cause of BMS, the general consensus, including that of the International Headache Society, is that the condition represents a neuropathy resulting in chronic pain.[7,21–23] Evidence in favor of this is seen both on histopathology and in neurologic testing. Current areas of debate regarding the etiology of BMS include its status as primarily a central or peripheral neuropathic phenomenon, and the role of dysguesia as a primary or secondary event. Also, the nature of associations between BMS, menopause, and psychiatric disease remains unclear. Finally, it is important to understand the wide variety of other conditions causing oral burning symptoms, ensuring that patients diagnosed with BMS are not in fact experiencing burning secondary to a potentially treatable mucosal or systemic condition.

Evidence for BMS as a Peripheral Neuropathy

BMS is associated with unique histopathologic findings and alterations of levels of salivary neuropeptides. Lauria and colleagues[24] evaluated the innervation of the epithelium of the anterolateral tongue in 12 patients with BMS present for at least 6 months using 3-mm punch biopsies of the region. In addition, samples were obtained from 9 normal patients as a control. Immunohistochemical and confocal microscopy colocalization studies were performed with cytoplasmatic, cytoskeletal, Schwann cell, and myelin markers for pathologic changes. Of note, BMS patients showed a significantly lower density of epithelial nerve fibers than controls, with a trend toward correlation with the duration of symptoms. There was no correlation between density of fibers and severity of symptoms. Epithelial and subpapillary nerve fibers also showed diffuse morphologic changes reflecting axonal degeneration, demonstrating that BMS is associated with a small-fiber sensory neuropathy or axonopathy of the tongue and that biopsy can be used to assess the diagnosis. The investigators note that these findings correlate with histologic findings in burning disorders of the lower limbs, and that the nociceptive stimulation of these fibers may be contributory to the accompanying dysguesia.[24] A recent study by Borelli and colleagues[25] examined the levels of salivary neuropeptides in 20 BMS patients and matched controls, and found significantly increased nerve growth factor peptide and tryptase activity in saliva of BMS subjects. Conversely, levels of substance P were shown to be significantly lower while neutrophil markers were unchanged. The investigators felt these substances might be useful biomarkers for diagnosis and monitoring of BMS.

There are alterations in trigeminal nerve function in BMS patients. Two studies by Jaaskelainen and colleagues examined alteration in function of the trigeminal nerve among BMS patients. Their 1997 article[23] reported on 11 patients with BMS for at least 1 year and 10 healthy controls. Following a thorough neurologic and laboratory evaluation to rule out any other contributory factors, the patients underwent electrophysiologic evaluation of the blink reflex and jaw reflex, and needle electromyographic evaluations of facial and masticatory muscles were performed on those with abnormal blink reflexes. Although all other testing was normal, there was a significant abnormality noted in the blink reflexes of patients with BMS, suggestive of trigeminal dysfunction. A follow-up study in 2002[21] confirmed the findings of abnormal blink reflexes in 52 BMS patients, and correlated them with quantitative thermal thresholds in 46 of the patients. Seventy-six percent of patients tested had thermal sensory abnormalities, the majority of those some variety of hypoesthesia. Less than 10% of all patients had entirely normal electrophysiological testing of the trigeminal nerve. Some potential mechanisms include neuropathy due to causes such as injury during procedures in the mouth and throat, and viral-induced neuropathy.

Evidence for BMS as a Central Neuropathy

Central neuropathic mechanisms are also felt to be involved in BMS. Albuquerque and colleagues[26] demonstrated differences in perception of trigeminal pain between BMS and normal patients on functional magnetic resonance imaging (fMRI) in a 2006 study. In follow-up to their aforementioned work in trigeminal abnormalities in BMS, Jaaskelainen and colleagues[27] evaluated the nigrostriatal dopaminergic pathway in 10 BMS patients and 14 controls using modified positron emission tomography (PET). Findings of decreased uptake in the right putamen indicated decreased dopaminergic inhibition in BMS patients. Another study by the same group in 2003 found alterations consistent with a decline in endogenous dopamine levels in the putamen in BMS patients.[28]

Evidence for BMS as a Phantom Pain

The role of dysguesia as a primary or secondary phenomenon in BMS remains a point of investigation. Whereas some have felt dysguesia is a secondary event arising from trigeminal dysfunction,[24] others question if loss of taste might be an inciting event, playing a primary role in the etiology of some cases of BMS.[29–31] It is hypothesized that BMS represents a central oral phantom pain secondary to damage to the gustatory system and disinhibition of central nociceptive regions.[29,31–34] Other taste phantoms may also be associated with a similar etiology.[35] Other supporting evidence is that anesthesia of the chorda tympani has been demonstrated to increase the contralateral pain response to capsaicin,[36] and that overlap exists between brain regions involved in taste and pain perception.[37] Supertasters, those with a genetic alteration causing increased number of fungiform papillae and an ability to taste the bitter compound phenylthiocarbamide,[38,39] may be at increased risk.[32,33] BMS patients may also have a higher likelihood of taking medications interfering with taste.[31] Evidence that BMS is a form of oral phantom pain is both tantalizing and revealing, given the challenges experienced in treating the most common phantom sensation in otolaryngology, namely, tinnitus. Like tinnitus, BMS has an association with psychopathology and central and peripheral factors, as well as limited success with current medical therapies and a need for careful counseling of those affected.

Evidence for BMS as Variable Disorder with Subcategories

One recent effort to investigate a central versus peripheral origin for BMS was a double-blind, randomized crossover trial comprising 20 patients with BMS. The patients underwent lidocaine and saline injection of the lingual nerve, and although the group overall showed no significant difference in response, central (n = 7) and peripheral (n = 13) subgroups were identified. In the peripheral group, there was a significant decrease in burning with lidocaine injection compared with saline, whereas the central group had a nonsignificant trend toward worse burning with lidocaine. In addition, the peripheral group had a trend toward improved response to clonazepam, and had significantly less evidence of concomitant psychiatric issues on a validated survey. The 2 groups identified in this small study should be considered in the design of future treatment trials.[40]

Contributions of Psychiatric and Hormonal Disturbances

Several studies have investigated relationships between BMS and psychiatric disease.[6,41–49] Indeed, for several years BMS was felt by some to be primarily psychological in origin,[24] although studies were unable to demonstrate a link between its onset and a stressful life event.[46] Similar to other chronic pain patients, one group found an Axis I diagnosis in more than 50% of BMS patients, with depression predominating. Anxiety, when present, had an additional marked impact.[43] Another study assessed Axis II diagnoses in 70 BMS patients compared with a normal population and a group of patients with somatoform disorders. Whereas only 24% of the normal group had a personality disorder, 86% of the BMS patients and 88% of the somatoform patients had an Axis II disorder, although interestingly Cluster A predominated among BMS patients whereas somatoform patients had a higher incidence of Cluster B disorders.[42] Other potential psychogenic factors may include obsessive-compulsive disorder, depression, anxiety, and cancerophobia.[13] Psychopathology may also increase the likelihood of the patient's presentation and worsen the severity of the complaint, as is the case in chronic pain in general. So while considerable psychiatric comorbidity is present among BMS patients, this is felt to be usually a concurrent or secondary factor rather than its primary cause.

Menopause also has a definite but unclear relationship with BMS.[6,18,20,22] As mentioned earlier, up to 90% of patients with BMS are perimenopausal women.[5] Suggested explanations for this finding have included age-related changes, estrogen-related decreased perception of bitter tastes,[33] coexistence of depression and anxiety, and subtle mucosal changes. Pisanty and colleagues[50] relate the lack of evidence regarding the effects of estrogens on oral mucosa. Woda and colleagues[51] recently proposed that at menopause, the drastic decrease in gonadal steroids leads to altered production of neuroactive steroids, resulting in neurodegenerative changes of small nerve fibers of the oral mucosa and/or some brain areas involved in oral somatic sensations. These investigators posit that these neuropathic changes become irreversible and precipitate the burning pain, dysguesia, and xerostomia associated with BMS, which all involve small nerve fibers.

Distinguishing BMS from Secondary Oral Burning

One difficulty in assessing the literature regarding BMS is that it is often unclear whether local and systemic underlying conditions have been adequately assessed and excluded. Danhauer and colleagues[52] examined patients with BMS and compared them with patients who had oral burning derived from other clinical abnormalities. These investigators concluded that although the 2 categories of patients may initially present with similar clinical and psychosocial features, they are distinguishable with careful diagnosis that often enables successful management of symptoms for each group. Failure to rule out secondary oral burning will result in inappropriate management strategies. Because of this, it is important to understand the potential causes of secondary oral burning and symptom presentation. In BMS, complaints of oral burning may decrease when eating or chewing; symptoms are typically bilateral in presentation and may be present at multiple oral sites. Secondary oral burning related to mucosal changes may be localized to areas of mucosal lesions, and is typically increased with eating, particularly spicy or acidic foods. Secondary oral burning associated with systemic conditions may be bilateral.

One classification divides etiology of secondary oral burning into factors related to the mouth (such as decreased salivary production), systemic factors, and psychological conditions.[12,49] Another article by Cerchiari and colleagues[13] goes into further detail and includes etiologic categories of local, systemic, psychogenic, and idiopathic. In cases identifying local or systemic factors, the definition of idiopathic BMS is not met. Local factors might include parafunctional behaviors such as tongue movements or habits causing mucosal irritation,[53] dental disease or galvanism, allergic reactions to dental materials, dentures, or other local factors,[54] stomatitis, and infectious conditions such as candidiasis. Possible systemic causes of secondary oral burning include salivary dysfunction, endocrine disturbances, nutritional disorders such as vitamin B complex, folate, iron, or zinc deficiencies, gastrointestinal disease including gastritis, reflux, or *Helicobacter pylori* infection, medication-related causes, other distinct cranial neuropathies, and possibly primary psychiatric disease.[13,31,55]

PROGNOSIS

Limited studies have been done thus far to assess prognosis.[56] A retrospective review in 2006 including 48 women and 5 men with a mean age of 67.7 years (range 33–82 years) demonstrated a complete spontaneous remission in 3% of the patients within 5 years after the onset of BMS and moderate improvement in fewer than 30% of the subjects.[57] Other investigators have noted the tendency of BMS to persist for many years.[6]

EVALUATION AND DIAGNOSIS

As mentioned earlier, the diagnosis of BMS is primarily one of exclusion. To that end, it is important to conduct a history and physical examination of a patient with the complaint of oral burning, with the goal of identifying any primary etiology. Laboratory studies should also be guided by this principle in a cost-effective manner. **Box 1** outlines components of a thorough evaluation for BMS.

TREATMENT

The idea that BMS represents a form of chronic neuropathy is reflected in the most common approaches to clinical management. Recent reviews have examined evidence for various therapeutic interventions, including a 2004 Cochrane review[58]

Box 1
Recommended evaluation for oral burning symptoms

History

    Characteristics of the burning, including location, quality, severity, onset, duration, course over the day, aggravating/relieving factors: work, stress, foods, talking

    Associated symptoms: taste disturbances, oral dryness

    Medical history including ear disease, dental or oral disease, dentures, zoster, menopause, diabetes, thyroid disease, peripheral neuropathy, depression/anxiety

    Surgical history including oral, ear, and intracranial surgery

    Medications: angiotensin-converting enzyme inhibitors, antiretrovirals, tricyclic antidepressants, others (review side effect profiles)

Physical Examination Highlights

    General: age, gender, affect/mood

    Head: evidence of radiation or previous trauma or tumor

    Ears: examine for middle ear disease or evidence of surgery that might have damaged the chorda tympani

    Oral cavity: evaluate mucosa, dental health, salivary production, taste testing, tenderness to palpation, local anesthetic testing

    Neck: evaluate for goiter, lipodystrophy secondary to antiretrovirals, evidence of radiation

    Neurologic: peripheral neuropathy, complete neurologic examination

Laboratory Evaluation

    Full blood count

    Random blood glucose, Fasting blood glucose, hemoglobin A1c

    Alanine and aspartate transaminase

    Thyroid function (T3/T4)

    Serum iron, ferritin, total IgE, vitamin B6, B12, D

    Serum antinuclear antibodies, erythrocyte sedimentation rate

    Serum antibodies to *H pylori*

    Oral swab for *Candida*

---

and a more recent review by Buchanan and Zakrzewska.[56] Strategies that have thus far been investigated for treatment of BMS include clonazepam, α-lipoic acid, lafutidine, hormone replacement therapy, antidepressants, a variety of topical applications, anticonvulsants, medications for neuropathic pain, and psychiatric therapies. There are limited data on treatment approaches; although most represent small cohort studies, they do provide some guidance in treatment. **Box 2** summarizes current recommendations regarding management of BMS.

α-Lipoic Acid

Three studies of α-lipoic acid (ALA) in BMS,[69–71] all by Femiano and colleagues, were included in the Cochrane review mentioned previously.[58] ALA is mitochondrial coenzyme with antioxidant effect that has been shown to be neuroprotective in previous studies of diabetic neuropathy.[64] The first study included 42 patients with BMS in

---

Box 2
Current approach to management of BMS

- Diagnosis: rule out local and systemic conditions that may cause oral burning; if present treat accordingly and assess outcome

  Treatment of hyposalivation or tongue/jaw habit if present[53]

- Medication trials

  First-line therapies

    Clonazepam[30,59,60]

    Paroxetine[61,62]

    Lafutidine if available (not currently approved by Food and Drug Administration [FDA])[55]

  Second-line therapies (poor evidence supporting)

    Sertraline[62]

    Amisulpride[62]

    Gabapentin[63]

  Not recommended: α-lipoic acid,[64–66] hormone replacement therapy[50]

- Counseling and possible referral for formal psychiatric intervention

  Cognitive behavioral therapy[67]

  Group psychotherapy[68]

---

an open placebo-controlled trial. Forty-two percent of patients in the ALA arm initially had "decided improvement" versus 0% of placebo, and overall 76% reported "any improvement" versus 14% of placebo. After the placebo arm was crossed over, 52% of those patients had "decided improvement" and 63% reported "any improvement."[70] The second study of ALA was done in a double-blind, randomized controlled fashion in 2002 and featured 60 patients split into 2 arms. After 2 months, there was "any improvement" in 97% of the ALA arm versus 40% of placebo, and "decided improvement or resolution" in 87% of the ALA arm versus 0% of placebo ($P<.0001$).[71] The third study compared ALA with bethanecol, Biotene, and placebo, using 4 groups of 20 patients with BMS. The study found ALA of remarkable benefit with minimal adverse effects as compared with the other arms. Further multi-institutional double-blind, randomized controlled trials were recommended.[69] It is unclear whether any of the patient data are duplicated in these 3 studies by the same authors published within a similar timeframe.[56]

Recently, 3 randomized, double-blinded, placebo-controlled studies of ALA for BMS have been published, all by investigators and institutions unrelated to the aforementioned studies and each other. The first recent study features 66 patients enrolled in a 3-arm trial (ALA, ALA with multivitamin, and placebo) with treatment of ALA, 400 mg twice daily for 2 months in both ALA groups.[65] Fifty-two patients completed the trial and responders were those who had at least a 50% decrease in pain scores measured by the Visual Analog Scale (VAS) at 2 and 4 months. The study showed a significant response to intervention in all 3 groups (including placebo), with about 30% of each group responding. A second recent study by Lopez-Jornet and colleagues[66] included 60 patients split into 2 groups (ALA 800 mg daily and placebo) with responses also measured on the VAS. Again, no significant difference was found with ALA versus placebo. A third trial completed by 31 patients also failed to demonstrate the effectiveness of ALA over placebo.[72] These 3 well-designed trials cast serious doubt on the efficacy of ALA in the treatment of BMS.

Antidepressants

Several studies have examined the use of antidepressant medications in BMS, although in a limited fashion. A single double-blind, randomized controlled trial of trazodone versus placebo has been reported.[73] This study, which was done in Finland in 1999, included 37 women and failed to show any effect over the 8-week trial period; the trazodone group showed significantly worse symptoms of drowsiness and dizziness versus placebo. An open-label, single-arm, dose-escalation pilot study of the effect of paroxetine (Paxil) in treatment of BMS reported 80% of patients with pain reduction after 12 weeks of paroxetine treatment, with only minor transient side effects. These results suggest that paroxetine may be useful in the treatment of patients with BMS.[61]

A third trial in 2002 compared 2 selective serotonin reuptake inhibitors, paroxetine and sertraline (Zoloft), and amisulpride, an atypical antipsychotic.[62] The study was single-blinded without a placebo arm. Overall, 76 patients without concurrent major depression were enrolled in the 8-week trial and assigned to sertraline 50 mg daily, paroxetine 20 mg daily, or amisulpride 50 mg daily. Results were assessed using a VAS as well as the Hamilton Rating Scale for Depression and the Hamilton Rating Scale for Anxiety. Overall, 69.6% to 72.2% of patients responded, with mean VAS pain scores decreasing in all 3 arms from an initial range of 7.2 to 7.0 to a final range of 3.3 to 2.8 at week 8 ($P<.001$). Although no adverse events were noted in any arm of the trial,[62] paroxetine may cause congenital malformations when given in the first trimester,[74] and patients who do have concurrent major depressive disorder should be managed in coordination with a physician with appropriate experience in psychiatry.[56] Again, the study was limited by lack of a placebo arm.

Clonazepam and Chlordiazepoxide

Inspired by earlier promising successful open-label studies of topical[59] and systemic[30] clonazepam (Klonopin) for BMS, a multicenter, double-blinded, randomized controlled trial of topical clonazepam versus placebo was conducted with 84 patients (40 women and 44 men) in France and published in 2004.[60] The prior studies assessed low-dose systemic clonazepam without topical contact and reported improvement in oral burning in the majority of patients. Patients in the study were instructed to suck a tablet (either 1 mg clonazepam or placebo) for 3 minutes and swishing the dissolved medicine around the painful oral sites without swallowing before expectorating the medicine. The therapy was given 3 times daily for a total of 2 weeks. Pain was rated on a standard zero to 10 numerical scale before and after the intervention. Pain scores decreased 2.4 ± 0.6 in the clonazepam group versus 0.6 ± 0.4 in the placebo group ($P = .014$). There was no significant difference in adverse events between placebo and control. Despite the finding in the same study that the swish and spit technique resulted in significantly lower blood levels of clonazepam versus swallowing a 1-mg tablet, Buchanan and Zakrzewska[56] remind physicians of the addictive potential of benzodiazepines.

One other study of lower quality that remains interesting is a large nonrandomized nonplacebo controlled trial of multiple medications in 130 BMS patients in 1991 that included 78 patients who were placed on chlordiazepoxide (Librium), a benzodiazepine relative.[11] Of these, 14% had complete resolution, 35% had marked benefit, 15% had slight benefit, and 36% showed no change. The study design, however, was poor. By contrast, the cohort studies of clonazepam show more positive outcomes.[30,60] Of note, although both drugs bind to benzodiazepine receptors and enhance the action of γ-aminobutyric acid, clonazepam is used in the treatment of neuralgias and neuropathies, whereas chlordiazepoxide is not.[75,76] Given the likely neuropathic nature of BMS, the greater efficacy of clonazepam is perhaps unsurprising.

Gabapentin

Gabapentin (Neurontin) has been of interest in BMS on account of the putative neuropathic nature of the illness (or some subset thereof), but evidence in the literature in support of its use is discouraging. A trial of gabapentin[34] cited by Grushka and colleagues[77] in one review article was unavailable through PubMed and the journal's Web site. Another article in support is a single case report.[78] More importantly, the only multipatient trial currently available is an open dose-escalation study, in which 15 patients took gabapentin at doses from 300 up to 2400 mg per day over a course of 3 weeks. No significant improvement in pain, mood scales, or Beck Depression Inventory scores was seen after the 3-week period. These data indicate that gabapentin should not be used for trials except after the failure of other medications. A larger randomized trial of this medication may confirm its lack of efficacy for BMS.[63]

Hormone Replacement Therapy

The most recent Cochrane review of BMS[58] reports one trial of hormone replacement therapy. Pisanty and colleagues[50] conducted a blinded trial of estrone cream versus estrone and progesterone cream versus placebo in 1975. The 3 arms of the trial had 6, 9, and 7 patients, respectively. The results of the trial showed minimal effect, with no more than 25% of patients in any arm reporting improvement in the burning sensation. Many aspects of the trial were unclear, including criteria for diagnosis, baseline characteristics of the 3 groups, and whether randomization was performed. Buchanan and Zakrzewska[56] identified 3 other similarly poor-quality studies with unclear implications.

Lafutidine

Lafutidine is a unique histamine H2-receptor antagonist (H2RA) that has a sensitizing effect on capsaicin-sensitive afferent neurons. Because of this it was felt to have potential for treatment of BMS, and in a randomized controlled trial 34 BMS patients switched blindly to lafutidine from their previous H2-blocker and 30 BMS controls remained on their original H2-blocker. Both groups also did azulene sulfonate rinses. Symptoms were scored using a VAS at 4, 8, and 12 weeks. The improvement rate was consistently higher in the lafutidine group than in the control group; the differences between the groups were significant ($P<.05$).[55] Lafutidine is not currently approved by the FDA and is not available in the United States at present.[79]

Other Medical Treatments

Other treatments studied in the literature with minimal findings have included topical anesthetics, topical anti-inflammatory medications, capsaicin, sucralfate (Carafate), and St John's wort, among others. Oral habit appliances have been mentioned for use in patients with evidence of active tongue habits and lingual fasciculations; however, no clinical data are available. The topical anesthetic dyclonine hydrochloride was studied by Formaker and colleagues[33] in an open noncontrolled study of 33 patients. Of those, 12 had increased burning, 14 had no change, and 7 had improvement. A single trial in 1999 of benzydamine hydrochloride, a topical anti-inflammatory, failed to show an effect.[80] Therefore, limited study to date does not support the use of locally applied anesthetic or analgesic agents for idiopathic BMS.

Two articles discuss the use of capsaicin in BMS,[81,82] but the results are unclear, as one article in Italian does not give any information about patient response to capsaicin in the English abstract,[82] while the other includes only 2 patients classified as BMS among many with neuropathic oral pain. Of those two patients who used the topical capsaicin 0.025% cream, one had symptom resolution and the other discontinued the study with minimal improvement.[81] A single small nonplacebo controlled study in 1997 of sucralfate found very mixed results in 14 patients with BMS, with improvement in 6 patients and worsening of symptoms in 4.[83] Another recent study investigated possible therapy for BMS with *Hypericum perforatum* (St John's wort) in a placebo-controlled, double-blind, randomized controlled trial comprising 39 patients.[84] Unfortunately, the study failed to show any significant reduction in pain with this treatment.

Although amitriptyline (Elavil) and nortripyline (Pamelor) have been cited as therapeutic options for BMS in the same review,[77] there does not appear to be any reason to support this beyond anecdotal evidence. Despite this, it seems to be a not unreasonable third-line medication to try with otherwise unresponsive patients, given the apparent neuropathic nature of the disease. The nonrandomized noncontrolled trial by Gorsky and colleagues[11] of BMS therapies mentioned earlier also included patients who were trialed on antifungal agents, amitriptyline, prednisone, pilocarpine, vitamin B complex, and diazepam. Aside from diazepam, on which 4 of 6 patients noted considerable improvement, the results of the other groups were uniformly poor.

Cognitive Behavioral Therapy and Group Psychotherapy

Although there are various case reports in the literature,[85,86] only one randomized controlled trial has investigated cognitive behavioral therapy (CBT) for BMS. This trial from Umea University in Sweden included 30 patients split into 2 equal groups. The first group received CBT in the form of 12 to 15 sessions for 1 hour per week and the second attention and placebo group (APG) received a similar number of sessions, but without the CBT techniques. Pain was measured with a VAS (scale of 1–7). Pretreatment scores were similar between the 2 groups (CBT = 5.0, APG = 4.3). After treatment the CBT group showed an average score decrease of 3.6 versus an increase of 0.4 for the APG ($P<.001$). Weaknesses of the study included minimal information provided about other characteristics of the 2 groups and the lack of a validated pain scale.[67]

A recent study by Miziara and colleagues[68] investigated group psychotherapy as an additional modality for treatment of BMS. Of 44 diagnosed patients, 24 underwent group psychotherapy while 20 had placebo therapy. Improvement occurred among 71% of patients in the treatment group versus 40% in the placebo group ($P = .04$).

New Directions

Several recent case reports and studies have emerged concerning possible novel therapies for BMS. A 2007 article describes a single patient with BMS who had adverse reactions to initial therapy with carbamazepine (Tegretol) and gabapentin, but resolved completely with topiramate (Topamax).[87] A noncontrolled trial was recently reported using levosulpiride, 100 mg daily for 8 weeks, in 44 patients.[88] Of the 39 patients who completed the study, 28 showed some improvement, although none had complete resolution. Those with improvement tended to be patients with a shorter history of symptoms. The study is limited by its lack of a control arm. A third report in 2008 describes a patient with severe BMS who failed multiple initial attempts at therapy but who responded to pramipexol (Mirapex).[89] This case seems unusual, however, because the patient had relief of symptoms with tongue motion. Similarity to documented modulation of tinnitus with head and neck motions is curious,[90–92] and may represent a subcategory of BMS patients able to modulate the burning sensation. These reports, though intriguing, will require further investigation before they could be recommended as possible alternative therapies.

SUMMARY

Patients who present for evaluation of oral burning symptoms require a thorough evaluation to distinguish between secondary oral burning and primary BMS. Ensuring that other confounding conditions have been addressed prior to diagnosis of BMS is key to preventing improper attempts at treatment. While the exact etiology of BMS remains unclear, it seems most likely a neuropathy, with variable central and peripheral contributions among individuals. It is hoped that future efforts for BMS will include larger randomized therapeutic trials of both medical and psychiatric therapies as well as continued research into its exact origin.

REFERENCES

1. Klasser GD, Fischer DJ, Epstein JB. Burning mouth syndrome: recognition, understanding, and management. Oral Maxillofac Surg Clin North Am 2008; 20(2):255–71, vii.
2. Maltsman-Tseikhin A, Moricca P, Niv D. Burning mouth syndrome: will better understanding yield better management? Pain Pract 2007;7(2):151–62.
3. Sardella A. An up-to-date view on burning mouth syndrome. Minerva Stomatol 2007;56(6):327–40.
4. Zakrzewska JM, Forssell H, Glenny AM. Interventions for the treatment of burning mouth syndrome: a systematic review. J Orofac Pain 2003;17(4):293–300.
5. Clark GT, Minakuchi H, Lotaif AC. Orofacial pain and sensory disorders in the elderly. Dent Clin North Am 2005;49(2):343–62.
6. Grushka M. Clinical features of burning mouth syndrome. Oral Surg Oral Med Oral Pathol 1987;63(1):30–6.
7. Society IH. The international classification of headache disorders, 2nd edition. Cephalalgia 2004;24(Suppl 1):1–160.
8. Fox H. Burning tongue glossodynia. N Y State J Med 1935;35:881–4.
9. Merskey BN, editor. Classification of chronic pain: descriptions of chronic pain syndromes and definitions of pain terms. 2nd edition. Seattle (WA): IASP Press; 1994. p. 74–5.
10. WHO. World health organization international classification of diseases and related health problems 2009. Available at: http://www.icd9data.com/2009/Volume1/520-579/520-529/529/default.htm. Accessed March 28, 2010.
11. Gorsky M, Silverman S Jr, Chinn H. Clinical characteristics and management outcome in the burning mouth syndrome. An open study of 130 patients. Oral Surg Oral Med Oral Pathol 1991;72(2):192–5.
12. Bergdahl M, Bergdahl J. Burning mouth syndrome: prevalence and associated factors. J Oral Pathol Med 1999;28(8):350–4.
13. Cerchiari DP, de Moricz RD, Sanjar FA, et al. Burning mouth syndrome: etiology. Braz J Otorhinolaryngol 2006;72(3):419–23.
14. Chimenos-Kustner E, Marques-Soares MS. Burning mouth and saliva. Med Oral 2002;7(4):244–53.

15. Just T, Steiner S, Pau HW. Oral pain perception and taste in burning mouth syndrome. J Oral Pathol Med 2009;4:4.
16. Lamey PJ, Lamb AB, Hughes A, et al. Type 3 burning mouth syndrome: psychological and allergic aspects. J Oral Pathol Med 1994;23(5):216–9.
17. Lipton JA, Ship JA, Larach-Robinson D. Estimated prevalence and distribution of reported orofacial pain in the United States. J Am Dent Assoc 1993;124(10):115–21.
18. Basker RM, Sturdee DW, Davenport JC. Patients with burning mouths. A clinical investigation of causative factors, including the climacteric and diabetes. Br Dent J 1978;145(1):9–16.
19. Tammiala-Salonen T, Hiidenkari T, Parvinen T. Burning mouth in a Finnish adult population. Community Dent Oral Epidemiol 1993;21(2):67–71.
20. Wardrop RW, Hailes J, Burger H, et al. Oral discomfort at menopause. Oral Surg Oral Med Oral Pathol 1989;67(5):535–40.
21. Forssell H, Jaaskelainen S, Tenovuo O, et al. Sensory dysfunction in burning mouth syndrome. Pain 2002;99(1–2):41–7.
22. Frutos R, Rodriguez S, Miralles-Jorda L, et al. Oral manifestations and dental treatment in menopause. Med Oral 2002;7(1):26–30, 31–5.
23. Jaaskelainen SK, Forssell H, Tenovuo O. Abnormalities of the blink reflex in burning mouth syndrome. Pain 1997;73(3):455–60.
24. Lauria G, Majorana A, Borgna M, et al. Trigeminal small-fiber sensory neuropathy causes burning mouth syndrome. Pain 2005;115(3):332–7.
25. Borelli V, Marchioli A, Di Taranto R, et al. Neuropeptides in saliva of subjects with burning mouth syndrome: a pilot study. Oral Dis 2010;16(4):365–74.
26. Albuquerque RJ, de Leeuw R, Carlson CR, et al. Cerebral activation during thermal stimulation of patients who have burning mouth disorder: an fMRI study. Pain 2006;122(3):223–34.
27. Jaaskelainen SK, Rinne JO, Forssell H, et al. Role of the dopaminergic system in chronic pain—a fluorodopa-PET study. Pain 2001;90(3):257–60.
28. Hagelberg N, Forssell H, Rinne JO, et al. Striatal dopamine D1 and D2 receptors in burning mouth syndrome. Pain 2003;101(1–2):149–54.
29. Bartoshuk LM, Snyder DJ, Grushka M, et al. Taste damage previously unsuspected consequences. Chem Senses 2005;30(Suppl 1):i218–9.
30. Grushka M, Epstein J, Mott A. An open-label, dose escalation pilot study of the effect of clonazepam in burning mouth syndrome. Oral Surg Oral Med Oral Pathol Oral Radiol Endod 1998;86(5):557–61 [Evidence Grade B].
31. Femiano F, Lanza A, Buonaiuto C, et al. Burning mouth disorder (BMD) and taste: a hypothesis. Med Oral Patol Oral Cir Bucal 2008;13(8):E470–4.
32. Eliav E, Kamran B, Schaham R, et al. Evidence of chorda tympani dysfunction in patients with burning mouth syndrome. J Am Dent Assoc 2007;138(5):628–33.
33. Formaker BK, Mott AE, Frank ME. The effects of topical anesthesia on oral burning in burning mouth syndrome. Ann N Y Acad Sci 1998;855:776–80.
34. Grushka M, Bartoshuk LM. Burning mouth syndrome and oral dysesthesias. Can J Diagnos 2000;17:99–109.
35. Bartoshuk LM, Kveton J, Lehman C. Peripheral source of taste phantom (i.e., dysgeusia) demonstrated by topical anesthesia. Chem Senses 1991;16(5):499–500.
36. Tie K, Fast K, Kveton J, et al. Anesthesia of chorda tympani nerve and effect on oral pain. Chem Senses 1999;24:609.
37. Small DM, Apkarian AV. Increased taste intensity perception exhibited by patients with chronic back pain. Pain 2006;120(1–2):124–30.
38. Fox AL. Six in ten "tasteblind" to bitter chemical. Sci News 1931;9:249.

39. Reed DR, Nanthakumar E, North M, et al. Localization of a gene for bitter-taste perception to human chromosome 5p15. Am J Hum Genet 1999;64(5):1478–80.
40. Gremeau-Richard C, Dubray C, Aublet-Cuvelier B, et al. Effect of lingual nerve block on burning mouth syndrome (stomatodynia): a randomized crossover trial. Pain 2010;149(1):27–32.
41. Lamey PJ, Lamb AB. The usefulness of the HAD scale in assessing anxiety and depression in patients with burning mouth syndrome. Oral Surg Oral Med Oral Pathol 1989;67(4):390–2.
42. Maina G, Albert U, Gandolfo S, et al. Personality disorders in patients with burning mouth syndrome. J Personal Disord 2005;19(1):84–93.
43. Rojo L, Silvestre FJ, Bagan JV, et al. Psychiatric morbidity in burning mouth syndrome. Psychiatric interview versus depression and anxiety scales. Oral Surg Oral Med Oral Pathol 1993;75(3):308–11.
44. Bogetto F, Maina G, Ferro G, et al. Psychiatric comorbidity in patients with burning mouth syndrome. Psychosom Med 1998;60(3):378–85.
45. Browning S, Hislop S, Scully C, et al. The association between burning mouth syndrome and psychosocial disorders. Oral Surg Oral Med Oral Pathol 1987; 64(2):171–4.
46. Eli I, Kleinhauz M, Baht R, et al. Antecedents of burning mouth syndrome (glossodynia)—recent life events vs. psychopathologic aspects. J Dent Res 1994; 73(2):567–72.
47. Feinmann C, Harris M, Eli I, et al. Psychogenic facial pain. Part 2: management and prognosis. Br Dent J 1984;156(6):205–8.
48. Feinmann C, Harris M, Eli I, et al. Psychogenic facial pain. Part 1: the clinical presentation. Br Dent J 1984;156(5):165–8.
49. Lamey PJ, Lewis MA. Oral medicine in practice: burning mouth syndrome. Br Dent J 1989;167(6):197–200.
50. Pisanty S, Rafaely B, Polishuk W. The effect of steroid hormones on buccal mucosa of menopausal women. Oral Surg Oral Med Oral Pathol 1975;40(3):346–53.
51. Woda A, Dao T, Gremeau-Richard C. Steroid dysregulation and stomatodynia (burning mouth syndrome). J Orofac Pain 2009;23(3):202–10.
52. Danhauer SC, Miller CS, Rhodus NL, et al. Impact of criteria-based diagnosis of burning mouth syndrome on treatment outcome. J Orofac Pain 2002;16(4): 305–11.
53. Kho HS, Lee JS, Lee EJ, et al. The effects of parafunctional habit control and topical lubricant on discomforts associated with burning mouth syndrome (BMS). Arch Gerontol Geriatr 2009;21:21 [Evidence Grade B].
54. Marino R, Capaccio P, Pignataro L, et al. Burning mouth syndrome: the role of contact hypersensitivity. Oral Dis 2009;15(4):255–8.
55. Toida M, Kato K, Makita H, et al. Palliative effect of lafutidine on oral burning sensation. J Oral Pathol Med 2009;38(3):262–8 [Evidence Grade A].
56. Buchanan J, Zakrzewska J. Burning mouth syndrome. Clin Evid (Online) 2008;3: 1301–7.
57. Sardella A, Lodi G, Demarosi F, et al. Burning mouth syndrome: a retrospective study investigating spontaneous remission and response to treatments. Oral Dis 2006;12(2):152–5.
58. Zakrzewska JM, Forssell H, Glenny AM. Interventions for the treatment of burning mouth syndrome. Cochrane Database Syst Rev 2005;1:CD002779.
59. Woda A, Navez ML, Picard P, et al. A possible therapeutic solution for stomatodynia (burning mouth syndrome). J Orofac Pain 1998;12(4):272–8 [Evidence Grade B].

60. Gremeau-Richard C, Woda A, Navez ML, et al. Topical clonazepam in stomato-dynia: a randomised placebo-controlled study. Pain 2004;108(1–2):51–7 [Evidence Grade A].

61. Yamazaki Y, Hata H, Kitamori S, et al. An open-label, noncomparative, dose escalation pilot study of the effect of paroxetine in treatment of burning mouth syndrome. Oral Surg Oral Med Oral Pathol Oral Radiol Endod 2009;107(1): e6–11 [Evidence Grade B].

62. Maina G, Vitalucci A, Gandolfo S, et al. Comparative efficacy of SSRIs and ami-sulpride in burning mouth syndrome: a single-blind study. J Clin Psychiatry 2002; 63(1):38–43 [Evidence Grade B].

63. Heckmann SM, Heckmann JG, Ungethum A, et al. Gabapentin has little or no effect in the treatment of burning mouth syndrome—results of an open-label pilot study. Eur J Neurol 2006;13(7):e6–7 [Evidence Grade B].

64. Ziegler D, Hanefeld M, Ruhnau KJ, et al. Treatment of symptomatic diabetic polyneuropathy with the antioxidant alpha-lipoic acid: a 7-month multicenter randomized controlled trial (ALADIN III Study). ALADIN III Study Group. Alpha-lipoic acid in diabetic neuropathy. Diabetes Care 1999;22(8): 1296–301.

65. Carbone M, Pentenero M, Carrozzo M, et al. Lack of efficacy of alpha-lipoic acid in burning mouth syndrome: a double-blind, randomized, placebo-controlled study. Eur J Pain 2009;120(1–2):492–6 [Evidence Grade A].

66. Lopez-Jornet P, Camacho-Alonso F, Leon-Espinosa S. Efficacy of alpha lipoic acid in burning mouth syndrome: a randomized, placebo-treatment study. J Oral Rehabil 2009;36(1):52–7 [Evidence Grade A].

67. Bergdahl J, Anneroth G, Perris H. Cognitive therapy in the treatment of patients with resistant burning mouth syndrome: a controlled study. J Oral Pathol Med 1995;24(5):213–5 [Evidence Grade B].

68. Miziara ID, Filho BC, Oliveira R, et al. Group psychotherapy: an additional approach to burning mouth syndrome. J Psychosom Res 2009;67(5):443–8 [Evidence Grade B].

69. Femiano F. Burning mouth syndrome (BMS): an open trial of comparative efficacy of alpha-lipoic acid (thioctic acid) with other therapies. Minerva Stomatol 2002; 51(9):405–9 [Evidence Grade B].

70. Femiano F, Gombos F, Scully C, et al. Burning mouth syndrome (BMS): controlled open trial of the efficacy of alpha-lipoic acid (thioctic acid) on symptomatology. Oral Dis 2000;6(5):274–7 [Evidence Grade B].

71. Femiano F, Scully C. Burning mouth syndrome (BMS): double blind controlled study of alpha-lipoic acid (thioctic acid) therapy. J Oral Pathol Med 2002;31(5): 267–9 [Evidence Grade A].

72. Cavalcanti DR, da Silveira FR. Alpha lipoic acid in burning mouth syndrome—a randomized double-blind placebo-controlled trial. J Oral Pathol Med 2009; 38(3):254–61 [Evidence Grade A].

73. Tammiala-Salonen T, Forssell H. Trazodone in burning mouth pain: a placebo-controlled, double-blind study. J Orofac Pain 1999;13(2):83–8 [Evidence Grade A].

74. Cole JA, Ephross SA, Cosmatos IS, et al. Paroxetine in the first trimester and the prevalence of congenital malformations. Pharmacoepidemiol Drug Saf 2007; 16(10):1075–85.

75. Epocrates. Clonazepam; 2010. Available at: https://online.epocrates.com/noFrame/showPage.do?method=drugs&MonographId=182. Accessed March 28, 2010.

76. Epocrates. Chlordiazepoxide; 2010. Available at: https://online.epocrates.com/noFrame/showPage.do?method=drugs&MonographId=171. Accessed March 28, 2010.

77. Grushka M, Epstein JB, Gorsky M. Burning mouth syndrome. Am Fam Physician 2002;65(4):615–20.

78. White TL, Kent PF, Kurtz DB, et al. Effectiveness of gabapentin for treatment of burning mouth syndrome. Arch Otolaryngol Head Neck Surg 2004;130(6):786–8.

79. FDA.Drugs@FDA. 2010. Available at: http://www.accessdata.fda.gov/scripts/cder/drugsatfda/index.cfm. Accessed March 28, 2010.

80. Sardella A, Uglietti D, Demarosi F, et al. Benzydamine hydrochloride oral rinses in management of burning mouth syndrome. A clinical trial. Oral Surg Oral Med Oral Pathol Oral Radiol Endod 1999;88(6):683–6.

81. Epstein JB, Marcoe JH. Topical application of capsaicin for treatment of oral neuropathic pain and trigeminal neuralgia. Oral Surg Oral Med Oral Pathol 1994;77(2):135–40.

82. Lauritano D, Spadari F, Formaglio F, et al. Etiopathogenic, clinical-diagnostic and therapeutic aspects of the burning mouth syndrome—research and treatment protocols in a patient group. Minerva Stomatol 1998;47(6):239–51.

83. Campisi G, Spadari F, Salvato A. [Sucralfate in odontostomatology. Clinical experience]. Minerva Stomatol 1997;46(6):297–305 [in Italian].

84. Sardella A, Lodi G, Demarosi F, et al. Hypericum perforatum extract in burning mouth syndrome: a randomized placebo-controlled study. J Oral Pathol Med 2008;37(7):395–401.

85. Bonfils P, Peignard P, Malinvaud D. Cognitive-behavioral therapy in the burning mouth syndrome—a new approach. Ann Otolaryngol Chir Cervicofac 2005; 122(3):146–9.

86. Humphris GM, Longman LP, Field EA. Cognitive-behavioural therapy for idiopathic burning mouth syndrome: a report of two cases. Br Dent J 1996;181(6): 204–8.

87. Siniscalchi A, Gallelli L, Marigliano NM, et al. Use of topiramate for glossodynia. Pain Med 2007;8(6):531–4.

88. Demarosi F, Tarozzi M, Lodi G, et al. The effect of levosulpiride in burning mouth syndrome. Minerva Stomatol 2007;56(1–2):21–6.

89. Stuginski-Barbosa J, Rodrigues GG, Bigal ME, et al. Burning mouth syndrome responsive to pramipexol. J Headache Pain 2008;9(1):43–5.

90. Bjorne A. Assessment of temporomandibular and cervical spine disorders in tinnitus patients. Prog Brain Res 2007;166:215–9.

91. Kaltenbach JA. The dorsal cochlear nucleus as a contributor to tinnitus: mechanisms underlying the induction of hyperactivity. Prog Brain Res 2007; 166:89–106.

92. Rocha CA, Sanchez TG. Myofascial trigger points: another way of modulating tinnitus. Prog Brain Res 2007;166:209–14.

Early Detection of Premalignant Lesions and Oral Cancer

Toby O. Steele, MD[a],*, Arlen Meyers, MD, MBA[b]

KEYWORDS

- Oral cancer/carcinoma • Oral premalignant lesions
- Optical detection technology • Spectroscopy
- Optical coherence tomography • Oral cancer screening

Oral cavity cancer accounts for approximately 3% of all malignancies and is a significant worldwide health problem.[1,2] The American Cancer Society estimates that there will be approximately 5300 deaths in the United States in 2010, with more than 23,000 new cases of oral cancer.[3] Oral cancer occurs most commonly in middle-aged and elderly individuals; however, recent evidence suggests these demographics may be changing. Surveillance, Epidemiology, and End Results (SEER) data demonstrated an increase in the incidence of tongue cancer in young individuals (aged <40 years), from 3% in 1973 to approximately 6% in 1993, and many of the affected individuals are without traditional risk factors. Additionally, research indicates that the traditional male predominance is less overt in young individuals with oral squamous cell carcinomas (SCC).[4]

The majority of oral malignancies occur as squamous cell carcinomas and despite remarkable advances in treatment modalities, the 5-year survival rate has not significantly improved over the past several decades, hovering at about 50% to 60%.[3] The unfavorable 5-year survival rate may be attributable to several factors. First, oral cancer is often diagnosed at a late stage, with late stage 5-year survival rates as low as 22%.[3] Additionally, the development of secondary primary tumors in patients with early stage disease has a major impact on survival.[5] The early detection and surveillance of oral cancer and premalignant lesions offers the promise to not only detect disease at early stages but also to improve the monitoring of disease progression or regression during treatment.

It is well accepted that many oral SCCs develop from premalignant conditions of the oral cavity.[6,7] A wide array of conditions have been implicated in the development of oral cancer, including leukoplakia; erythroplakia; palatal lesion of reverse cigar smoking;

[a] Department of Otolaryngology, Head and Neck Surgery, University of California Davis, 2521 Stockton Boulevard, Suite 7200, Sacramento, CA 95817, USA
[b] Department of Otolaryngology, Dentistry, and Engineering, University of Colorado Denver, 12631 East 17th Avenue, B205 Aurora, CO 80045, USA
* Corresponding author.
E-mail address: Tosteele@ucdavis.edu

Otolaryngol Clin N Am 44 (2011) 221–229
doi:10.1016/j.otc.2010.10.002
0030-6665/11/$ – see front matter © 2011 Published by Elsevier Inc.

oto.theclinics.com

oral lichen planus; oral submucous fibrosis; discoid lupus erythematosus; and heredi-tary disorders, such as dyskeratosis congenital and epidermolysis bullosa.[8] Much of the published information describing the prevalence of potentially malignant disorders varies by geographic location and population studied. Despite this limitation, a generally accepted prevalence rate ranges between 1% and 5%.[9] The majority of affected patients are middle-aged or elderly men. Potentially malignant disorders are discovered most commonly on the buccal mucosa, lower gingiva, tongue, and floor of the mouth, with the remaining cases distributed throughout the remainder of the oral cavity.[9]

Although it is generally accepted that early detection and screening for oral cancer has the potential to decrease the morbidity and mortality of disease, methods for screening have yet to be proven successful. The United States Preventive Services Task Force found no new good quality evidence that screening for oral cancer leads to improved health outcomes for either high-risk adults (ie, those over the age of 50 who use tobacco) or for average- risk adults in the general population.[10] Additionally, a recent Cochrane review stated "there is insufficient evidence to support or refute the use of a visual examination as a method of screening for oral cancer using a visual examination in the general population. Furthermore, no robust evidence exists to suggest that other methods of screening, toluidine blue, fluorescence imaging or brush biopsy, are either beneficial or harmful".[11] The following text provides a review of several of the investigated techniques for oral cancer detection, as well as an intro-duction to optical techniques for oral cancer detection.

THE EARLY DETECTION OF ORAL CANCER

With the development and success of screening programs for breast, cervical, and colon cancer, the potential to reduce the morbidity and mortality of oral cancer through early detection modalities is of critical importance. Data indicates that the diagnosis of oral squamous cell carcinoma at an early stage of disease allows for less aggressive treatment, improves quality of life, and improves the overall 5-year survival rate when compared with SCCs diagnosed at late stages.[3] The major modal-ities designed to reduce this burden include oral cavity examination, supravital stain-ing, oral cytology, and optical detection systems.

ORAL CAVITY EXAMINATION

The examination of the oral cavity has traditionally been the preferred approach for the detection of oral mucosal abnormalities. As a noninvasive technique, the oral cavity examination can be performed quickly, is without additional diagnostic expense to patients, and may be performed by health care professionals across a multitude of disci-plines. The evidence regarding oral examination as an effective screening technique, however, remains controversial. In a recently published randomized controlled trial with nearly 130,000 participants, investigators concluded that there was insufficient evidence to support or refute the use of oral examination as a screening program. However, this study, performed by the Kerala group in India, demonstrated improved survival rates at 9 years among men with high-risk habits (tobacco use).[12] Although there was no increase in survival for the overall population, this study was the first to clearly support the efficacy of an oral cancer screening program in a high-risk population.

SUPRAVITAL STAINING

Toluidine blue (TB) is an acidophilic dye designed to stain acidic cellular components, such as DNA and RNA. Its use in the detection of precancerous/cancerous tissue is based on the fact that dysplastic tissue contains quantitatively more DNA and RNA than nondysplastic tissue. To perform the staining, a 1% solution is placed on the oral mucosa and removed after 1 to 2 minutes with 2% acetic acid. The clinician then examines the oral mucosa for areas of increased cellular staining.[13] In the evaluation of a potentially malignant oral lesion, TB staining may provide better demarcation of lesion margins, guide biopsy site selection, and is thought to be valuable in identification and visualization of lesions in high-risk patients.[14–16] Though useful as an adjunct to clinical examination, the specificity of TB staining is limited as cells undergoing inflammatory changes and benign hyperplasia may also retain dye leading to false-positive results. Overall, the sensitivity of TB staining ranges from 0.78 to 1.00 and the specificity from 0.31 to 1.00.[14]

ORAL CYTOLOGY

Oral cytology describes a diagnostic technique employed to sample oral tissue for histomorphologic analysis. To obtain a tissue sample, the clinician applies a stiff brush to the oral mucosa with enough pressure to induce pinpoint bleeding which ensures a full-thickness or trans-epithelial tissue sample. These cellular samples can then be analyzed by a variety of unique diagnostic measures, including cytomorphometry, DNA cytometry, and immunocytochemical analysis.[13,17]

Computerized image analysis of brush biopsy samples (OralCDx Laboratories Suffern, NY, USA) uses a computer program to perform morphologic and cytologic analysis of tissue samples. The computerized analysis ranks cells based on the amount of abnormal morphology, which are then presented to a pathologist for further distinction and classification. The sensitivity of the OralCDx ranges from 0.71 to 1.00 and specificity as low as 0.32.[13]

DNA cytometry uses a DNA specific Feulgen dye to quantify and identify deviations in DNA content in sampled tissue. Although data are still limited, the addition of DNA measurements to cytologic analysis has been shown to increase the sensitivity and specificity of brush biopsies.[11]

The use of oral cytology in the detection of dysplastic lesions shows considerable promise, but has been limited thus far by variable false-positive and false-negative results.[13,14,16,17]

THE OPTICAL DETECTION OF ORAL CANCER

The field of optical diagnostics comprises a variety of techniques designed to characterize the relationship between the optical and biologic properties of tissue. Through the detection of changes in light after interaction with tissue, optical technologies provide information on the physiologic condition of the tissue at a molecular level. Early research in optical diagnostics suggested that alterations in light-tissue interactions can be used to differentiate normal from malignant tissue.[18] Subsequent advances in molecular biology, genomics, and proteomics, have vastly improved our scientific understanding of the complex biochemical and morphologic changes that occur as tissue undergoes the transformation from normal to neoplasia. Many of these early biologic events have been shown to alter the optical properties of precancerous and cancerous tissue. Light-based detection systems identify these optical signatures created during tissue transformation to provide a real-time assessment of tissue structure and metabolism.

Although the pathways responsible for the development of cancer are complex, it is widely accepted that cancer arises through the accumulation of DNA mutations that lead to unregulated proliferation. The proliferation of squamous cell cancer cells forms a morphologically distinctive spectrum of disease ranging from mild dysplasia to invasive carcinoma.[19] The current identification and diagnosis of precancerous and cancerous lesions relies on the histologic and cytologic examination performed by a pathologist after suspicious tissue is biopsied. Although these methods represent the gold standard for cancer diagnosis, they have several limitations. Tissue biopsy is invasive, expensive, and often time consuming. The diagnostic interpretation of the tissue sample has been shown to vary among pathologists, and the pathologic criteria for the identification of precancerous lesions are not well defined.[20] In addition, early precancerous changes are frequently undetectable by conventional visual inspection, leading to missed opportunities for diagnosis. Optical technologies have the potential to improve these limitations in several ways. Although the benefits provided vary with each technology, optical techniques offering objective data analysis may reduce the variation in pathologic diagnosis. Furthermore, optical technologies show the potential to provide a real-time tissue assessment through a minimally invasive route, eliminating lengthy waits and the need for tissue biopsy. Although the benefits of optical technologies are currently limited in clinical practice, the achievement of a highly sensitive and specific optically determined histopathologic diagnosis, an optical biopsy, has the potential to revolutionize medical practice.

TECHNIQUES FOR THE OPTICAL DETECTION OF CANCER
Spectroscopy

The use of spectroscopic techniques for the detection of cancerous and precancerous lesions is based on the analysis of specific light-tissue interactions to assess the state of biologic tissue. As tissue undergoes the carcinogenic sequence from normal to neoplasia, complex morphologic and molecular transformations occur that modify the manner in which light is absorbed and reflected in the tissue. With the delivery of specific wavelengths of light to tissue through an optical probe, a spectral pattern is collected that contains diagnostic information for tissue classification. Using histologically confirmed tissue specimens from benign and neoplastic tissue, scientists have assembled a spectral database of known light-tissue interactions. The spectra collected from an unknown tissue sample can then be analyzed through various empirical and statistical techniques to produce a histologic diagnosis. Spectroscopic techniques, such as fluorescence spectroscopy, light scattering spectroscopy, and Raman spectroscopy, use the unique spectral patterns that are created as tissue progresses toward cancer to offer the potential to detect diseased tissue during the initial stages of carcinogenesis.[21]

Fluorescence Spectroscopy

Fluorescence spectroscopy is based on the biologic emission of fluorescent light from tissue exposed to ultraviolet (UV) or short wavelength visible (VIS) light. To better understand fluorescence, a brief review of the interaction of light and tissue is warranted. Light is formed by packages of energy termed photons. When tissue is exposed to light, photons may be absorbed, reflected, or scattered by specific molecules within the tissue. As light illuminates the targeted tissue, these biomolecules, termed fluorophores, absorb the energy in the illuminating light and respond by emitting fluorescent light of lower energy (and longer wavelength). The change in wavelength then allows fluorescent light to be differentiated from illuminating light (UV or VIS light). Each group of fluorophores will respond to specific excitation wavelengths, and in turn, emit a different range of wavelengths resulting in a spectral pattern that ideally represents the biochemical and metabolic status of the tissue undergoing optical interrogation.[21–24]

Fluorescent light may be generated by the administration of an exogenous agent, such as in drug-induced fluorescence, or by the excitation of endogenous fluorophores (autofluorescence). As tissue undergoes the biochemical and morphologic progression to neoplasia, the concentration and distribution of the fluorophores are transformed. Known fluorophores include components of the connective matrix (collagen, elastin), metabolic coenzymes (reduced nicotinamide adenine dinucleotide, flavin adenine dinucleotide, flavin mononucleotide), aromatic amino acids (tryptophan, tyrosine, phenylalanine), byproducts of the heme biosynthetic pathway (porphyrins) and lipopigments (lipofuscin, ceroids). Factors influencing tissue autofluorescence include tissue architecture, light absorption and scattering properties of each tissue layer, the distribution and concentration of the fluorophores in the different tissue layers, the biochemical environment, and the metabolic status of the tissue. Though complex, tissue autofluorescence patterns reflect changes in tissue composition and have been shown to be capable of distinguishing benign from malignant tissue.[21–25]

Elastic Scattering (Reflectance) Spectroscopy

Elastic scattering spectroscopy, also known as diffuse reflectance spectroscopy, uses the principle of white light (400–700 um) reflectance to determine the structural characteristics of illuminated tissue. Elastic scattering occurs when photons from visible light are reflected from tissue constituents without a change in wavelength (or energy). The intensity of this back scattered light is measured resulting in a reflectance spectrum that describes the interaction of white light with tissue following multiple scattering events. As tissue transitions to dysplasia or neoplasia, the relative concentrations, density, and size of endogenous scatterers is affected. The measurement of the intensity of back scattered light is then influenced by the characteristics of the scatterers (ie, nuclei, mitochondria, connective tissue) and absorbers (ie, hemoglobin). For example, dysplastic change is often characterized by enlarged nuclei, crowding, and hyperchromaticity. These changes lead to characteristic reflectance spectra used to identify the structural composition of tissue and aid in clinical diagnosis.[21–25]

Raman Spectroscopy

Raman spectroscopy is a novel optical technique employed to provide detailed information about the molecular composition of tissue. In contrast to elastic scattering spectroscopy, Raman spectra are generated from the molecule-specific inelastic scattering of light. Following exposure to a light source (generally near-infrared light 700–1300 um), a minute fraction of the scattered light undergoes a wavelength shift caused by the energy transfer between incident photons and tissue molecules. The wavelength shift (and change in energy) is achieved when the incident photon alters the vibrational state of an intramolecular bond. A Raman emission spectrum is generated from the combination of the wavelengths scattered by the molecules in a tissue sample. These spectral features provide detailed and specific information about the molecular composition of tissue. Although Raman spectroscopy is sensitive to a wide range of specific biomolecules, such as proteins, lipids, and nucleic acids, the Raman effect only compromises a small fraction (1 in 1 million) of scattering events and signals may be weak and difficult to implement.[22,24,26] Other modifications of the Raman technique, such as surface enhancing Raman spectroscopy and coherent antistokes Raman scattering, are designed to amplify the signal.

Fluorescence Imaging

Fluorescent imaging systems use spectroscopic principles to capture fluorescence emission spectra from a larger tissue sampling area than is possible with point spectroscopy. The acquisition of an image requires tissue illumination with a light source, often in the near-UV to green range. The subsequent fluorescence produced from the absorption and scattering events is recorded with a camera and results in a real-time image. In addition, fluorescence imaging systems are capable of sampling larger tissue areas and provide 2-dimensional information allowing for the detection of lesion-specific features, such as homogeneities.[27]

Optical Coherence Tomography

Optical coherence tomography (OCT) is an innovative optical imaging technique designed to provide high-resolution (approximately 10 to 20 um), cross-sectional images of microscopic subsurface tissue structures. As the optical analog of high-frequency, B-scan ultrasonography, an imaging technique that detects back scattered sound waves, OCT images are generated by measuring the intensity of back scattered light after the tissue is probed with a low-power, near-infrared light source (wavelengths ranging from 750 to 1300 um). Based on the principle of low-coherence interferometry, OCT is able to provide real-time images at a resolution 10 times greater than endoscopic ultrasound, thereby allowing for the identification of microscopic tissue features, such as villi, glands, crypts, lymphatic aggregates, and blood vessels. Despite this high resolution, OCT imaging is limited by a depth of penetration of 1 to 3 mm.

To obtain images, infrared light is delivered to tissue through an optical probe, typically 2.0 to 2.4 mm in diameter. Various OCT system designs allow for tissue to be scanned in a linear, transverse, or radial fashion and are easily interfaced with endoscopes, laparoscopes, catheters, and hand-held probes. Initially applied to obtain images in the field of ophthalmology, technological advancements have resulted in the clinical application of OCT imaging in a diverse set of medical specialties, including gastroenterology, dermatology, cardiology, and oncology.[28]

Narrow-Band Imaging

Narrow-band imaging (NBI) is a recently developed optical technique designed to enhance the visualization of microvasculature on the mucosal surface. Developed to improve the quality of endoscopic images, NBI systems limit the depth of light penetration into tissue through red, green, and blue optical interference filters. These 3 filters divide the visible wavelength ranges into 3 shorter wavelength bands, while increasing the relative contribution of blue filtered light. The increased contribution of blue light is fundamental to creating a narrow-band image because blue light corresponds to the peak absorption of hemoglobin. The resulting image demonstrates preferential enhancement of the vascular network of the superficial mucosa. To differentiate normal from dysplastic tissue, the microvascular patterns present in the narrow-band image are analyzed. Areas of nondysplastic tissue generally have fine capillary patterns of normal size and distribution; whereas, areas harboring dysplasia demonstrate abnormal capillary patterns with increased size, number, and dilation. The clear visualization of vascular patterns through NBI has been shown to enhance the diagnostic capability of endoscopy and offers promise for the early detection of cancer.[24,29]

Multimodal Optical Imaging

Advances in bioengineering and the continued refinement of optical detection techniques have led to the development of multimodal optical detection systems. These multimodal devices often function in real time to provide complementary diagnostic information and wide tissue surveillance capability. The ultimate goal of the optical detection systems centers on the achievement of an optical biopsy. This achievement would allow clinicians to determine a tissue diagnosis based on in-vivo optical measurements and would eliminate the need for conventional biopsy and histopathologic interpretation. Furthermore, the reliable detection of malignant change through the optical biopsy will provide the clinician the ability to immediately determine definitive treatment and optimally improve patient outcomes.

THE APPLICATION OF OPTICAL DIAGNOSTIC TECHNOLOGY IN THE ORAL CAVITY

As the most thoroughly investigated optical techniques for the detection and characterization of oral lesions, autofluorescence spectroscopy and imaging systems are capable of distinguishing normal oral mucosa from cancerous lesions. In addition, research suggests that autofluorescence techniques are capable of discriminating between lesion types, although sensitivities and specificities reported by researchers have varied. Research suggests that autofluorescence spectroscopy is exceedingly accurate in distinguishing lesions from healthy oral mucosa (sensitivity 82%–100%, specificity 63%–100%), although there is a lack of compelling evidence for the discrimination between lesion types.[27] Autofluorescence imaging systems, such as the commercially available (VELscope LED Dental, White Rock, British Columbia, Canada), allow the clinician to probe oral cavity tissue for the direct visualization of precancerous and cancerous lesions. Studies demonstrate that oral cancer and precancerous lesions show a characteristic decrease in green fluorescence when probed with autofluorescent imaging systems. This fluorescent pattern allows for the clinician to visualize malignant changes of oral tissue that manifest as darkened areas surrounded by healthy, green fluorescent tissue.[30]

In addition to fluorescence spectroscopy and imaging techniques, several additional optical diagnostic systems have demonstrated potential for the successful evaluation of the oral cavity. A recent study using a multispectral imaging system (fluorescence, narrow-band imaging, and orthogonal polarized reflectance) demonstrated that oral lesion borders change with each imaging modality, suggesting that multimodal imaging can provide important diagnostic information not available through conventional white light examination or through the use of a single imaging mode alone.[31] Trimodal spectroscopy (fluorescence spectroscopy, elastic scattering spectroscopy, Raman spectroscopy) has been shown to be capable of diagnosing malignant/precancerous tissue with a sensitivity and specificity of 96%.[25] Despite the diagnostic advantages created by the combination of optical technologies, these complementary techniques may prove to be time consuming and expensive, limiting clinical utility.

The application of optical coherence tomography for the evaluation of oral cavity disease began as early as 1998 when researchers obtained images of the human tooth and oral mucosa.[32,33] In 2004, OCT images captured from varying states of pathology in hamster cheek mucosa were used to study the feasibility of OCT scanning for oral disease diagnosis.[34] Recent improvements in OCT technology have led researchers to study the clinical utility of OCT for oral cancer diagnosis. Images obtained from in-vivo benign and malignant oral tissue demonstrated that OCT is capable of recognizing differences in mucosal and submucosal tissue structures, allowing for image correlation with known histologic features.[35] As OCT technology continues to evolve, faster scanning speeds and higher-resolution images will improve characterization of tissue structure with the hope that this optical modality could improve the detection and management of early stage oral disease.

SUMMARY

Even with remarkable technological advancements and extraordinary efforts from cancer advocates, scientists, and clinicians, the diagnosis of oral cancer often occurs at a late stage conferring a dismal prognosis. Importantly, the improvement of patient outcomes is related to the detection and surveillance of cancerous or precancerous lesions at early stages of disease. Although many of these techniques have only recently been implemented in medical settings, they offer scientists a highly sought after method for the early detection of cancer. Many of the optical diagnostic techniques are still in the research and development stage and before they can be implemented in widespread clinical practice, further research in large clinical trials must confirm the initial experimental data provided by researchers across the globe.

REFERENCES

1. Kademani D. Oral cancer. Mayo Clin Proc 2007;82(7):878–87.
2. Silverman S Jr. Demographics and occurrence of oral and pharyngeal cancers. The outcome, the trends, the challenge. J Am Dent Assoc 2001;132:7S–11S.
3. Ries LAG, Melbert D, Krapcho M, et al, editors. SEER cancer statistics review, 1975–2005. Bethesda (MD): National Cancer Institute; 2008. Available at: http://seer.cancer.gov/csr/1975_2005/. Accessed November 2007.
4. Llewellyn CD, Johnson NW, Warnakulasuriya KA. Risk factors for squamous cell carcinoma of the oral cavity in young people – A comprehensive literature review. Oral Oncol 2001;37:401–18.
5. Rennemo E, Zatterstrom U, Boysen M. Impact of second primary tumors on survival in head and neck cancer: an analysis of 2,063 cases. Laryngoscope 2008;118:1350–6.
6. Silverman S Jr, Gorsky M, Lozada F. Oral leukoplakia and malignant transformation: a follow-up study of 257 patients. Cancer 1984;53:563–8.
7. Silverman S Jr. Observations on the clinical characteristics and natural history of leukoplakia. J Am Dent Assoc 1968;76:772–7.
8. Warnakulasuriya S, Johnson NW, van der Waal I. Nomenclature and classification of potentially malignant disorders of the oral mucosa. J Oral Pathol Med 2007;36: 575–80.
9. Napier Seamus S, Speight PM. Natural history of potentially malignant oral lesions and conditions: an overview of the literature. J Oral Pathol Med 2008;37:1–10.
10. Screening for Oral Cancer. U.S. Preventive Services Task Force. 2004. Available at: http://www.uspreventiveservicestaskforce.org/uspstf/uspsoral.htm. Accessed October 7, 2010.
11. Kujan O, Glenny AM, Oliver RJ, et al. Screening programmes for the early detection and prevention of oral cancer. Cochrane Database Syst Rev 2006;3:CD004150.
12. Sankaranarayanan R, Ramadas K, Thomas G, et al. Effect of screening on oral cancer mortality in Kerala, India: a cluster-randomised controlled trial. Lancet 2005;365(9475):1927–33.
13. Driemel O, Kunkel M, Hullman M, et al. Diagnosis of oral squamous cell carcinoma and its precursor lesions. J Dtsch Dermatol Ges 2007;5:1095–100.
14. Lingen MW, Kalmar JR, Karrison T, et al. Critical evaluation of diagnostic aids for the detection of oral cancer. Oral Oncol 2008;44:10–22.
15. Epstein JB, Sciubba J, Silverman S Jr, et al. Utility of toluidine blue in oral premalignant lesions and squamous cell carcinoma: continuing research and implications for clinical practice. Head Neck 2007;29(10):948–58.

16. Patton LL, Epstein JB, Kerr AR. Adjunctive techniques for oral cancer examination and lesion diagnosis. J Am Dent Assoc 2008;139(7):896–905.
17. Mehrotra R, Gupta A, Singh M, et al. Application of cytology and molecular biology in diagnosing premalignant or malignant oral lesions. Mol Cancer 2006;5:11.
18. Lycette RM, Leslie RB. Fluorescence of malignant tissue. Lancet 1965;40:436.
19. Lodish HF, Berk A, Matsudaira P, et al. Molecular cell biology. 5th edition. New York: W.H. Freeman and Company; 2003.
20. Xin-Hua Hu, JQ Lu. Optical detection of cancers. Encyclopedia of biomaterials and bioengineering. Taylor & Francis; 2005.
21. Sokolov K, Follen M, Richards-Kortum R. Optical spectroscopy for detection of neoplasia. Curr Opin Chem Biol 2002;6:651–8.
22. Crow P, Stone N, Kendall CA, et al. Optical diagnostics in urology: current applications and future prospects. BJU Int 2003;92:400–7.
23. DaCosta RS, Wilson BC, Marcon NE. Photodiagnostic techniques for the endoscopic detection of premalignant gastrointestinal lesions. Dig Endosc 2003;15: 153–73.
24. Wong Kee Song LM, Wilson BC. Endoscopic detection of early upper GI cancers. Best Pract Res Clin Gastroenterol 2005;19:833–56.
25. Swinson B, Jerjes W, El-Maaytah M, et al. Optical techniques in diagnosis of head and neck malignancy. Oral Oncol 2006;42(3):221–8.
26. Wong Kee Song LM, Molckovsky A, Wang KK, et al. Diagnostic potential of raman spectroscopy in Barrett's esophagus. Proc SPIE 2005;5692:140–6.
27. De Veld DCG, Witjes MJH, Sterenborg HJCM, et al. The status of in vivo autofluorescence spectroscopy and imaging for oral oncology. Oral Oncol 2005;41: 117–31.
28. Zysk AM, Nguyen FT, Oldenburg AL, et al. Optical coherence tomography: a review of clinical development from bench to bedside. J Biomed Opt 2007; 12:051403.
29. Watanabe A, Tsujie H, Taniguchi M, et al. Laryngoscopic detection of pharyngeal carcinoma in situ with narrowband imaging. Laryngoscope 2006;116:650–4.
30. Lane PM, Gilhuly T, Whitehead P, et al. Simple device for the direct visualization of oral-cavity tissue fluorescence. J Biomed Opt 2006;11(2):024006.
31. Roblyer D, Richards-Kortum R, Sokolov K, et al. Multispectral optical imaging device for in vivo detection of oral neoplasia. J Biomed Opt 2008;13(2):024019.
32. Colston BW Jr, Everett MJ, Da Silva LB, et al. Imaging of hard and soft-tissue structure in the oral cavity by optical coherence tomography. Appl Opt 1998; 37:3582–5.
33. Colston BW Jr, Everett MG, Sathyam US, et al. Imaging of the oral cavity using optical coherence tomography. Monogr Oral Sci 2000;17:32–55.
34. Matheny E, Hanna N, Jung W, et al. Optical coherence tomography of malignancy in hamster cheek pouches. J Biomed Opt 2004;9:978–81.
35. Ridgway JM, Armstrong WB, Guo S, et al. In vivo optical coherence tomography of the human oral cavity and oropharynx. Arch Otolaryngol Head Neck Surg 2006;132:1074–81.

Diagnosis and Management of Oral Candidiasis

Peter J. Giannini, DDS, MS[a],*, Kishore V. Shetty, BDS, DDS, MS, MRCS[b]

KEYWORDS

- Candidiasis • Oral • Clinical presentation
- Immunocompromised • Diagnosis • Management

Candidiasis is the most common oral fungal infection. Fungal infections of the oral cavity are caused by a group of saprophytic fungi that includes 8 species of the genus *Candida*.[1] *Candida albicans* is the most common candidal species residing in the oral cavity of humans, accounting for 70% to 80% of oral isolates.[2–5] *Candida glabrata* and *Candida tropicalis* account for approximately 5% and 8% of oral isolates, respectively.[5] *C albicans* is a dimorphic fungus existing in both yeast and hyphal forms; however, only the hyphal form is associated with oral candidiasis. It may be a component of the normal oral microflora in approximately 30% to 50% of the population.

PREDISPOSING FACTORS

There are various predisposing factors for oral candidiasis, including systemic diseases that affect the immune status of the host, the local oral mucosal environment, and the specific strain of *C albicans*.[6] Recurrent oral candidiasis is noted in patients with poorly controlled diabetes mellitus, human immunodeficiency virus (HIV)-positive patients (especially those with a CD4 cell count $<200/\mu L$), and patients with xerostomia. In one study, oral candidiasis was evident in 28.6% of HIV-positive patients and was the most common oral manifestation of HIV infection.[7] The use of medications, especially among the elderly population, is one of the most common causes of xerostomia. Medications that are commonly associated with predisposition to xerostomia include antidepressants, diuretics, and those that possess

Financial disclosures/conflicts of interest: The authors have nothing to disclose.
[a] Department of Oral Biology, Cruzan Center for Dental Research, University of Nebraska Medical Center College of Dentistry, 40th and Holdrege Streets, Box 830740, Lincoln, NE 68583-0740, USA
[b] Private Dental Practice, Denver, CO, USA
* Corresponding author.
E-mail address: pgiannini@unmc.edu

Otolaryngol Clin N Am 44 (2011) 231–240
doi:10.1016/j.otc.2010.09.010
0030-6665/11/$ – see front matter

oto.theclinics.com

anticholinergic effects. Other causes of xerostomia include radiation treatment to the head and neck region and Sjögren's syndrome. A decrease in the salivary flow leads to a reduction in the cleansing capability of the saliva, in addition to a decrease in secretory immunoglobulin A levels, creating an environment that is more conducive to the growth of *C albicans*.[8–10]

Additional predisposing factors for oral candidiasis include the use of broad-spectrum antibiotics that alter the normal microflora, corticosteroid medications, removable prostheses, and physical disabilities that impair proper oral hygiene or nutrition.[11] The use of topical corticosteroids (eg, clobetasol), steroid inhalers, and systemic steroids are common iatrogenic causes of oral candidiasis.[12]

CLINICAL MANIFESTATIONS

Patients with oral candidiasis may be asymptomatic or complain of a burning sensation or stomatodynia. They also occasionally report the presence of a metallic taste. Although the symptom of burning is a common complaint in patients with candidiasis, additional causes of oral burning should also be considered. These include xerostomia, as well as iron, vitamin B_{12}, or zinc deficiency. If no definitive cause for the burning sensation is elucidated, a diagnosis of burning mouth syndrome is often rendered. Burning mouth syndrome is considered to be a diagnosis of exclusion once all other potential causes of burning mouth have been excluded.

The clinical presentation of oral candidiasis is variable and includes both white and erythematous forms. The white forms include pseudomembranous and hyperplastic candidiasis (candidal leukoplakia). The erythematous forms of the disease occur more commonly than the pseudomembranous or hyperplastic subtypes.

Pseudomembranous Candidiasis

Pseudomembranous candidiasis, also known as thrush, is the most commonly recognized form of candidiasis. It presents as adherent white wipeable plaques resembling curdled milk. The plaques occur anywhere on the oral mucosa, including the tongue, buccal mucosa, and hard palate. When the plaques are wiped off, the underlying mucosa often exhibits an erythematous appearance. This form of candidiasis is most commonly observed in infants and immunocompromised patients, including those who are HIV positive or who have undergone organ or tissue transplants.[1] In patients with a compromised immune system, pseudomembranous candidiasis also affects regions other than the oral cavity, including the oropharynx and esophagus.[13] Pseudomembranous candidiasis is the second most common AIDS-defining opportunistic infection following *Pneumocystis carinii* pneumonia, and results in significant morbidity in terms of weight loss, malaise, and reduced quality of life.[14,15]

Erythematous Candidiasis

Erythematous candidiasis is the most common form of oral candidiasis and is categorized into several different forms depending on the cause and site of involvement. Causes include the use of medications, wearing removable prosthetic appliances for an extended period, and xerostomia. Erythematous candidiasis is categorized into the following subtypes: acute atrophic, chronic atrophic, angular cheilitis, median rhomboid glossitis, and chronic multifocal.

Acute atrophic candidiasis

Acute atrophic candidiasis has also been referred to as antibiotic sore mouth, as this subtype results from the use of broad-spectrum antibiotics. The clinical presentation is typically that of erythema of the involved tissues, including atrophy of the dorsal tongue papillae. Patients often present with a chief complaint of an oral burning sensation. The use of broad-spectrum antibiotics facilitates the overgrowth of C albicans by suppressing the normal oral bacterial microflora. The clinical presentation of an erythematous burning tongue demonstrating papillary atrophy also occurs in association with other disorders, including iron deficiency anemia, vitamin B_{12} deficiency, and poorly controlled diabetes mellitus.

Chronic atrophic candidiasis

This form of candidiasis is commonly designated denture stomatitis, and as the name suggests, is noted in patients who wear primarily poorly fitting removable prosthetic appliances for extended periods, for example, by not removing them at night (**Fig. 1**). Patients are most often asymptomatic and clinically present with erythema and petechiae of the mucosa coinciding with the denture-bearing area of the prosthesis. Denture stomatitis is primarily noted on the palatal denture-bearing mucosa where natural salivary flow is restricted.[16]

Denture stomatitis is classified into 3 clinical subtypes or Newton classifications: (1) type I consists of localized inflammation or pinpoint petechial hemorrhages, (2) type II is a more diffuse erythema involving either a portion or the entire denture-bearing mucosa, and (3) type III is erythema in association with papillary hyperplasia of the denture-bearing mucosa.[17] Culturing the tissue surface of the denture and the denture-bearing palatal mucosa often reveals a significantly greater extent of candidal growth from the denture itself. The acrylic porosities on the tissue surface of the denture provide an ideal environment for the growth of C albicans.[18] Much of the observed erythematous tissue reaction is the result of the by-products of C albicans in contact with the mucosa. Petechial hemorrhages and papillary mucosal hyperplasia result from long-term irritation of the poorly fitting denture. In addition, patients with denture stomatitis often present with associated angular cheilitis.

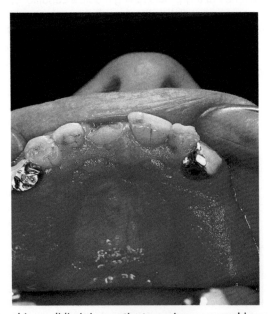

Fig. 1. Chronic atrophic candidiasis in a patient wearing a removable prosthesis.

Angular cheilitis

This variant of candidiasis most commonly represents a combination of fungal and bacterial infections (**Fig. 2**). Most cases of angular cheilitis are caused by both *C albicans* and *Staphylococcus aureus*, and the remaining by either *C albicans* or *S aureus*. The clinical presentation consists of soreness along with erythema and fissuring at the commissures, most often bilaterally. Angular cheilitis is often noted in patients who are denture wearers, especially those with an old poorly fitting prosthesis. Over time, as alveolar bone recedes, there is a resultant decreased vertical dimension of occlusion, thereby allowing for the pooling and accumulation of saliva at the commissures. Thus, a favorable environment for the growth of *C albicans* and *S aureus* exists. Less common contributing factors for the development of angular cheilitis include nutritional deficiencies such as iron, vitamin B_{12}, folic acid, thiamine, and riboflavin.[19] Angular cheilitis is also seen in younger dentate patients who are HIV positive, most likely as a result of decreased immunity.[20]

Median rhomboid glossitis

Median rhomboid glossitis is also known as central papillary atrophy. The clinical presentation consists of a well-demarcated, rhomboid region of atrophy of the dorsal tongue papillae localized to the midline posterior aspect of the tongue anterior to the circumvallate papillae. In some cases, an associated "kissing lesion" is present on the hard palate, resulting from direct inoculation that occurs when the dorsal tongue makes contact with the hard palate during deglutition. Median rhomboid glossitis was originally thought to be a developmental anomaly before being considered a variant of oral candidiasis.[21]

Chronic multifocal candidiasis

Chronic multifocal candidiasis is defined as the presentation of candidiasis in more than one clinical location, such as concurrent denture stomatitis and angular cheilitis. Additional clinical criteria for this condition include the presence of lesions for more than 4 weeks, the absence of any predisposing medical conditions, and the exclusion of patients who have received radiation therapy; drugs such as antibiotics, antiinflammatory medications, or immunosuppressive drugs; and cytotoxic or psychotropic agents.[22]

Hyperplastic Candidiasis

Hyperplastic candidiasis, also known as chronic hyperplastic candidiasis or candidal leukoplakia, presents clinically as a well-defined, white nonwipeable lesion most

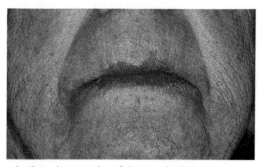

Fig. 2. Mild angular cheilitis along with exfoliative cheilitis.

commonly on the buccal mucosa involving the commissural region and less frequently on the palate and lateral tongue. Clinically, hyperplastic candidiasis cannot be distinguished from leukoplakia. Leukoplakia is defined as the presence of a white nonwipeable well-defined lesion that cannot be characterized clinically or pathologically as any other disease entity and has no known etiology except tobacco and/or alcohol.[23] If the lesion does not resolve after antifungal treatment, leukoplakia should be considered as a possible clinical diagnosis and it should be biopsied to rule out dysplasia or squamous cell carcinoma.

Hyperplastic candidiasis is the least common variant of oral candidiasis and remains somewhat controversial. Some consider it to be a preexisting leukoplakia that is colonized by candidal organisms. In other situations, *Candida* is determined to be the sole cause of the lesion, given that it resolves after antifungal treatment. Although many of these cases present as white lesions, occasionally there are focal areas of erythema in association with the white areas. Therefore, speckled leukoplakia, or erythroleukoplakia, should also be included in the differential diagnosis. Such lesions should be biopsied promptly because of the significantly increased frequency of the presence of either dysplasia or squamous cell carcinoma in lesions that demonstrate an erythematous clinical presentation.[21]

Candidiasis and the Immunocompromised Host

Chronic candidiasis may present in immunocompromised patients with an inherited immune defect, such as chronic mucocutaneous candidiasis, or in patients who are immunocompromised as a result of an underlying disease process, including HIV infection, hematologic malignancies, and impaired immune status secondary to chemotherapy for cancer or immunosuppression subsequent to a transplant.

Chronic Mucocutaneous Candidiasis

This form of candidiasis presents as a long-term involvement of the mucosa, skin, and nails exhibiting a poor response to treatment with topical antifungal agents.[24] The oral lesions are usually of the hyperplastic type, although other forms of candidiasis may be observed. Generally, the severity of the candidal infection correlates with the degree of immune dysfunction. Most cases are sporadic; however, an autosomal recessive inheritance pattern has been noted. Candidal infections usually present within the first few years of life.[21] The underlying immune defect is thought to be cell mediated. Previous studies have shown that it may involve a defect in cytokine production in response to candidal and bacterial antigens.[25]

Chronic mucocutaneous candidiasis has also been associated with various endocrinopathies, including endocrine-candidiasis syndrome and autoimmune polyendocrinopathy-candidiasis-ectodermal dystrophy (APECED) syndrome, in addition to iron deficiency anemia. The endocrine abnormalities that have been noted include hypothyroidism, hypoparathyroidism, Addison disease, and diabetes mellitus. The endocrine disturbance often develops months or years after the onset of the candidal infection.[21] In a study by Rautemaa and colleagues,[26] an increased prevalence of oral and esophageal carcinoma was noted in patients with APECED syndrome, with 10% of adult patients affected by these malignancies.

HIV-Associated Candidiasis

Oral candidiasis is one of the most common opportunistic infections in HIV-positive patients. Studies have shown that more than 90% of HIV-positive individuals develop oral candidiasis some time during the course of their disease.[20,27,28] It is also the most common oral fungal infection associated with HIV disease.[29,30] HIV-associated oral candidiasis presents clinically as pseudomembranous, erythematous, or hyperplastic variants.[4,31] The pseudomembranous form most frequently involves the tongue, hard and soft palate, and buccal mucosa, although any region of the oral mucosa may be involved.[32] The erythematous form more often presents as an early oral manifestation of HIV infection, usually involving the palate and dorsal tongue.[4,31]

Another form of HIV-associated oral candidiasis is linear gingival erythema. It is a nonplaque-induced gingivitis that presents as an erythematous band along the marginal gingiva and can be diffuse or generalized. Linear gingival erythema does not respond to the typical treatment regimen for gingivitis, which consists of scaling, professional tooth polishing with prophylaxis paste, and improved oral hygiene. It often results from a combination of candidal and bacterial infections. Linear gingival erythema is considered to be an oral manifestation of HIV infection; however, it is also noted in patients who are HIV-negative, although at a much lower frequency.[33]

DIAGNOSIS

The diagnosis of oral candidiasis is often made based on the clinical signs and symptoms. When the clinical presentation is suggestive of oral candidiasis, the clinician often empirically treats the patient with an antifungal medication. Resolution of the fungal infection confirms the diagnosis. Additional adjunctive methods for the diagnosis of oral candidiasis include exfoliative cytology, biopsy, and culture.

Samples for exfoliative cytology are obtained by the use of a moistened wooden tongue blade to scrape the candidal organisms along with the superficial keratinocytes. This method yields the best results with the pseudomembranous form of candidiasis, in which there are greater numbers of fungal hyphae. The sample is then smeared onto a glass microscope slide. It ideally should be fixed with an alcohol fixative; however, it can also be allowed to air dry. The specimen is sent to the laboratory and stained by the periodic acid-Schiff (PAS) method. The PAS stain preferentially stains glycogen in the fungal cell wall and thus renders the candidal organisms magenta in color. Alternatively, a chairside diagnostic procedure can be performed instead of submitting the sample to the laboratory. For this method, a drop of 10% potassium hydroxide (KOH) is placed onto the slide. KOH lyses the keratinocytes, thus allowing the candidal organisms to be more readily seen under the microscope. The main disadvantage of the KOH preparation compared with the PAS-stained slide is the lack of a permanent record.

The diagnosis of oral candidiasis can also be made based on a mucosal biopsy specimen. After the specimen is obtained, it is placed in 10% formalin to allow for proper fixation. The tissue is then processed, embedded in paraffin, cut into 4- to 6-μm sections, and placed on a glass microscope slide. Staining with the PAS method highlights the candidal hyphae (**Figs. 3** and **4**). Because oral candidiasis is a superficial mucosal infection in the immunocompetent population, the hyphal organisms are noted within the parakeratin layer of the epithelium.

Culture, using Sabouraud dextrose agar, represents an additional adjunctive diagnostic modality and is useful in a qualitative manner to determine the presence or absence of C albicans. A sterile cotton swab is placed in contact with the involved mucosa, after which it is used to inoculate a Sabouraud agar plate or slant containing cycloheximide and chloramphenicol. The agar is incubated at 25°C to 30°C for 48 to 72 hours.[34] The presence of creamy white colonies indicates a positive culture result.

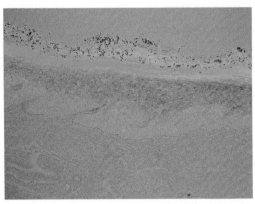

Fig. 3. *C albicans* within the parakeratin layer (PAS stain, original magnification ×10).

A sample from one of the colonies is smeared onto a slide and viewed under the microscope to confirm the diagnosis.

A quantitative assessment of *C albicans* can be performed by determining the number of colony-forming units (CFUs) per 1 mL of unstimulated whole saliva. A 0.01-mL sterile loop is used to obtain a sample of the collected saliva, which is then used to inoculate a Sabouraud agar plate. The number of CFUs on the agar plate is determined after incubation for 48 to 72 hours at 25°C to 30°C.[35] In healthy individuals, candidal CFU counts range from 0 to 1000/mL. In patients with oral candidiasis, the counts may be as high as 50,000/mL.[34] However, because there are no known established criteria to differentiate candidal commensalism from disease, the presence of candidal organisms by cytology or culture along with the presence of clinical signs and symptoms remains the fundamental basis for diagnosing oral candidiasis.[9,36–39]

MANAGEMENT

There are different treatment modalities to manage oral candidiasis using antifungal agents. The mechanism of action involves an alteration of RNA and DNA metabolism or an intracellular accumulation of peroxide, which is toxic to the fungal cell.[21,39] It is

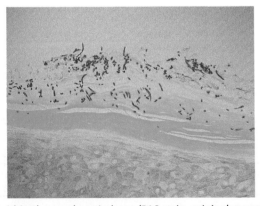

Fig. 4. *C albicans* within the parakeratin layer (PAS stain, original magnification ×20).

Table 1
Topical antifungal agents for oral candidiasis

Agents	Form	Dosage	Comments
Clotrimazole Troche	Lozenge	10 mg dissolved po 5 times a day for 2 wk	Alters cell membrane and antistaphylococcal activity
Miconazole (Oravig)	Buccal tablet	50 mg dissolved each morning for 2 wk	For the treatment of oropharyngeal candidiasis
Nystatin Oral Suspension	Suspension	400,000–600,000 U po; swish and swallow 4–5 times a day	Fungicidal and fungistatic antibiotic obtained from *Streptomyces noursei*
Nystatin Pastilles	Pastilles	200,000–400,000 U po 4–5 times a day	Changes permeability of fungal cell membrane after binding to cell membrane sterols
Amphotericin B (Fungilin)	Suspension	100–200 mg po; swish and swallow qid	Fungistatic and/or fungicidal
Gentian Violet	Solution	2% solution bid	Efficacious for refractory localized candidiasis
Ketoconazole	Cream	2% cream bid	May cause nausea, vomiting, rashes, and pruritus

Adapted from various sources.

important to evaluate the chronicity and severity of the candidal infection with appropriate clinical laboratory and serologic studies. Earlier options involved the use of a topical polyene agent (nystatin and amphotericin B), and over time, there has been a shift to using systemic azoles (fluconazole, ketoconazole, and itraconazole). However, there has been an emergence of drug-resistant fungi, such as *C glabrata*, *C krusei*, *C tropicalis*, and *C dubliniensis*, especially during long-term administration.[21,28] **Tables 1** and **2** detail the most commonly used topical and systemic antifungal drugs in the management of oral candidiasis, respectively.

Future research in diagnostic technology relating to the clinical and laboratory markers of *Candida* colonization will definitely help to formulate an accurate colonization profile, leading to effective antifungal therapeutics.

Table 2
Systemic antifungal agents for oral candidiasis

Agents	Form	Dosage	Comments
Fluconazole (Diflucan)	Capsules	50 or 100 mg qd	Interferes with cell membrane and is eliminated via renal pathway; fungistatic activity with excellent bioavailability
Ketoconazole (Nizoral)	Tablets	200 or 400 mg qd	Contraindicated in liver disease and pregnancy
Miconazole (Daktarin)	Tablets	50 mg qd	Damages fungal cell wall membrane by inhibiting biosynthesis of ergosterol
Itraconazole (Sporanox)	Capsules	100 mg qd	Contraindicated in liver disease and pregnancy

Adapted from various sources.

REFERENCES

1. Mohammad AR, Giannini PJ. Oral candidiasis: current concepts in the diagnosis and management in the institutionalized elderly patient. A review. Dental Forum 2005;33(2):65–70.
2. Samaranayake LP, MacFarlane TW. Oral candidosis. London: Wright; 1990.
3. Zegarelli DJ. Fungal infections of the oral cavity. Otolaryngol Clin North Am 1993; 26:1069–89.
4. Silverman S, Gallo JW, McKnight ML, et al. Clinical characteristics and management responses in 85 HIV-infected patients with oral candidiasis. Oral Surg Oral Med Oral Pathol Oral Radiol Endod 1996;82:402–7.
5. Vazquez JA, Sobel JD. Mucosal candidiasis. Infect Dis Clin North Am 2002;16(4): 793–820.
6. Neville BW, Damm DD, Allen CM, et al. Fungal and protozoal diseases. In: Oral and maxillofacial pathology. 1st edition. Philadelphia: WB Saunders; 1995. p. 166–7.
7. Pinheiro A, Marcenes W, Zakrzewska JM, et al. Dental and oral lesions in HIV-infected patients: a study in Brazil. Int Dent J 2004;54(3):131–7.
8. Ghannoum MA, Radwan SS. Candida adherence to epithelial cells. Boca Raton (FL): CRC Press Inc; 1990.
9. Rossie KM, Taylor J, Beck FM, et al. Influence of radiation therapy on oral *Candida albicans* colonization: a quantitative assessment. Oral Surg Oral Med Oral Pathol 1987;64:698–701.
10. Silverman S, Luangjarmekorn L, Greenspan D. Occurrence of oral *Candida* in irradiated head and neck cancer patients. J Oral Med 1984;39:194–6.
11. Lockhart SR, Joly S, Vargas K, et al. Natural defenses against *Candida* colonization breakdown in the oral cavities of the elderly. J Dent Res 1999;78(4):857–68.
12. Epstein JB, Komiyama K, Duncan D. Oral topical steroids and secondary oral candidiasis. J Oral Med 1986;41:223–7.
13. Bonacini M, Young T, Laine L. The causes of esophageal symptoms in human immunodeficiency virus infection: a prospective study of 110 patients. Arch Intern Med 1991;151:1567–72.
14. Farizo KM, Buehler JW, Chamberland ME, et al. Spectrum of disease in persons with human immunodeficiency virus infection in the United States. JAMA 1992; 267:1798–805.
15. Rabeneck L, Laine L. Esophageal candidiasis in patients infected with the human immunodeficiency virus. Arch Intern Med 1994;154:2705–10.
16. Budtz-Jorjenson E. Oral candidosis. In: Samaranayake LP, MacFarlane TW, editors. *Candida*-associated denture stomatitis and angular cheilitis. London: Wright; 1990. p. 156–83.
17. Newton AV. Denture sore mouth: a possible aetiology. Br Dent J 1962;112: 357–60.
18. Glass RT, Bullard JW, Hadley CS, et al. Partial spectrum of microorganisms found in dentures and possible disease implications. J Am Osteopath Assoc 2001; 101(2):92–4.
19. Rose JA. Folic-acid deficiency as a cause of angular cheilosis. Lancet 1971; 2(7722):453–4.
20. Samaranayake LP, Holmstrup P. Oral candidiasis and human immunodeficiency virus infection. J Oral Pathol Med 1989;18:554–64.
21. Neville BW, Damm DD, Allen CM, et al. Fungal and protozoal diseases. In: Oral and maxillofacial pathology. 3rd edition. Philadelphia: WB Saunders; 2009. p. 216–9.

22. Holmstrup P, Bessermann M. Clinical, therapeutic and pathogenic aspects of chronic oral multifocal candidiasis. Oral Surg Oral Med Oral Pathol 1983;56: 388–95.
23. World Health Organization. Adenoid squamous cell carcinoma. In: Pindborg JJ, Reichart PA, Smith CJ, et al, editors. Histological typing of cancer and precancer of the oral mucosa. 2nd edition. Berlin: Springer-Verlag; 1997. p. 21–31.
24. Kirkpatrick CH. Candidiasis, pathogenesis, diagnosis and treatment. In: Bodey GP, editor. Chronic mucocutaneous candidosis. New York: Raven Press Ltd; 1993. p. 167–83.
25. Lilic D, Cant AJ, Abinum M, et al. Chronic mucocutaneous candidiasis. I. Altered antigen-stimulated IL-2, IL-4, IL-6 and interferon-gamma (IFN-gamma) production. Clin Exp Immunol 1996;105:205–12.
26. Rautemaa R, Hietanen J, Niissalo S, et al. Oral and esophageal squamous cell carcinoma—a complication or component of autoimmune polyendocrinopathy-candidiasis-ectodermal dystrophy (APECED, APS-1). Oral Oncol 2007;43: 607–13.
27. Feigal DW, Katz MH, Greenspan D. The prevalence of oral lesions in HIV-infected homosexual and bisexual men: three San Francisco epidemiological cohorts. AIDS 1991;5:519–25.
28. Greenspan D. Treatment of oropharyngeal candidosis in HIV-positive patients. J Am Acad Dermatol 1994;31:S51–5.
29. Begg MD, Panageas KS, Mitchell-Lewis D, et al. Oral lesions as markers of severe immunosuppression in HIV-infected homosexual men and injection drug users. Oral Surg Oral Med Oral Pathol Oral Radiol Endod 1996;82:276–83.
30. Arendorf TM, Bredekamp B, Cloete CA, et al. Oral manifestations of HIV infection in 600 South African patients. J Oral Pathol Med 1998;27:176–9.
31. Kolokotronis A, Kioses V, Antoniades D, et al. Immunologic status in patients infected with HIV and oral candidiasis and hairy leukoplakia and median rhomboid glossitis. An oral manifestation in patients infected with HIV. Oral Surg Oral Med Oral Pathol Oral Radiol Endod 1994;78:36–46.
32. Ellepola AN, Samaranayake LP. Oral candidal infections and actinomycotics. Crit Rev Oral Biol Med 2000;11(2):172–98.
33. Umadevi M, Adeyemi O, Patel M, et al. Periodontal diseases and other bacterial infections. Adv Dent Res 2006;19:139–45.
34. Mohammad AR. Physical evaluation, diagnosis and management of oral conditions in the elderly patient. In: Geriatric dentistry. 6th edition. 2010. p. 237–8.
35. Williams DW, Lewis MA. Isolation and identification of Candida from the oral cavity. Oral Dis 2000;6:3–11.
36. Lamey PJ, Darwaza A, Fisher BM, et al. Secretor status, candidal carriage and candidal infection in patients with diabetes mellitus. J Oral Pathol 1988;17:354–7.
37. Johnston RD, Chick EW, Johnston NS, et al. Asymptomatic quantitative increase of Candida albicans in the oral cavity: predisposing conditions. South Med J 1967;43:903.
38. Epstein JB, Pearsall NN, Truelove EJ. Quantitative relationships between Candida albicans in saliva and the clinical status of human subjects. J Clin Microbiol 1980; 12:475–6.
39. Kauffman CA, Jones PG. Candidiasis (a diagnostic and therapeutic challenge). Postgrad Med J 1986;180:129–33.

Index

Note: Page numbers of article titles are in **boldface** type.

Otolaryngol Clin N Am 44 (2011) 241–250
doi:10.1016/S0030-6665(10)00229-X
0030-6665/11/$ – see front matter © 2011 Elsevier Inc. All rights reserved.

oto.theclinics.com

Moving?

Make sure your subscription moves with you!

To notify us of your new address, find your **Clinics Account Number** (located on your mailing label above your name), and contact customer service at:

Email: journalscustomerservice-usa@elsevier.com

800-654-2452 (subscribers in the U.S. & Canada)
314-447-8871 (subscribers outside of the U.S. & Canada)

Fax number: 314-447-8029

Elsevier Health Sciences Division
Subscription Customer Service
3251 Riverport Lane
Maryland Heights, MO 63043

*To ensure uninterrupted delivery of your subscription, please notify us at least 4 weeks in advance of move.

Printed and bound by CPI Group (UK) Ltd, Croydon, CR0 4YY

03/10/2024

01040453-0007